Precision Medicine: Applied Concepts of Pharmacogenomics in Patients with Various Diseases and Polypharmacy

Precision Medicine: Applied Concepts of Pharmacogenomics in Patients with Various Diseases and Polypharmacy

Editors

Jacques Turgeon
Veronique Michaud

MDPI • Basel • Beijing • Wuhan • Barcelona • Belgrade • Manchester • Tokyo • Cluj • Tianjin

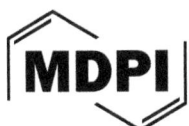

Editors
Jacques Turgeon
Tabula Rasa HealthCare
USA
Université de Montréal
Canada

Veronique Michaud
Tabula Rasa HealthCare,
Precision Pharmacotherapy
Research and Development
Institute
USA
Université de Montréal
Canada

Editorial Office
MDPI
St. Alban-Anlage 66
4052 Basel, Switzerland

This is a reprint of articles from the Special Issue published online in the open access journal *Pharmaceutics* (ISSN 1999-4923) (available at: https://www.mdpi.com/journal/water/special_issues/hydraulics_numerical_methods).

For citation purposes, cite each article independently as indicated on the article page online and as indicated below:

LastName, A.A.; LastName, B.B.; LastName, C.C. Article Title. *Journal Name* **Year**, *Volume Number*, Page Range.

ISBN 978-3-0365-1026-2 (Hbk)
ISBN 978-3-0365-1027-9 (PDF)

Cover image courtesy of Shutterstock, Inc.

© 2022 by the authors. Articles in this book are Open Access and distributed under the Creative Commons Attribution (CC BY) license, which allows users to download, copy and build upon published articles, as long as the author and publisher are properly credited, which ensures maximum dissemination and a wider impact of our publications.
The book as a whole is distributed by MDPI under the terms and conditions of the Creative Commons license CC BY-NC-ND.

Contents

About the Editors vii

Preface to "Precision Medicine: Applied Concepts of Pharmacogenomics in Patients with Various Diseases and Polypharmacy" ix

Veronique Michaud and Jacques Turgeon
Precision Medicine: Applied Concepts of Pharmacogenomics in Patients with Various Diseases and Polypharmacy
Reprinted from: *Pharmaceutics* **2021**, *13*, 197, doi:10.3390/pharmaceutics13020197 1

Kristina A. Malsagova, Tatyana V. Butkova, Arthur T. Kopylov, Alexander A. Izotov, Natalia V. Potoldykova, Dmitry V. Enikeev, Vagarshak Grigoryan, Alexander Tarasov, Alexander A. Stepanov and Anna L. Kaysheva
Pharmacogenetic Testing: A Tool for Personalized Drug Therapy Optimization
Reprinted from: *Pharmaceutics* **2020**, *12*, 1240, doi:10.3390/pharmaceutics12121240 5

Emiliene B. Tata, Melvin A. Ambele and Michael S. Pepper
Barriers to Implementing Clinical Pharmacogenetics Testing in Sub-Saharan Africa. A Critical Review
Reprinted from: *Pharmaceutics* **2020**, *12*, 809, doi:10.3390/pharmaceutics12090809 29

Dan Li, April Hui Xie, Zhichao Liu, Dongying Li, Baitang Ning, Shraddha Thakkar, Weida Tong and Joshua Xu
Linking Pharmacogenomic Information on Drug Safety and Efficacy with Ethnic Minority Populations
Reprinted from: *Pharmaceutics* **2020**, *12*, 1021, doi:10.3390/pharmaceutics12111021 49

Eloy Almenar-Pérez, Teresa Sánchez-Fito, Tamara Ovejero, Lubov Nathanson and Elisa Oltra
Impact of Polypharmacy on Candidate Biomarker miRNomes for the Diagnosis of Fibromyalgia and Myalgic Encephalomyelitis/Chronic Fatigue Syndrome: Striking Back on Treatments
Reprinted from: *Pharmaceutics* **2019**, *11*, 126, doi:10.3390/pharmaceutics11030126 59

Theodore J. Wigle, Elena V. Tsvetkova, Stephen A. Welch and Richard B. Kim
DPYD and Fluorouracil-Based Chemotherapy: Mini Review and Case Report
Reprinted from: *Pharmaceutics* **2019**, *5*, 199, doi:10.3390/pharmaceutics11050199 81

Veronique Michaud, My Tran, Benoit Pronovost, Philippe Bouchard, Sarah Bilodeau, Karine Alain, Barbara Vadnais, Martin Franco, François Bélanger and Jacques Turgeon
Impact of *GSTA1* Polymorphisms on Busulfan Oral Clearance in Adult Patients Undergoing Hematopoietic Stem Cell Transplantation
Reprinted from: *Pharmaceutics* **2019**, *11*, 440, doi:10.3390/pharmaceutics11090440 99

Vladislav Suntsov, Filip Jovanovic, Emilija Knezevic, Kenneth D. Candido and Nebojsa Nick Knezevic
Can Implementation of Genetics and Pharmacogenomics Improve Treatment of Chronic Low Back Pain?
Reprinted from: *Pharmaceutics* **2020**, *12*, 894, doi:10.3390/pharmaceutics12090894 111

Jefferson Antonio Buendía, Esteban Halac, Andrea Bosaleh, María T. Garcia de Davila, Oscar Imvertasa and Guillermo Bramuglia
Frequency of CYP3A5 Genetic Polymorphisms and Tacrolimus Pharmacokinetics in Pediatric Liver Transplantation
Reprinted from: *Pharmaceutics* **2020**, *12*, 898, doi:10.3390/pharmaceutics12090898 . . . . **133**

Sara Salvador-Martín, Bartosz Kaczmarczyk, Rebeca Álvarez, Víctor Manuel Navas-López, Carmen Gallego-Fernández, Ana Moreno-Álvarez, Alfonso Solar-Boga, Cesar Sánchez, Mar Tolin, Marta Velasco, Rosana Muñoz-Codoceo, Alejandro Rodriguez-Martinez, Concepción A. Vayo, Ferrán Bossacoma, Gemma Pujol-Muncunill, María J. Fobelo, Antonio Millán-Jiménez, Lorena Magallares, Eva Martínez-Ojinaga, Inés Loverdos, Francisco J. Eizaguirre, José A. Blanca-García, Susana Clemente, Ruth García-Romero, Vicente Merino-Bohórquez, Rafael González de Caldas, Enrique Vázquez, Ana Dopazo, María Sanjurjo-Sáez and Luis A. López-Fernández
Whole Transcription Profile of Responders to Anti-TNF Drugs in Pediatric Inflammatory Bowel Disease
Reprinted from: *Pharmaceutics* **2021**, *13*, 77, doi:10.3390/pharmaceutics13010077 . . . . **141**

About the Editors

Jacques Turgeon B.Pharm., Ph.D., is the Chief Scientific Officer, Tabula Rasa HealthCare. He is recognized internationally for his excellence in research and pharmacy education, has received >USD 70 million in research awards and mentored >70 students. He has authored >170 peer-reviewed articles, made >375 presentations scientific meetings, and his work has been cited, on average, more than 400 times per year with a H-index at 45. His research interests focus on studying factors responsible for the intersubject variability in drug response. He is renowned for his expertise on the cytochrome P450 system and pharmacogenetics. Dr. Turgeon has held numerous leadership roles, including serving as Dean of the School of Pharmacy and Vice Rector of Research at the University of Montreal; Director of the University of Montreal Hospital Research Centre; Chief Executive Officer of the University of Montreal Hospital; Associate Dean of the College of Pharmacy, University of Florida. Dr. Turgeon is Professor Emeritus from University of Montreal, a fellow of the Canadian Academy of Health Sciences and an international fellow of the Académie Nationale de Médecine in France.

Veronique Michaud B.Pharm., PhD, is the Chief Operating Officer of the Tabula Rasa Healthcare Scientific Precision Pharmacotherapy Research & Development Institute in Orlando. The institute aims to develop advanced clinical decision support systems to optimize medication safety. She is an adjunct professor, Faculty of Pharmacy, Université de Montréal, and has directed a pharmacokinetic and bioanalytic core facility at the CRCHUM. Her research investigates the contribution of CYP450 drug-metabolizing enzymes in drug disposition, with special attention to the role of disease states (focusing on type 2 diabetes), the role of pharmacogenomics and drug–drug interactions, while attempting to better understand and predict variation in drug responses. She has earned more than USD 22 million in research awards, published more than 46 peer-reviewed journal articles, published more than 110 scientific abstracts and mentored graduate students and PharmD residents. Her work has been cited more than 865 times since 2015. She completed fellowships at Indiana University and McGill University and earned her Ph.D. and M.Sc. degrees from the Université de Montréal.

Preface to "Precision Medicine: Applied Concepts of Pharmacogenomics in Patients with Various Diseases and Polypharmacy"

The entire pharmacotherapy system needs to be made personalized, precise, and, above all, science based. The clinical implementation of pharmacogenomic (PGx) testing is an obvious answer to this need.

The silent pandemic of preventable Adverse Drug Events (ADEs), which is exacerbated by the proliferation of polypharmacy, aging populations, and direct-to-consumer advertising of prescription medications, continues unabated. Why is this such a societal plague? The opaque underlying issue is the universal lack of pharmacotherapy science at the point of prescribing and/or dispensing. Prescribing decisions continue to be preference-based (i.e., what the prescriber thinks) or evidence based (e.g., population-harvested guidelines). These anachronistic practice methods have not and will not attenuate the ravage of ADEs, which continue to manifest as significant avoidable morbidity and pre-mature mortality. There are three obvious tailwinds to finally achieve broad-based implementation of PGx in clinical practice.

First, about a decade ago, we saw the initial publications regarding clopidogrel and CYP2C19 slow metabolizers, followed by an FDA Black Box warning; yet the widespread use of PGx to avoid this preventable ADE interaction (and to save lives) never materialized. This year, however, we see the first of many judgments when a court in Hawaii ordered two drug companies to pay more than USD 834 million to the state for failing to warn non-white patients properly of health risks from clopidogrel. This bellwether decision will be transformationally prescient to foster the use of applied PGx in practice.

Aside from judicial pressure, the second tailwind to propel the use of PGx in practice is the strong pivot towards value-based care models for financially at-risk outcomes. Governmental incentives abound, fueling the move from fee-for-service provider payments to outcomes-for-service compensation. This effort goes beyond in United States models such as Medicare and Medicaid, and now is penetrating commercial insurers. This bodes as an astute paradigm shift from: *the more one does, the more one invoices*; to a construct of, *first comes outcome, then comes income*.

The third tailwind for PGx appropriation is the march toward personalization of pharmacotherapy. There are two underlying rationale here. The first argument is that it is the right thing to do. The prescriptive approach must change from preference-based and evidence-based to recognizing that each person is different, both in their combinatorial medication regimen and the underlying diseases that affect drug metabolism. The second argument is that the science is real, tested, deep, still evolving, and ought to be applied at point of care. There is no rational ethical case to continue with trial-and-error pharmacotherapy practice.

The solution to rampant ADEs is at hand. You will find both PGx contextual insight and persuasive exemplary applications herein. In that spirit, let us begin the exploration.

Calvin H. Knowlton, BSc Pharm, MDiv, PhD, CEO Tabula Rasa HealthCare
Editors

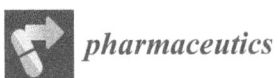

Editorial

Precision Medicine: Applied Concepts of Pharmacogenomics in Patients with Various Diseases and Polypharmacy

Veronique Michaud [1,2] and Jacques Turgeon [1,2,*]

1. Precision Pharmacotherapy Research and Development Institute, Tabula Rasa Health Care, Lake Nona, Orlando, FL 32827, USA; vmichaud@trhc.com or veronique.michaud@umontreal.ca
2. Faculty of Pharmacy, Université de Montréal, Montréal, QC H3C 3J7, Canada
* Correspondence: jturgeon@trhc.com or jacques.turgeon@umontreal.ca; Tel.: +1-407-454-9934

Received: 22 January 2021; Accepted: 25 January 2021; Published: 2 February 2021

Over the last century, the process of choosing medications to treat certain diseases has evolved significantly. In the early days of our pharmacological armamentarium, prescribers were selecting medications mostly by Preference whenever more than one option was available. With the venue of evidence-based medicine and the surge of clinical trials, drug selection became more standardized among prescribers as they paid more attention to patient characteristics and disease treatment guidelines. This brought us to the era of Personalized treatments. This is not to say that physicians were not paying attention to each patient prior this time, but as of then, drug selection was established on more sound and solid clinical evidence, running away from the "one-size-fits-all" approach.

On 16 April 1999, a short article appeared in *The Wall Street Journal* entitled "Genetic Mapping Ushers In New Era Of Profitable Personal Medicines". At this time, the public was introduced to the term "Personalized Medicine", and the article, written by Robert Langreth and Michael Waldholz, described the formation of the Single Nucleotide Polymorphism Consortium, an initiative leading to a large collaboration between several pharmaceutical companies [1]. This occurred as the Human Genome Project, launched in 1990, was to reach completion 4 years later [2,3]. Although the term "Personalized" was used at that time, several scientists now prefer to describe the use of genetics and other technologies to established treatment as "Precision" pharmacotherapy. Eventually, the use of preemptive testing favors more Predictive, Preventive, and Participatory medicine or pharmacotherapy, such that several versions of P(N) Medicine or P(N) Pharmacotherapy toponomy have been proposed [4].

In this colligated Special Issue of *Pharmaceutics* on "Precision Medicine: Applied Concepts of Pharmacogenomics in Patients with Various Diseases and Polypharmacy", our objective is to offer the reader a series of articles that describe the concept of "Precision Medicine", discuss its implementation process and limitations, demonstrate its value by illustrating some clinical cases, and open the door to new and more sophisticated techniques and applications.

In their review, Malsagova et al. lead the reader through the general concept of pharmacogenomics (PGx) and related issues of PGx testing efficiency, personal data security, and health safety at a current clinical level. The authors present a short history of PGx, describe various drug-metabolizing enzyme phenotypes, and illustrate the PGx testing cycle. They identify most relevant conditions and drugs where PGx testing could be applicable and also provide a list of PGx companies and services [5].

In a second article, Tata et al. describe the difficulties encountered in the implementation of PGx testing in sub-Saharan African countries. The authors recognize that PGx testing can significantly improve healthcare delivery considering the high incidence of communicable diseases, the increasing incidence of non-communicable diseases, and the high degree of genetic diversity in these populations. Among the limitations identified, the authors discuss under-resourced clinical care logistics, a paucity of PGx clinical trials, scientific and technical barriers to genotyping, and socio-cultural as well as ethical issues regarding healthcare stakeholders [6].

Third, Li et al. discuss the challenges encountered while trying to link PGx information on drug safety and efficacy in ethnic minority populations. They bring to light the notion that several clinical studies on PGx markers and related drug dose adjustments are often not conducted in diverse ethnic populations. To address this challenge, they initiated a bioinformatic project where PGx information is gathered from drug labels, extracted data on the allele frequency information of genetic variants in ethnic minority groups, and collected published research articles on PGx biomarkers to construct a new PGx database [7].

In the "applied section" of this Special Issue, six articles are presented to illustrate the clinical application and relevance of PGx testing and "Precision Medicine" for the diagnosis and treatment of various diseases under various conditions. Almenar-Pérez et al. present the study, "Impact of polypharmacy on candidate biomarker miRNomes for the diagnosis of fibromyalgia and myalgic encephalomyelitis/chronic fatigue syndrome: striking back on treatment". Their study demonstrates that miRNomes could help refine PGx/pharmacoepigenomic analysis to elevate future personalized and precision medicine programs in the clinic [8]. Wigle et al. provide a focused review of 5-fluorouracil (5-FU) metabolism and efforts to improve predictive dosing through screening for dihydropyrimidine dehydrogenase (DPD) deficiency, a single enzyme largely responsible for the metabolism of 5-FU. Using a patient case related to an orthotopic liver transplant recipient, they highlight some limitations of PGx testing but suggest that such case supports the development of robust multimodality precision medicine services [9]. Michaud et al. provide compelling results on the role of glutathione S-transferase A1 (*GSTA1*) gene variants on busulfan oral clearance in a population of patients undergoing hematopoietic stem cell transplantations. They demonstrate that homozygote patients for *GSTA1*B/*B* exhibit much lower busulfan oral clearance than patients with a **A/*A* genotype: after the first standard dose, 2/3 of *GSTA1*B/*B* patients had plasma levels above the therapeutic levels [10]. In their review, Suntsov et al. discuss how an individual's genotype could affect their response to therapy, as well as how genetic polymorphisms in CYP450 and other enzymes are crucial for affecting the metabolic profile of drugs used for the treatment of chronic lower back pain. They suggest that implementation of gene-focused pharmacotherapy has the potential to deliver select, more efficacious drugs and avoid unnecessary polypharmacy-related adverse events in many painful conditions [11]. Buendia et al. report on the clinical value of PGx in special populations such as children undergoing liver transplantation. Their study demonstrates that the frequency of *CYP3A5*1* expression for recipients was 37.1% and was 32.2% for donors. Patients who received an expresser organ showed a lower concentration/dose ratio, especially in the 90 days following the surgery. They conclude that the role of each polymorphism is different according to the number of days after the transplant. They also suggest that such polymorphism be considered to optimize the benefits of tacrolimus therapy during the post-transplant induction and maintenance phases [12]. Finally, in their study, Salvador-Martin et al. aimed to identify PGx markers that could predict early response to anti-tumor necrosis factor (TNF) drugs in pediatric patients with inflammatory bowel disease. They characterized whole-gene expression profiles from the total RNA of their patients and demonstrated overexpression of FCGR1A, FCGR1B, and GBP1 in non-responders to treatment [13].

We are convinced that this Special Issue on "Precision Medicine" will provide clinicians and scientists a perspective on the potential of PGx. We have paid special attention to colligate articles addressing implementation, limitations, applicability, and value, using clinical cases to inspire the scientific community in future development around precision medicine.

Author Contributions: Writing—original draft preparation, V.M. and J.T.; writing—review and editing, V.M. and J.T. All authors have read and agreed to the published version of the manuscript.

Funding: This research received no external funding.

Institutional Review Board Statement: Not applicable.

Informed Consent Statement: Not applicable.

Acknowledgments: We want to thank Pamela Dow, for her support and review of this editorial.

Conflicts of Interest: V.M. and J.T. are employees and shareholders of Tabula Rasa HealthCare. The authors declare no conflict of interest.

References

1. Langreth, R.; Waldholz, M. Genetic Mapping Ushers in New Era of Profitable Personal Medicines. *Wall Str. J.* **1999**, *16*. Available online: https://www.wsj.com/articles/SB924225073307249185 (accessed on 19 January 2021).
2. National Human Genome Institute. All Goals Achieved; New Vision for Genome Research Unveiled. Available online: https://www.genome.gov/11006929/2003-release-international-consortium-completes-hgp#:~{}:text=BETHESDA%2C%20Md.%2C%20April%2014,two%20years%20ahead%20of%20schedule (accessed on 19 January 2021).
3. International Human Genome Sequencing Consortium. Finishing the euchromatic sequence of the human genome. *Nature* **2004**, *431*, 931–945. [CrossRef] [PubMed]
4. Flores, M.; Glusman, G.; Brogaard, K.; Price, N.D.; Hood, L. P4 medicine: How systems medicine will transform the healthcare sector and society. *Per. Med.* **2013**, *10*, 565–576. [CrossRef] [PubMed]
5. Malsagova, K.A.; Butkova, T.V.; Kopylov, A.T.; Izotov, A.A.; Potoldykova, N.V.; Enikeev, D.V.; Grigoryan, V.; Tarasov, A.; Stepanov, A.A.; Kaysheva, A.L. Pharmacogenetic Testing: A Tool for Personalized Drug Therapy Optimization. *Pharmaceutics* **2020**, *12*, 1240. [CrossRef] [PubMed]
6. Tata, E.B.; Ambele, M.A.; Pepper, M.S. Barriers to Implementing Clinical Pharmacogenetics Testing in Sub-Saharan Africa. A Critical Review. *Pharmaceutics* **2020**, *12*, 809. [CrossRef] [PubMed]
7. Li, D.; Xie, A.H.; Liu, Z.; Li, D.; Ning, B.; Thakkar, S.; Tong, W.; Xu, J. Linking Pharmacogenomic Information on Drug Safety and Efficacy with Ethnic Minority Populations. *Pharmaceutics* **2020**, *12*, 1021. [CrossRef] [PubMed]
8. Almenar-Pérez, E.; Sánchez-Fito, T.; Ovejero, T.; Nathanson, L.; Oltra, E. Impact of Polypharmacy on Candidate Biomarker miRNomes for the Diagnosis of Fibromyalgia and Myalgic Encephalomyelitis/Chronic Fatigue Syndrome: Striking Back on Treatments. *Pharmaceutics* **2019**, *11*, 126. [CrossRef]
9. Wigle, T.J.; Tsvetkova, E.V.; Welch, S.A.; Kim, R.B. DPYD and Fluorouracil-Based Chemotherapy: Mini Review and Case Report. *Pharmaceutics* **2019**, *11*, 199. [CrossRef] [PubMed]
10. Michaud, V.; Tran, M.; Pronovost, B.; Bouchard, P.; Bilodeau, S.; Alain, K.; Vadnais, B.; Franco, M.; Bélanger, F.; Turgeon, J. Impact of GSTA1 Polymorphisms on Busulfan Oral Clearance in Adult Patients Undergoing Hematopoietic Stem Cell Transplantation. *Pharmaceutics* **2019**, *11*, 440. [CrossRef] [PubMed]
11. Suntsov, V.; Jovanovic, F.; Knezevic, E.; Candido, K.D.; Knezevic, N.N. Can Implementation of Genetics and Pharmacogenomics Improve Treatment of Chronic Low Back Pain? *Pharmaceutics* **2020**, *12*, 894. [CrossRef] [PubMed]
12. Buendía, J.A.; Halac, E.; Bosaleh, A.; de Davila, M.T.G.; Imvertasa, O.; Bramuglia, G. Frequency of CYP3A5 Genetic Polymorphisms and Tacrolimus Pharmacokinetics in Pediatric Liver Transplantation. *Pharmaceutics* **2020**, *12*, 898. [CrossRef] [PubMed]

13. Salvador-Martín, S.; Kaczmarczyk, B.; Álvarez, R.; Navas-López, V.M.; Gallego-Fernández, C.; Moreno-Álvarez, A.; Solar-Boga, A.; Sánchez, C.; Tolín, M.; Velasco, M.; et al. Whole Transcription Profile of Responders to Anti-TNF Drugs in Pediatric Inflammatory Bowel Disease. *Pharmaceutics* **2021**, *13*, 77. [CrossRef] [PubMed]

Publisher's Note: MDPI stays neutral with regard to jurisdictional claims in published maps and institutional affiliations.

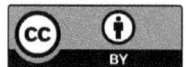

© 2021 by the authors. Licensee MDPI, Basel, Switzerland. This article is an open access article distributed under the terms and conditions of the Creative Commons Attribution (CC BY) license (http://creativecommons.org/licenses/by/4.0/).

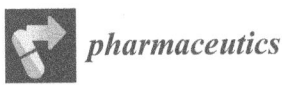

Review

Pharmacogenetic Testing: A Tool for Personalized Drug Therapy Optimization

Kristina A. Malsagova [1,*], Tatyana V. Butkova [1], Arthur T. Kopylov [1], Alexander A. Izotov [1], Natalia V. Potoldykova [2], Dmitry V. Enikeev [2], Vagarshak Grigoryan [2], Alexander Tarasov [3], Alexander A. Stepanov [1] and Anna L. Kaysheva [1]

[1] Biobanking Group, Branch of Institute of Biomedical Chemistry "Scientific and Education Center", 109028 Moscow, Russia; t.butkova@gmail.com (T.V.B.); a.t.kopylov@gmail.com (A.T.K.); farmsale@yandex.ru (A.A.I.); aleks.a.stepanov@gmail.com (A.A.S.); kaysheva1@gmail.com (A.L.K.)
[2] Institute of Urology and Reproductive Health, Sechenov University, 119992 Moscow, Russia; potoldykovanv@gmail.com (N.V.P.); enikeev_dv@mail.ru (D.V.E.); nii-uronephrology@yandex.ru (V.G.)
[3] Institute of Linguistics and Intercultural Communication, Sechenov University, 119992 Moscow, Russia; alexgarmisch@yandex.ru
* Correspondence: kristina.malsagova86@gmail.com; Tel.: +7-499-764-9878

Received: 2 November 2020; Accepted: 17 December 2020; Published: 19 December 2020

Abstract: Pharmacogenomics is a study of how the genome background is associated with drug resistance and how therapy strategy can be modified for a certain person to achieve benefit. The pharmacogenomics (PGx) testing becomes of great opportunity for physicians to make the proper decision regarding each non-trivial patient that does not respond to therapy. Although pharmacogenomics has become of growing interest to the healthcare market during the past five to ten years the exact mechanisms linking the genetic polymorphisms and observable responses to drug therapy are not always clear. Therefore, the success of PGx testing depends on the physician's ability to understand the obtained results in a standardized way for each particular patient. The review aims to lead the reader through the general conception of PGx and related issues of PGx testing efficiency, personal data security, and health safety at a current clinical level.

Keywords: pharmacogenetics; pharmacogenetic test; personalized medicine; genetic polymorphism

1. Introduction

P4-medicine represents an actively developing field of modern medical science. The P4 conception is based on a personalized approach to human health (Personalization, Prediction, Prevention, and Participation). Modern diagnostic kits allow the identification of human metabolic characteristics at the molecular level, thus enabling the revelation of a personal, genetically determined predisposition to a disease or certain metabolic disorders in particular individuals [1]. Personalized medicine involves drug therapy to improve the patient's condition and minimize any adverse effects, thus increasing the quality of life at both the individual and socioeconomic levels.

Pharmacogenetics goes back to 1959 when Vogel coined this term to designate severe adverse drug reactions in a small number of patients reported by the pharmacologists [2]. The adverse reactions, which followed the administration of primaquine, succinylcholine, and isoniazid, were anemia, apnea, and peripheral neuropathy, respectively [3,4].

Pharmacogenetics is purposed to study the response to the drug therapy depending on the genetic background. Response to drugs is frequently governed by genes encoding drug-metabolizing proteins, thus, regulating drug transformation, pharmacokinetics, and pharmacodynamics [5].

PGx may support the investigation of the effect of vitamins [6,7] and additives/supplements and, to some degree [8], homeopathic preparations. However, there is no strong evidence regarding the interaction between genes and vitamins/supplements/homeopathies.

The majority of the related assays in PGx are erroneous or misinterpreted due to biases in the design of the experiment, small sampling, small size of the population, and insufficient time of observation. So far, it is obligatory to provide more correct experiments and researches to observe the suggested effects, otherwise, most of the discussion about the possible influence of non-pharmacological compounds on the genome could be considered doubtful.

In clinical practice, a physician follows the national standards of specialized medical care, based on the evidence from fundamental research and clinical trials of drugs. However, to a greater extent, the therapy process remains a creative task [9].

In addition to adverse drug reactions, the body can demonstrate immunity and/or just partial response to the treatment [10]. Despite the underlying causes of drug resistance remain unclear; however, one can suppose that this is connected with genetic factors. Moreover, aside from the predisposition to diseases, various body metabolic functions are also determined genetically. Namely, genetic variations probably determine the rates of synthesis and decay of multiple biomolecules in the body, the effect of pharmaceuticals, the metabolism of nutrients, etc. [11]. However, answers to these questions have not yet been received.

Nevertheless, genetic testing is slowly finding its niche in drug therapy selection—this process is followed by improving care to a widening range of patients. Pharmacogenomic Biomarkers in Drug Labeling Food and Drug Administration (FDA) provides data about 297 drugs for 100 molecular biomarkers (www.fda.gov/drugs/science-and-research-drugs/table-pharmacogenomic-biomarkers-drug-labeling). Several companies offer genetic testing for adverse drug reactions in patients.

The main goal of this paper is to review current and the latest (up to the latest five years) achievement and progression in PGx relevant to human healthcare and personalized medicine (excluding animal models). The review summarizes general information about pharmacogenomics and trends based on the current level of PGx testing and clinical application for the past decade. The review aims to outline the main approaches used in PGx and provide a brief overview of the related issues and criticism of shortcomings

2. Pharmacogenetic Studies of Drugs

The success of the "Human Genome" project gave impetus to molecular medicine, representing a new branch of medicine focused on the genetic marker panel. Genetic markers represent point nucleotide polymorphisms, which are individual for each person, and reflect his/her personal characteristics.

Even though the growing amount of available data on single nucleotide polymorphisms (SNPs) and other types of genetic mutations makes a significant contribution to the revelation of genome structural variability, the functional importance of these pharmacogenetic variations remains unclear.

Gene variants–alleles- are designated with an "asterisk" followed by a number (e.g., * 1, * 5, * 13) and include one or more SNPs, which are inherited together. Alleles have various levels of activity identified by number, where * 1 (haplotype) denotes a "wild type" or lack of any detected variation [12].

Pairs of these stellate alleles (diplotypes) are subdivided into phenotypes based on their enzymatic activity:

- poor metabolism (PM): a type of alleles that carry the mutated gene(s) encoding important metabolizing enzyme that participates in drug transformation and exhibition of drug activity. Such mutations cause the synthesis of either an insufficient amount of enzyme or produce its inactive gene product which entails decreasing of enzymatic activity and even complete loss of activity. They are much slower to eliminate various drugs metabolized by the same enzyme. Therefore, the patient runs a risk to reach a high plasma concentration of the drug, causing dose-dependent adverse effects. In this regard, slow metabolizers require a careful drug dose selection:

- Extensive metabolizers (EM): they provide a regular rate of drug biotransformation. They usually have two active allelic genes or one functional and one partially active allele;
- Intermediate metabolizers (IM): heterozygous carriers of the mutation (with an autosomal recessive inheritance). To achieve an optimal therapeutic effect, they may require a lower pharmacological dosage than the usual one;
- Ultra-fast metabolizers (UM): they are characterized with an increased gene expression—owing to the presence of three or more functional alleles following the duplication or multiple duplications of a functional allele (e.g., duplication of the CYP2D6 gene). Ultra-fast metabolizers may require a higher drug dose for an optimal effect (Figure 1).

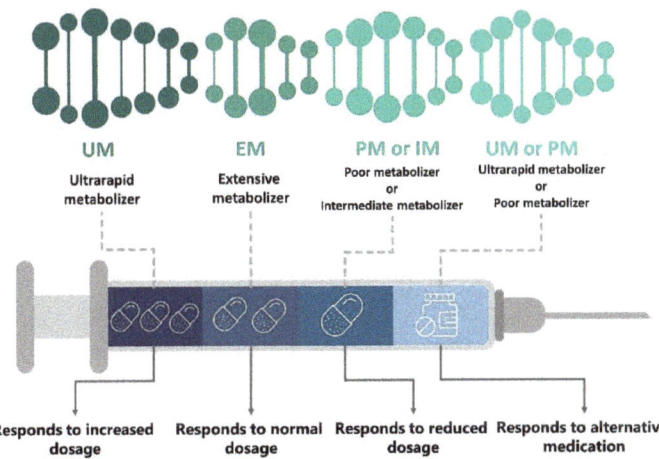

Figure 1. Genetic variation in metabolic phenotype. Depending on the pharmacogenomics (PGx) testing of genes encoding enzymes that are involved in the drug transport and transformation activity, the examined person can be attributed to either of the defined phenotype (ultra-fast metabolizers (UM), extensive metabolizers (EM), poor metabolism (PM), or intermediate metabolizers (IM)) which, in turn, indicates a personal response to dosage and the certain medication.

UM and PM metabolizers represent the groups connected with the most significant risk of therapy ineffectiveness or adverse effects [13].

Even though clinical sites and laboratory centers have an individual approach to the need for PGx testing and the workflow, there are four main stages. These steps include: (1) patient identification, (2) taking the biomaterial for the PGx testing, (3) sending the biomaterial to the laboratory to perform the selected PGx test, (4) analyzing the obtained results, and (5) review the results by a professional physician together with a curated patient to, (6) eventually, elaborate the treatment strategy (Figure 2).

These steps are not meant to be exhaustive or set out in guidelines. Hospitals can adapt the steps outlined to their individual practice structure, patient needs, and clinical priorities.

Planning a personalized medicine study design depends on the goal. The first stage of the planning involves searching for candidate genes-genes whose transcription products affect the pharmacokinetics or pharmacodynamics of drugs. Typically, this stage includes a literature review. Most of the candidate genes are known and are being actively studied. If there is no data in the literature on the effect of genetic polymorphisms on the investigated drug's efficacy and safety, it is necessary to conduct its research.

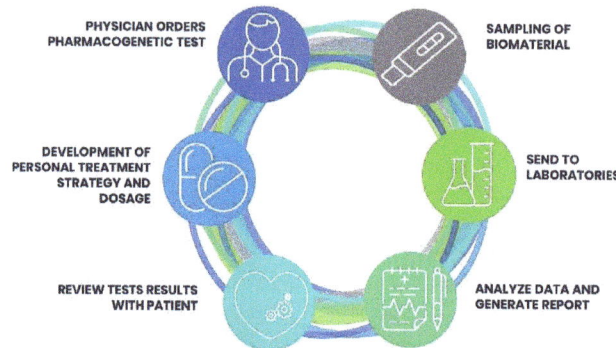

Figure 2. Schematic representation of PGx testing steps. Initially, the physician orders the PGx testing to the curated patient. The test is usually performed on saliva or peripheral blood and requires a small amount of biomaterial, and does not require special preparation for the test. After the testing, the physician reviews the obtained report and discuss it with the curated patient to find out whether certain medication can be effective and what is the best dosage for the treatment therapy. The results may also include the prediction of possible side-effect from the prescribed medication.

2.1. Comparative Cohort Study with Posterior Analysis

Posterior research is the most common pharmacogenetic analysis design where patients with a specific nosology are selected based on the studied drug's indication. The control group is either the "placebo" group or the group provided therapy with an alternative medication. Simultaneously, the parameters of the effectiveness and safety of treatment in the comparison groups are evaluated. The study ends with an analysis of the association of the patient's genotype for the studied polymorphic marker with the results of therapy. It is possible to establish a possible association between the presence of a polymorphic gene variant and the impact of pharmacotherapy. The genotyping of a sample of the already completed study is performed to implement this design. The main disadvantage is that it is impossible to influence the number of carriers of the polymorphic variant, which may be insufficient for statistical analysis [14,15].

2.2. Comparative Cohort Study with Genotyping of Participants before Inclusion

The study can be carried out in two versions:

1. Posterior analysis, in which genotyping is carried out before inclusion in the study to form subgroups of equal number with the "wild" genotype and polymorphic variant and does not affect the appointment of pharmacotherapy;
2. The assignment of pharmacotherapy is carried out depending on genotype to determine whether a study drug actually has an advantage in this patient population over an alternative (or placebo) [14,16].

2.3. Comparative Study of the Pharmacogenetic Approach

A comparative study of two approaches, traditional and pharmacogenetic, is conducted if rigorous evidence about the influence of genetic polymorphisms on a particular drug's efficacy and safety exists. This is the final stage before the introduction of pharmacogenetic testing into clinical practice. The population includes patients with indications for the study drug. The drug dose selection is carried out based on the results of pharmacogenetic testing, and the traditional selection of the dose of the given drug serves as a control. As a result of the study, the advantages of a personalized approach are assessed in comparison with an empirical one [14]. This study alone is not enough. To achieve the highest level of evidence, a meta-analysis of several studies with this design is required.

It is important to determine the mechanism underlying the variability of drug response and drug efficiency, to establish the starting point that can support the identification of genes that produce the necessary pharmacogenetic effect. Therefore, many instances in pharmacogenetics relate to the personal assimilation, metabolism, or elimination of a drug. Other features contributing to the variable drug responses include distinctions in drug target molecules or disease pathways. In some cases, variants in several genes are implicated ("combinatorial pharmacogenetics") in the determination of variable response. Recently, searches for previously unexpected relationships between phenotypes and thousands of common polymorphic sites in the genome (an unbiased approach) have been utilized to address the problem of variable drug action [17].

3. Prospects for the Introduction of a Pharmacogenetic Test into the Clinic

Nowadays, personalized medicine becomes more and more important [18]. Ongoing clinical trials can result in the introduction of pharmacogenetic testing into practice. This may accelerate the approval of distinct medication with no obligation to be tested on a PGx matter, which makes their market entry faster and more cost-effective. Typically, genomic information related to individual patients is made available to those who prescribe therapy. By 2017, the UK planned to perform the sequencing of 100,000 genomes of cancer patients and patients suffering from occasional or most dangerous infectious diseases (HIV, hepatitis C, tuberculosis), and to provide the pharmacogenetic information about the patients admitted in the study by the National Health Service [19]. Company 23andMe (Sunnyvale, CA, USA) (www.23andme.com) also provides pharmacogenetic information to guide the treatment directly upon customer request [20]. The FDA approved the first pharmacogenetic test in 2005. That was AmpliChip CYP450 test system manufactured by Affymetrix (Santa Clara, CA, USA) and Third Wave Technologies (Madison, WI, USA) Invader UGT1A1 (UDP-glucuronosyltransferase) Molecular Assay. The approval procedure was endorsed by clinicians, general healthcare systems, insurance companies, and concerned patients to determine the best way to integrate these tests into clinical practice [21]. At the same time, the critical questions raised were as to whom the tests should be applied and what are the most appropriate circumstances for their application, what evidence is required for the application of these tests, and how the results of the tests must be stored in electronic health data depositaries [22]? Haga and Kantor [23] reviewed laboratories, which offer clinical PGx testing in the United States. Of the 111 reviewed laboratories, 76 offered PGx testing services. Of these laboratories, 31 laboratories offered tests for only specific genes; 30 laboratories offered tests for multiple genes, while only 15 laboratories offered both types of tests. A total of 45 laboratories offered 114 multigene panel tests that cover 295 genes. However, no clinical guidelines were available for most of these tests [23]. In the industry, there is a trend towards multiplex tests intended to detect polymorphisms in a large number of genes. In 2005, the FDA-approved AmpliChip test (Roche, Basel, Switzerland) was designed to analyze two genes [24]. In 2010, Affymetrix introduced the DMET chip to diagnose 225 genes; the latter number is now expanded to 231 genes [23,25]. In 2012, researchers from Stanford University and the University of Florida developed a panel containing an SNP array of 120 genes including 25 genes responsible for drug metabolism and 12 drug carrier genes [26]. In 2014, the PGRN-Seq capture test for the analysis of 84 pharmacogens was developed [27]. The variety of gene panels is not limited to the examples mentioned above. Other types of pharmacological tests are available or are under development [28,29].

Currently, the clinical relevance of multigene panels mainly depends on a few well-studied and classical genes. Using the 84 gene PGRN-Seq capture panel, the examination of only five genes among ca. 5000 patients indicated that 99% of tested patients carried at least one clinically valid variant or one known variant relevant to decide about their treatment [30]. However, the clinical significance of large multiplex panels can mainly be determined by a certain task to be solved. For instance, PGx testing can be arranged as an immediate decision on treatment based on a panel of genes with a high level of evidence for a particular drug. However, the most common type of multigenic complex panel PGx test without specific clinical indications can be performed for a forward-looking patient. Such tests can be warranted since alternative drugs can be further used, and the clinical relevance of the data can increase with time. Despite the absence of consensus on the preventive PGx testing [31,32], many healthcare organizations implemented such testing programs to obtain valuable information regarding clinical validity and usefulness [27,33].

3.1. Audience for PGx Testing

Currently, PGx tests exist in various areas of medicine, including, but not limited to, psychiatry, cardiology, anesthesia, and oncology. Some clinical guidelines for PGx tests are accessible for the prediction of tricyclic antidepressants (TCAs) and selective serotonin reuptake inhibitor (SSRI) efficacy based on CYP2D6 and CYP2C19 activity [34,35]. Recent studies revealed reduced adverse effects and improved scores in depressed patients after PGx-based antidepressant therapy [36]. PGx testing is particularly attractive given the time frame required. For instance, the estimation of the complete therapeutic response to SSRIs can require 4 to 6 weeks [37]. The patient and the healthcare provider can spend several months adjusting the dose and/or prescribing new medications before it becomes clear that the therapy does not lead to the therapeutic effect. PGx testing can allow a physician to determine the best drug for a given situation in a much shorter time.

PGx testing applicability, to a certain extent, depends on the intensity of potential adverse reactions to the drug. For instance, Abacavir, used for HIV treatment, can produce severe cutaneous adverse reactions (SCAR) [38]. Generally, the risk is low, but HLA-B*57:01 variation is related to much more pronounced SCAR after Abacavir intake. Thus, this drug is contraindicated for HLA-B*57:01- positive patients [38].

The use of PGx testing is relevant to the selection of the Warfarin dose. Intake of dietary vitamin K, health and social conditions, and genetic variations were also found to affect Warfarin therapy [39]. Changes in CYP2C9 can disrupt the metabolism of Warfarin, and alterations in VKORC1 (vitamin K epoxide reductase) can increase the drug susceptibility of a patient [38,39].

The use of codeine was limited to adult patients after the evidence of a risk of increased adverse effects in pediatric patients. The study revealed adverse reactions in infants whose breastfeeding mothers underwent codeine therapy [40]. These reactions resulted from codeine conversion to morphine, performed mainly by CYP2D6 protein [41]. Similar reactions can occur with other CYP2D6-mediated pain relievers—such as tramadol, oxycodone, and hydrocodone [42].

The high interest of patients in PGx testing was revealed [43,44]. The patients are particularly interested in the possibility of using recommendations based on PGx test results to reduce adverse drug effects and to choose proper therapy [45]. However, the cost of the tests, the insurance coverage, and the availability of testing results represent the limitations for PGx testing [46,47]. Some questions are still relayed uncertain after PGx testing. Thus, patients should be appropriately informed about the capabilities of PGx testing [48].

For this reason, one should understand that PGx testing allows the identification of (1) drugs with an increased risk of causing adverse effects, (2) drugs with a narrow therapeutic index. Besides that, PGx testing can reduce the set of drugs for therapy and predict the drug dosage [48,49]. At the same time, PGx testing will not be efficient for predicting: (1) occurrence of all possible adverse reactions with a drug, (2) the risk of a specific adverse effect for all drugs, 3) the risk of occurrence of complications [49].

The PGx testing provides an opportunity in decision making of whether the chosen medication and treatment strategy is of advantage and gives the proper results over the expectations based on the obtained profile of patients. That is exactly what opens the door for personalized medicine, that is what should happen when a person has a choice: to be healed but not at a cost of health deterioration, not in awaiting while inappropriate drug boosts dire consequences instead of a satisfying outcome.

3.2. Resources in the Pharmacogenetic Sector

Due to the ever-changing nature of genetic medicine, one should be aware of further changes in testing guidelines or results interpretation. This task can be simplified with the use of currently available Internet resources (Table 1).

Table 1. The most visited and popular internet resources in the pharmacogenetic sector.

Resource	Description	Reference
Coursera	Online personalized medicine course that provides short educational courses in genetics and mechanisms determining the variability of response to drugs; development of ethical issues and objections related to implementation and introduction of wide-scale genome-sequencing into clinical practice.	https://www.coursera.org/learn/personalizedmed
CPIC	An international consortium that specializes in publishing genotype-based drug guidelines to help clinicians understand the usability of the available genetic test results in optimizing drug therapy.	https://www.cpicpgx.org [50,51]
eMERGE	Funded by the NIH. This network brings together researchers with a wide range of expertise in genomics, statistics, ethics, informatics, and clinical medicine from leading medical research institutions across the country to research in genomics including the discovery, clinical implementation, and public resources.	https://www.emerge-network.org
GTR	Free of charge resource that provides generalized datastore of the exhaustive information about genetic tests which is provided and supported by vendors; main auditory is clinicians and researchers.	https://www.ncbi.nlm.nih.gov/gtr [52]
IGNITE	Was developed to enhance the use of genomic medicine by supporting the incorporation of genomic information into clinical practice and exploring methods for effective implementation, diffusion, and sustainability in various clinical settings.	https://www.gmkb.org
My Drug Genome	A portal to study how genetics affects drug response and how results of genetic testing can be implemented into healthcare.	https://www.mydruggenome.org
PharmGKB	Online knowledge base responsible for the aggregation, curation, integration, and distribution of data on the influence of genetic variation on the drug response in humans.	https://www.pharmgkb.org [53]

CPIC—Clinical Pharmacogenetics Implementation Consortium; eMERGE—Electronic Medical Records and Genomics Network; GTR—Genetic Testing Registry; IGNITE—GeNomics In pracTicE; NIH—National Institutes of Health; PharmGKB—Pharmacogenetic Knowledge Base.

Besides, there are also fewer known resources that merit attention. Among them, the Mayo Clinic portal that published numerous "AskMayoExpert" educational materials for both physicians and patients to enhance general knowledge and practice [54]. St. Jude Children's Research Hospital allows tracking the website-integrated gene or drug information and implementation-specific publications and presentations [55]. Ubiquitous Pharmacogenomics (U-PGx) developed an e-learning platform to disseminate general knowledge of pharmacology, suitable for physicians and pharmacists (https://upgx.eu/) [56].

Support and development of these resources can be a valuable tool for studying the upcoming or less known pharmacogenetic interactions. Several organizations are currently providing integration with PGx programs and updating the current data [51,57].

3.3. Choice of PGx Testing

PGx testing can be carried out either as a single gene analysis or as a multiplex panel of ten or more genes. Early testing mostly involves analyzing multiple variants of the same gene, targeting the most common and most effective variants. Novel technologies significantly increased the number of genes and variations covered by a single test. Most PGx tests analyze a variety of clinically relevant SNPs. During the determination of the best test or panel for a patient (or a population), one should consider the therapeutic indication. For instance, testing for CYP2D6 and CYP2C19 is required for antidepressant therapy. In addition, it will also be useful to consider whether the patient would benefit from a PGx test for cardiovascular and pain-killing drugs [58]. A panel test can be more expensive than a single gene assay, but it ensures that co-prescribed drugs are also tested.

Panel PGx tests are heterogeneous and vary in volume and scope [59,60]. Most of the panels cover several of the best-studied and most potent genes. The panel can contain SNP combinations based on a literature review of prospective studies. A panel that includes many genes may not necessarily provide additional value to the patient, as not all options offer the same clinical relevance. Some variants can be extremely rare outside of certain populations but can be quite common within a certain group. For instance, the HLA-B * 15: 02 variant, associated with an increased risk of SCAR in patients prescribed carbamazepine, has an allele frequency of 0.04% in patients of European descent and 6.88% in patients of East Asian descent [61]. A panel can be more beneficial to the patient if it analyzes options that match their ethnic origin more closely.

One should keep in mind available alternatives or special analyses. Multiple copies of the CYP2D6 gene (e.g., duplications) occur in about 1 in 8 patients, and this number may be even higher in black and Asian patients [62]. Gene duplication can cause increased enzymatic activity and can be clinically relevant. However, not all panels can reveal the presence or degree of gene duplication.

In addition to the panel contents, one should consider such factors as the type of biomaterial (buccal smear, saliva, or blood, etc.) since the way of biomaterial sampling can pose a problem for the patient. The access to results and the methods of their obtaining also represent the factors that should be considered. Several panels provide nothing but raw genetic data, while others are fully integrated into the electronic health record and enable sophisticated clinical decision support systems (CDS). Finally, one should consider the potential cost of PGx testing. Patients vary in ways and means to pay for testing.

3.4. Interpreting PGx Test Results

When prescribing PGx testing, one should keep in mind that the result obtained represents only a part of the overall picture of the patient's condition. Therefore, to determine the therapy risks and benefits, the PGx test results should be used and interpreted by taking into account the state of all the patient's systems, concomitant medications, and current pathological conditions. When the "best" drug is identified with the PGx test, this does not necessarily mean that it should be used in therapy since the patient may have a history of severe adverse reactions to the drug. Conversely, the PGx test identification of an increased risk of therapeutic failure should not lead to drug discontinuation if the current therapy is effective. Different result structures can be used, depending on the gene and protein in question [63]. Some genes can be described in terms of metabolic activity, some by their general function, and others only as present or absent. Several PGx test results describe general gene function—such as SLCO1B1 (solute carrier organic anion transporter family member 1B1), associated with simvastatin; VKORC1 (vitamin K epoxide reductase complex subunit 1), associated with Warfarin; OPRM1 (opioid receptor Mu 1), associated with opioids [63]. Results for these genes can be reported as normal, intermediate, or low function. For instance, a "normal gene function" result indicates that no change in the patient's dosage regimen is required. In other cases (decreased or poor function), the physician's recommendations will be based on the information on a reduced functional activity (or complete inactivity) of the analyzed genes.

PGx test results can be "positive" or "negative" [57]. For instance, human leukocyte antigen (HLA) genes produce essential components of the immune system. Patients who are positive for HLA-B * 58: 01, run an increased risk of hypersensitivity to allopurinol; patients, who are positive for HLA-B * 15: 02, run an increased risk of SCAR with carbamazepine or oxcarbazepine [64,65].

The way the results are presented can vary considerably from one report to another. The results can be delivered either as raw genetic data or as the ultimate therapeutic recommendation. In the reports, a proprietary iconography can be used for the description of results. This iconography can use specific symbols to indicate patients in which an increased risk of adverse effects or therapy ineffectiveness is expected. Other reports can use a traffic light view with three main drug categories: green for normal risk, yellow for use with caution, and red for exclusion. Results displayed in any format can cause the provider to oversimplify the PGx test results, ignoring additional clinical considerations.

Below (Figure 3) is an example of an abbreviated PGx test performed by AyassBioScience (Frisco, TX, USA). (the full report can be found at https://ayassbioscience.com/wp-content/uploads/2020/02/PGX-Medical-ManagementPrint-Fit-on-Page.pdf).

	REPORT DETAILS	
Ayass bioscience	Name: XXXX XXXXXX DOB: XX/XX/1970 ACC #: XXXXXX	
Pharmacogenetic Test Summary		
ABCB1	3435C>T C/C	Variant Allele Not Present
ANKK1/DRD2	DRD2:Taq1A G/G	Unaltered DRD2 function
Apolipoprotein E	ε3/ε3	Normal APOE function
COMT	Val158Met G/G	High/Normal COMT Activity
CYP1A2	*1L/*1L	Unknown Phenotype
CYP2B6	*1/*6	Intermediate Metabolizer
CYP2C19	*1/*17	Rapid Metabolizer
CYP2C9	*1/*1	Normal Metabolizer
CYP2D6	*1/*2 XN	Ultra-Rapid Metabolizer
CYP3A4	*1/*1	Normal Metabolizer
CYP3A5	*1/*6	Intermediate Metabolizer
Factor II	20210G>A GG	Normal Thrombosis Risk
Factor V Leiden	1691G>A GG	Normal Thrombosis Risk
MTHFR	1298A>C AC	Reduced MTHFR Activity
MTHFR	677C>T CC	Normal MTHFR Activity
OPRM1	A118G A/A	Normal OPRM1 Function
SLCO1B1	521T>C T/T	Normal Function
VKORC1	-1639G>A G/G	Low Warfarin Sensitivity

For a complete report contact Ayass BioScience LLC
www.AyassBioScience.com — Powered By Translational

Figure 3. Samples of PGx test at AyassBioScience: The report is featured with color-coded information for easier navigation and attention. The greed color indicates that the medication can be prescribed according to standard regimens, and the risk for the indicated condition is not increased; yellow color—indicated that dosage adjusting is required, there is an increased vigilance or the patient has a moderate risk for the indicated condition; red color designates that medication has potentially reduced efficacy and increased toxicity or the patient has an increased risk for the indicated condition. In the exemplified results, the patient has a normal response to Apixaban (the drug is a substrate for the efflux transport proteins P-gp (ABCB1) and BCRP (ABCG2) and, possibly, decreased response to Bupropion. Bupropion is metabolized to its active metabolite hydroxybupropion by CYP2B6. This metabolite contributes to the therapeutic effects of bupropion when used as a smoking cessation agent or as an antidepressant. The patient has also increased response to Codeine, which is converted into its active metabolite morphine by CYP2D6. Since this patient is the ultra-rapid metabolizer (UM), a greatly increased morphine level is expected, and the patient is at high risk of toxicity when taking codeine.

A variety of ways of presenting the information can be used in the report. Since each way is different, one should be careful to ensure a complete understanding of the meaning of each categorization [49].

3.5. Automation Tools for Integrating PGx Testing into the Clinic

Rapidly developing new technologies of DNA sequencing enabled quick and efficient identification of the genomic characteristics of organisms. The main result of the genomic and post-genomic technologies development was a significant expansion of the capabilities to study the genetic nature of a whole spectrum of human diseases. A genome-wide association study (GWAS) of clinical samples generated data on the genetic makeup featured for the specific groups (families or populations) to elaborate a personalized treatment approach. In this regard, to date, the research into the mechanisms of genetic predisposition to multifactorial diseases and the identification of specific genetic markers are of particular relevance. Such methods are widely used internationally and in Russia, where modern sequencing technologies are gradually introduced into medical research and medical practice to personify the treatment strategy.

Next-generation sequencing (NGS) is used for in-depth (multiple) reading of genetic material, which is necessary, for instance, for re-sequencing and assembly of new genomes (de novo), transcriptome, and epigenomic studies. This method allows one to reveal rare variations and to understand the genetic function better. However, the avalanche of new data will also make problems for researchers and clinicians, giving many "options of unknown importance" in the absence of clear indications [49]. Modifications of CDS are required to ensure the storage and use of new data architecture and new data availability programs. This, in turn, will identify significant opportunities in the coming years. Several healthcare systems use CDS tools to integrate PGx test data into clinical decision-making and provide information to end-users [66]. CDS systems can be used to administer high-risk drugs and provide automated recommendations indicating why certain modifications should be applied to a selected drug or dose.

The U-PGx PREPARE study developed solutions for sites with limited electronic health record infrastructure. The "Safety-Code" card is part of a mobile CDS, and with a quick response code, a medical professional is directed to a website with dosing recommendations customized for the patient [67]. This card also provides an overview of the most relevant PGx test results with a list of drugs with existing (known) recommendations [68].

Such CDS tools will be necessary, as PGx tests become more common due to the emergence of new results and test formats. One can also focus on developing patient-centered applications and portals, through which the patient can interact with his or her service providers and receive a consultation based on outcomes.

The increase in providers' and patients' awareness can stimulate the use of PGx testing. Consequently, laboratories will adjust the scope and type of available clinical PGx tests based on clinical requirements. The expected increase in the development of multigene panel PGx tests follows the advances in oncology, microbiology, and other fields. However, the proper clinical use of such tests appears to be more involved, requiring the support and participation of multiple interested parties.

4. Side Effects of Drugs and Safety

Adverse drug reactions (ADRs) are a significant cause of iatrogenic morbidity, mortality, and high cost [69]. They are one of the most common causes of death [70]. Today PGx is not a routine in clinical practice which may explain the lack of statistically significant data about the underlying reasons for ADRs-caused mortality. However, it is well known that the majority of ADRs are dose-dependent while the rest are related to allergy or idiosyncratic [71]. Usage of anticoagulants, opioids, or immunosuppressants is the most frequent reason for the lethal outcome [71]. At the same time, lethality indicator strictly correlates with the age, race, and urbanization level [72–75].

ADRs can result from inappropriate drug prescription, toxic effects of drug chemicals, impaired absorption, distribution, metabolism, and elimination of drugs related to age and sex, drug-drug interactions in combination therapy, or when a patient is treated with different medications for comorbid disorders [70]. This is especially important in chronic diseases that require long-term treatment and the treatment of the elderly, who, in 50% of cases or more, take several types of drugs daily [70]. To mitigate side effects, a large number of drug information resources and drug interactions have been developed over the past two decades to provide support to clinicians in making appropriate drug prescription decisions [70]. However, few resources include PGx as a practical tool for clinical use [70].

It is essential to develop interventional approaches to identify patients at risk of side effects to achieve favorable treatment results. Although the risk of developing ADRs may depend on clinical characteristics (organ functions of patients, their age, or the use of potentially interacting drugs), up to 10–20% of ADRs can be caused by genetic factors [69]. For example, genetic polymorphism can lead to metabolic disorders, which leads to the accumulation of drugs or toxic metabolites, and as a consequence to immune-mediated ADRs that can be potentially fatal [69].

The study [44,76,77] showed that women are more receptive to the ADRs. This may be related to gender differences in the pharmacokinetics and pharmacodynamics of drugs [78]. Also, the incidence of ADRs is higher in elderly patients, which has also been confirmed by other studies [79,80].

It is quite challenging to control and manage the development of ADRs. The occurrence of ADRs can increase treatment costs due to an increase in the period of hospitalization and additional clinical trials. In addition, ADRs can often lead to cascading processes where new drugs are prescribed for conditions that result from the use of another drug. Although some of the side effects are considered non-preventable, recent developments show that these reactions can be avoided by individualizing drug therapy based on genetic information obtained from pharmacological testing. For example, dihydropyrimidine dehydrogenase (DPD) was an enzyme involved in the detoxification of 5-fluorouracil, a crucial anti-cancer agent. Studies have shown that an inherited DPD defect can lead to severe toxicity associated with 5-fluorouracil, such as myelotoxicity, gastrointestinal toxicity, and neurotoxicity in cancer patients [81].

In the treatment of HIV, the drug Abacavir is prescribed, and one of the ADRs is hypersensitivity syndrome (HSS) [69]. HSS leads to systemic disease that manifests itself as fever and maculopapular rash. ADRs usually disappear after discontinuation of Abacavir, but can also be fatal if, despite the response, the drug is continued.

The pharmacogenetic test HLA-B * 57: 01 administered before the initiation of Abacavir effectively eliminated the HSS previously observed in approximately 5% of the treated European population [69].

The effectiveness of the HLA-B * 57: 01 test is explained by its high negative predictive value [82]. Patients lacking regular alleles are more suspicious to develop immunological hypersensitivity to Abacavir, strong evidence of clinical efficacy [83], and cost-effectiveness [84].

5. Obstacles on the Way to the Introduction of Pharmacogenetic Tests into Clinical Practice

PGx testing aims to personalize drug therapy to improve the effectiveness of drug prescription and minimize adverse effects. Despite the potential benefits, PGx testing applications are limited mainly to the use in specialized medical centers or laboratories. The large-scale dissemination and implementation of PGx tests in the typical laboratory and clinical practice are limited by several problems, including legal and ethical issues, scarce data on the effectiveness, validity, and prospects of clinical use, provision of hands-on training for clinicians, testing simplicity and the availability of alternative methods for drug reactions prediction [85,86].

Despite the PGx test constitutes a relatively new approach requiring additional investigations to be introduced in clinical practice population-wide, many companies actively develop in this direction (Table 2).

Table 2. Pharmacogenomic companies and services.

Companies	Main Activity	Reference
Ayass BioScience	A disease monitoring system for implementation in modern molecular medicine and daily clinical practice. Emphasizes genetic, epigenetic, proteomic, and metabolomic profiling, for data collection and interpretation using bioinformatics and biostatistics.	https://ayassbioscience.com
Biocerna	This company elaborated a PGx360™ test which is a panel of 22 genes and 62 associated variants to provide an opportunity for clinicians in the selecting of a proper drug. "Biocerna" also provides specific testing of translocations used to monitor a patient's response to chemotherapy strategy.	http://www.biocerna.com
Coriell Life Science (Gene Dose)	Provides data analysis of and reports on clinical laboratory pharmacogenomic assays. Coriell Life Sciences PGx elucidates results of PGx assays in association with drug-related risks to improve patient health to provide a complete, safe, and personalized drug therapy strategy.	https://www.coriell.com
Diatech Pharmacogenetics	Develops pharmacogenetic tests for precision cancer medicine and produces two groups of cancer therapy products: (1) pyrosequencing technology in pharmacogenetics of anti-EGFR therapy, and (2) pyrosequencing technology in pharmacogenetics of chemo- and radiotherapy.	https://www.diatechpharmacogenetics.com
Dynamic DNA Laboratories	This company provides a wide variety of gene testing services, including pharmacogenomic testing, drug discovery, DNA expression, and also some customized testing and DNA testing services. The main PGx product is the predictive Comprehensive PGx Test for over 150 different drugs.	https://dynamicdnalabs.com
Eurofins Genomics	Leader in food, environmental, pharmaceutical, and cosmetic testing. Specializes in pharmacogenetics and PGx research, offers a comprehensive package of services for the drug development process.	https://www.eurofins.com
Exceltox Laboratories	A CAP and CLIA accredited laboratory that offers advanced clinical, PGx, and toxicological analysis.	http://exceltox.com
GeneDx	Leader in genomics, including research on rare genetic diseases. PharmacoDx targets sequence variants in genes that contribute to drug metabolism. PharmacoDx is a comprehensive pharmacogenetic panel with over 100 genetic variants.	https://www.genedx.com
Genentech	A biotechnology company that pioneers research in and develops medications for patients with severe and life-threatening diseases.	https://www.gene.com
Genewiz	A leading international company that offers a wide range of services in genomic technologies, including NGS, classic Sanger sequencing, elaboration of synthetic genes, and bioinformatic data analysis support.	https://www.genewiz.com/en-GB

Table 2. Cont.

Companies	Main Activity	Reference
HudsonAlpha Institute for Biotechnology	Initiation and support of scientific research programs related to human health and well-being; supports the introduction of genomic medicine into clinical practice and promotes entrepreneurship in life sciences. Developing of work programs for specialists in genomics. Conducting extensive elaboration in the pharmacogenetic testing platform in collaboration with Kailos Genetics.	https://hudsonalpha.org
Integrated DNA Technologies	Develops and manufactures nucleic acid products. Areas of activity include scientific and commercial research, agriculture, medical diagnostics, pharmaceutical development, and synthetic biology.	https://www.idtdna.com
Myriad Genetics	Pioneering researches and innovations in molecular diagnostic testing aimed to improve personalized medicine.	https://myriad.com
Pathway Genomics	A company private that offers customized tests for the screening of diet, weight loss, and metabolic response to numerous commonly prescribed medications. The information can be securely delivered to patients and physicians through any mobile device in a comprehensive form using the in-house developed application. The company produces several PGx products, including "OmePsychiatricMeds" (genetic test for mental health medication efficacy) and "OmePainMeds" (genetic test for pain management medication efficacy).	https://www.pathway.com/about
Phenomics Health	This is a bioinformatic platform for precision medicine that transforms large health data sets of patients and even populations into certain products and services to support decision-making about pharmacological treatment.	https://www.phenomicshealth.com/
Quantigen	Development of gene expression and gene variation tests, methods validation, and other services related to clinical assays and PGx researches.	http://www.quantigen.com
RxGenomix	Developed a new highly secured and compatible data-concentrator RxGenomix that provides genomic data exchange through distinct healthcare IT services including laboratory management systems, electronic clinical records, and pharmacy operation systems.	https://www.rxgenomix.com
Sema4	This is an interdisciplinary partnership of scientists, clinicians, engineers, and genetic consultants. It is a unique consortium with a solid basis of more than 160 years of clinical experience, world-class academic research, and groundbreaking information technology.	https://sema4.com

Table 2. Cont.

Companies	Main Activity	Reference
Sorenson Genomics	This company is mainly focused on DNA testing in forensic and research projects. The main areas of interest are DNA genotyping, DNA sequencing and analysis of fragments in population genetics, and human genotyping. Offers: LEAD Local Entry Access DNA Database—a reliable, proven software that allows fast and secure storage, search, and analysis of millions of DNA profiles.	https://sorensongenomics.com
Transgenomic	Development of molecular technologies for personalized medicine specifically in cardiology and oncology. This company is an international leader in pharmacogenetic testing and offers a variety of products designed to detect specific mutations in a certain gene that can indicate a specific heart disease and risk of heart failure.	http://www.transgenomic.com
Translational Software	A leader in the use of genetic data purposed to support decision-making in precision medicine. Developed software that enables laboratories and clinicians to incorporate PGx data into treatment strategies to improve a personalized approach such as "PGxAPI"—a knowledge base purposed to include PGx data into healthcare and laboratory systems. PGxPortal offers an HL7 interface for receiving data and checking the quality of test results. This portal enables clinicians to deliver better patient care by providing clinically relevant pharmacogenomic information.	https://www.translationalsoftware.com
Xact Laboratories	A molecular diagnostics laboratory with a sophisticated research approach that provides a wide range of custom-centered distinctive tests for clinicians and healthcare providers.	https://xactlaboratories.com
23andMe	A biotechnology company that provides customers with information on their disease susceptibility. Pharmacogenetic studies include analysis of CYP2C19, DPYD, SLCO1B1.	https://www.23andme.com

CAP—College of American Pathologists; CLIA—Clinical Laboratory Improvement Amendments; CYP2C19—cytochrome P450 2C19; DPYD—dihydropyrimidine dehydrogenase; SLCO1B1—solute carrier organic anion transporter family member 1B1.

However, it should be kept in mind that the integration of PGx tests into clinical practice is primarily determined by the fact that the test's value and relevance depend on whether the test improves clinical outcomes, e.g., decreases morbidity, mortality, and ADRs [87,88].

The 2000 ACCE (analytical validity, clinical validity, clinical utility, and associated ethical, legal and social implications) project by the US Office of Public Health Genomics (OPHG) aims at the evaluation of genetic tests in the Centers for Disease Control and Prevention [89].

The sensitivity and specificity of the test determine the analytical and clinical validity of PGx testing. The analytical validity measures the ability of a test to identify the genotype of interest. At the same time, the clinical one determines the strength of the relationship between the genotype and the endpoint. Test results provide the data on the clinical utility. The latter improves the clinical outcomes and increases the testing value—compared to the absence of a test or standard treatment [89–91].

Later, the OPHG assigned the Evaluation of Genomic Applications in Practice and Prevention (EGAPP) working group, which expanded and refined the ACCE model. EGAPP supports the development of the systematic assessment of available data regarding the validity of genetic tests and their usefulness in clinical practice, works out recommendations for healthcare professionals [92], and evaluates the widely used genetic tests [93]. The EGAPP Working Group has developed three evidence-based guidelines for PGx tests: (1) genotyping of UGT1A1 for the prediction of response to irinotecan therapy in metastatic colorectal cancer (mCRC), (2) testing tumor tissue on EGFR persistence to choose anti-EGFR therapy for mCRC patients, (3) testing for cytochrome (CYP) P450 polymorphism in adults, suffering from non-psychotic depression, for the prediction of response to selective inhibitors of serotonin reuptake. As a rule, guidelines to these tests indicate insufficient evidence in favor of (or against) doing the test. CPIC develops guidelines for clinicians to help them understand how to use the results of genetic testing for improvement of the drug therapy effectiveness and acceleration of the pharmacogenetic knowledge uptake as a result [94].

The reproducibility and reliability of the data obtained represent a common problem of pharmacological testing [14]. The clinical validity of research can be determined by classical methods such as meta-analysis [95], which represents a systematic review of the literature to evaluate and synthesize all available data on a specific issue [96]. A meta-analysis demonstrated that individual or pioneer studies could provide inconsistent or contradictory results [31]. At the same time, research collaborations allow one to combine the results and to consider all available data (both non-published and published) in the meta-analysis. This provides a larger sample size, yielding a more accurate estimation of the association [97]. However, summarizing and processing large amounts of data can be very complicated and time-consuming [98].

Another problem limiting the PGx test integration into practice is the lack of (or insufficient) evidence to support the usefulness of the test. Randomized controlled trials (RCTs) usually give compelling evidence that preventive and predictive testing improves clinical outcomes with drug therapy. However, if the influence of the genotype is insignificant or the pathological condition is rare, an RCT may require extensive samples, engaged for decades or more [14,99]. In addition, RCTs are expensive, thus being difficult to find funding sources for, especially for low-cost or generic drugs [100]. The PGx test design also represents another restraint for using RCTs: the tests involve a limited number of polymorphisms in specific candidate genes. For instance, the response to depression drugs has a very polygenic architecture [101]. Each polymorphism is assumed to result in a 2–3% variance in the response [102]. Another problem is that the test should take into account polymorphism interaction. The most recent reviews indicate that published studies provided limited cost/benefit data for the available PGx tests. In some cases, the studies found limited (or the absence of) clinical benefit (improved response or remission, decreased adverse effects) [103–105].

There is certainly controversy about the evidence which will be reliable and, at the same time, really feasible to identify the PGx tests' clinical usefulness [91,106]. Many authors believe that a combination of retrospective and prospective studies will do the job; however, the recommendations will require considering the limitations of each research method [86,90].

In addition to scientific evidence, guidelines, and regulations developed, healthcare workers' willingness and ability to use the proposed tests determine the PGx tests scale-up [14,107]. Some time ago, healthcare professionals were reluctant to accept pharmacogenetics, although this position may have changed over time [108]. It may be difficult for specialists to change the tactics of treatment using the usual drugs since they already have a practice of leveling the side effects of the drugs used [109,110].

Most clinicians still lack confidence in PGx testing and subsequent data interpretation, indicating insufficient knowledge in this field [86,90]. The literature emphasizes the need to improve literacy among healthcare professionals regarding expertise in and understanding of PGx testing [14,111].

Lack of awareness of practitioners about the possibilities of pharmacogenetics and poor or insufficient explanation of the test results also reduce personalization technologies for patients. In addition to the development of thematic training courses at medical universities, the inclusion of educational cycles in continuing professional education systems, free placement of information for practicing doctors are required: educational internet portals, webinars, etc. A clinical pharmacologist plays a crucial role in the implementation of pharmacogenetic testing. The competence of a clinical pharmacologist in the field of pharmacogenetics is critical: he or she is the one who organizes the application of genotyping in clinical practice, interprets tests, informs doctors about the possibilities of pharmacogenetics for patients with specific nosologies, that is, acts as the main link between the scientific world, the healthcare system and practicing physicians in the process of introducing pharmacogenetics [14,112].

Currently, algorithms for the interpretation of the results of pharmacogenetic testing are mentioned in the

- Instructions for the medical use of a medicinal product (FDA and European Medicines Agency (EMA)), recommendations of international and national professional scientific public organizations (Recommendations of the experts of the European Science Foundation (ESF), discussed and approved by the participants European Conference on Pharmacogenetics and Pharmacogenomics in Barcelona in June 2010 (published in March 2011) [113],
- Expert recommendations of the Pharmacogenetics Working Group of the Royal Dutch Pharmaceutical Association (published in March 2011) [50],
- Expert guidance of the CPIC, beginning of publication—January 2011) [104].

Disclosure of genetic information to insurance companies is considered an essential socioeconomic issue. This may lead to an increase in health insurance rates for certain patient groups [114]. This problem is deemed to be ethical. It is necessary to determine the group of people who have access to the results of genotyping and formulate the possible consequences for the patient.

The cost of pharmacogenetic testing is another unresolved issue. Even though there are positive results of pharmacoeconomic studies, where the use of pharmacogenetic testing made it possible to reduce the cost of treatment by reducing the cost of correcting the consequences of therapy ineffectiveness or unwanted ADRs, not all insurance companies and health systems are ready to include genotyping in their programs. The cost of genetic tests is decreasing every year, but testing is still available to a wide range of patients with an average income [115].

6. Conclusions

We are on the verge of a new era in human genetic analysis. Deciphering the human genome, together with the development of high-throughput genetic analysis methods, provided a unique opportunity for the identification of complex genetic changes, resulting in the development of new branches of pharmacy: pharmacogenetics and pharmacogenomics. The genomic profiling of patients became a new diagnostic tool, enabling personalized drug therapy with higher effectiveness and fewer adverse effects. The pharmacogenetic tests can help select a specific drug with a specific dosage and administration regime, which will meet the requirements for the treatment of a particular patient in a specific setting, allowing one to avoid time-consuming dose adjustment inevitably associated with adverse effects.

Although PGx testing represents a significant therapeutic advance, it is just a healthcare professional's arsenal tool of the future, increasing therapy effectiveness. The technological breakthrough will never override a physician's experience and logic. This is a small paradigm shift towards the personalization of treatment.

PGx testing development inevitably will stimulate the progress in methods of data storage and data analysis, which are required for the integration of modern information technologies into routine clinical practice. However, the improvement in digital technologies, the increase in the volume and accessibility of databases is not the only problem in integrating genetic testing into the healthcare continuum. This, in turn, requires changes in the interaction between an individual patient and the healthcare system since the ultimate goal is the patient's recovery or control of the disease, regardless of what laboratory techniques and data analysis technologies are employed. In other words, the treatment should take into account both the patient's requirements and the test results. Today pharmacogenetics is in its infancy. A large pool of experimental, but mostly pilot, studies in this area have been accumulated; however, this information can barely be classified as systemic, which makes it difficult to explain the observed correlations between the presence of polymorphisms of a separate gene and epigenetic factors, or the severity of the course of the disease/resistance to therapy. The authors do not aspect information on congenital/acquired polymorphisms, even for the genetically determined diseases, such as cardiovascular diseases and diabetes mellitus. So far, pharmacogenetics provides mosaic information related to the association between the response to drug therapy depending on the genetic background. The next stage is expected to be the research on a larger group of participants, study the contribution of epigenetic factors, and providing clinical guidelines for adjusting or selecting the therapy based on the personal characteristics of the patient. Nevertheless, the field of pharmacogenetics is being actively developed and discussed, and the current demand for end-products in medicine is unusually high. We expect that soon researchers find answers to many questions that are still controversial.

Author Contributions: All authors contributed to the study conception and design. Material preparation, data collection, and analysis were performed by K.A.M., A.L.K., A.T.K., A.A.S., and A.T. The first draft of the manuscript was written by K.A.M., T.V.B., A.A.I., N.V.P., D.V.E., and V.G., and all authors commented on previous versions of the manuscript. All authors have read and agreed to the published version of the manuscript.

Funding: The research was carried out with financial support from the Russian Science Foundation, grant no. 19-14-00298.

Conflicts of Interest: The authors declare no conflict of interest. The funders had no role in the design of the study; in the collection, analyses, or interpretation of data; in the writing of the manuscript, or in the decision to publish the results.

References

1. Alonso, S.G.; de la Torre Díez, I.; Zapiraín, B.G. Predictive, Personalized, Preventive and Participatory (4P) Medicine Applied to Telemedicine and EHealth in the Literature. *J. Med. Syst.* **2019**, *43*, 140. [CrossRef] [PubMed]
2. Vogel, F. Moderne Probleme der Humangenetik. In *Ergebnisse der Inneren Medizin und Kinderheilkunde*; Heilmeyer, L., Schoen, R., de Rudder, B., Eds.; Springer: Berlin/Heidelberg, Germany, 1959; pp. 52–125. [CrossRef]
3. Meyer, U.A. Pharmacogenetics—Five Decades of Therapeutic Lessons from Genetic Diversity. *Nat. Rev. Genet.* **2004**, *5*, 669–676. [CrossRef] [PubMed]
4. Caldwell, J. Drug Metabolism and Pharmacogenetics: The British Contribution to Fields of International Significance. *Br. J. Pharmacol.* **2006**, *147* (Suppl. 1), S89–S99. [CrossRef] [PubMed]
5. Hassan, R.; Allali, I.; Agamah, F.E.; Elsheikh, S.S.M.; Thomford, N.E.; Dandara, C.; Chimusa, E.R. Drug Response in Association with Pharmacogenomics and Pharmacomicrobiomics: Towards a Better Personalized Medicine. *Brief. Bioinform.* **2020**, bbaa292. [CrossRef] [PubMed]
6. Testa, R.; Bonfigli, A.R.; Sirolla, C.; Boemi, M.; Manfrini, S.; Mari, D.; Testa, I.; Sacchi, E.; Franceschi, C. Effect of 4G/5G PAI-1 Polymorphism on the Response of PAI-1 Activity to Vitamin E Supplementation in Type 2 Diabetic Patients. *Diabetes Nutr. Metab.* **2004**, *17*, 217–221. [PubMed]
7. He, H.-Y.; Liu, M.-Z.; Zhang, Y.-L.; Zhang, W. Vitamin Pharmacogenomics: New Insight into Individual Differences in Diseases and Drug Responses. *Genom. Proteom. Bioinform.* **2017**, *15*, 94–100. [CrossRef]
8. Awh, C.C.; Lane, A.-M.; Hawken, S.; Zanke, B.; Kim, I.K. CFH and ARMS2 Genetic Polymorphisms Predict Response to Antioxidants and Zinc in Patients with Age-Related Macular Degeneration. *Ophthalmology* **2013**, *120*, 2317–2323. [CrossRef]
9. Mosolov, S.N. (Ed.) *Biological Methods of Therapy for Mental Disorders*; Sociopolitical thought (Socialno-politicheskaya mysl): Moscow, Russia, 2012. (In Russian)
10. Fabbri, C.; Zohar, J.; Serretti, A. Pharmacogenetic Tests to Guide Drug Treatment in Depression: Comparison of the Available Testing Kits and Clinical Trials. *Prog. Neuropsychopharmacol. Biol. Psychiatry* **2018**, *86*, 36–44. [CrossRef]
11. Carter, C.A.; Frischmeyer-Guerrerio, P.A. The Genetics of Food Allergy. *Curr. Allergy Asthma Rep.* **2018**, *18*, 2. [CrossRef]

12. Noble J., A.; Valdes A., M. Genetics of the HLA Region in the Prediction of Type 1 Diabetes. *Curr. Diabetes Rep.* **2011**, *11*, 533–542. [CrossRef]
13. Schaeffeler, E.; Schwab, M.; Eichelbaum, M.; Zanger, U.M. CYP2D6 Genotyping Strategy Based on Gene Copy Number Determination by TaqMan Real-Time PCR. *Hum. Mutat.* **2003**, *22*, 476–485. [CrossRef] [PubMed]
14. Lam, Y.W.F. Scientific Challenges and Implementation Barriers to Translation of Pharmacogenomics in Clinical Practice. *ISRN Pharmacol.* **2013**, *2013*, 641089. [CrossRef] [PubMed]
15. Stingl (formerly Kirchheiner), J.; Brockmöller, J. Study Designs in Clinical Pharmacogenetic and Pharmacogenomic Research. In *Pharmacogenomics*; Elsevier: Amsterdam, the Netherlands, 2013; pp. 309–341. [CrossRef]
16. Matsui, S. Genomic Biomarkers for Personalized Medicine: Development and Validation in Clinical Studies. *Comput. Math. Methods Med.* **2013**, *2013*, 865980. [CrossRef] [PubMed]
17. Roden, D.M.; Wilke, R.A.; Kroemer, H.K.; Stein, C.M. Pharmacogenomics: The Genetics of Variable Drug Responses. *Circulation* **2011**, *123*, 1661–1670. [CrossRef] [PubMed]
18. Cardon, L.R.; Harris, T. Precision Medicine, Genomics and Drug Discovery. *Hum. Mol. Genet.* **2016**, *25*, R166–R172. [CrossRef]
19. Marx, V. The DNA of a Nation. *Nature* **2015**, *524*, 503–505. [CrossRef]
20. Lu, M.; Lewis, C.M.; Traylor, M. Pharmacogenetic testing through the direct-to-consumer genetic testing company 23andMe. *BMC Med. Genomics* **2017**, *10*, 47. [CrossRef]
21. Crews, K.R.; Hicks, J.K.; Pui, C.-H.; Relling, M.V.; Evans, W.E. Pharmacogenomics and Individualized Medicine: Translating Science into Practice. *Clin. Pharmacol. Ther.* **2012**, *92*, 467–475. [CrossRef]
22. Veenstra, D.L. The Value of Routine Pharmacogenomic Screening—Are We There yet? A Perspective on the Costs and Benefits of Routine Screening—Shouldn't Everyone Have This Done? *Clin. Pharmacol. Ther.* **2016**, *99*, 164–166. [CrossRef]
23. Haga, S.B.; Kantor, A. Horizon Scan of Clinical Laboratories Offering Pharmacogenetic Testing. *Health Aff.* **2018**, *37*, 717–723. [CrossRef]
24. de Leon, J.; Susce, M.T.; Murray-Carmichael, E. The AmpliChip CYP450 Genotyping Test: Integrating a New Clinical Tool. *Mol. Diagn. Ther.* **2006**, *10*, 135–151. [CrossRef] [PubMed]
25. Burmester, J.K.; Sedova, M.; Shapero, M.H.; Mansfield, E. DMET Microarray Technology for Pharmacogenomics-Based Personalized Medicine. *Methods Mol. Biol.* **2010**, *632*, 99–124. [CrossRef] [PubMed]
26. Johnson, J.A.; Burkley, B.M.; Langaee, T.Y.; Clare-Salzler, M.J.; Klein, T.E.; Altman, R.B. Implementing Personalized Medicine: Development of a Cost-Effective Customized Pharmacogenetics Genotyping Array. *Clin. Pharmacol. Ther.* **2012**, *92*, 437–439. [CrossRef] [PubMed]
27. Bielinski, S.J.; Olson, J.E.; Pathak, J.; Weinshilboum, R.M.; Wang, L.; Lyke, K.J.; Ryu, E.; Targonski, P.V.; Van Norstrand, M.D.; Hathcock, M.A.; et al. Preemptive Genotyping for Personalized Medicine: Design of the Right Drug, Right Dose, Right Time-Using Genomic Data to Individualize Treatment Protocol. *Mayo Clin. Proc.* **2014**, *89*, 25–33. [CrossRef] [PubMed]
28. Chambers, C.; Jansen, L.A.; Dhamija, R. Review of Commercially Available Epilepsy Genetic Panels. *J. Genet. Couns.* **2016**, *25*, 213–217. [CrossRef] [PubMed]
29. Platt, J.; Cox, R.; Enns, G.M. Points to Consider in the Clinical Use of NGS Panels for Mitochondrial Disease: An Analysis of Gene Inclusion and Consent Forms. *J. Genet. Couns.* **2014**, *23*, 594–603. [CrossRef] [PubMed]
30. Bush, W.S.; Crosslin, D.R.; Owusu-Obeng, A.; Wallace, J.; Almoguera, B.; Basford, M.A.; Bielinski, S.J.; Carrell, D.S.; Connolly, J.J.; Crawford, D.; et al. Genetic Variation among 82 Pharmacogenes: The PGRNseq Data from the EMERGE Network. *Clin. Pharmacol. Ther.* **2016**, *100*, 160–169. [CrossRef]
31. Janssens, A.C.J.W.; Deverka, P.A. Useless Until Proven Effective: The Clinical Utility of Preemptive Pharmacogenetic Testing. *Clin. Pharmacol. Ther.* **2014**, *96*, 652–654. [CrossRef]
32. Lazaridis, K.N. Improving Therapeutic Odyssey: Preemptive Pharmacogenomics Utility in Patient Care. *Clin. Pharmacol. Ther.* **2017**, *101*, 39–41. [CrossRef]
33. Dunnenberger, H.M.; Crews, K.R.; Hoffman, J.M.; Caudle, K.E.; Broeckel, U.; Howard, S.C.; Hunkler, R.J.; Klein, T.E.; Evans, W.E.; Relling, M.V. Preemptive Clinical Pharmacogenetics Implementation: Current Programs in Five US Medical Centers. *Annu. Rev. Pharmacol. Toxicol.* **2015**, *55*, 89–106. [CrossRef]

34. Hicks, J.K.; Sangkuhl, K.; Swen, J.J.; Ellingrod, V.L.; Müller, D.J.; Shimoda, K.; Bishop, J.R.; Kharasch, E.D.; Skaar, T.C.; Gaedigk, A.; et al. Clinical Pharmacogenetics Implementation Consortium Guideline (CPIC) for CYP2D6 and CYP2C19 Genotypes and Dosing of Tricyclic Antidepressants: 2016 Update. *Clin. Pharmacol. Ther.* **2017**, *102*, 37–44. [CrossRef] [PubMed]
35. Hicks, J.K.; Bishop, J.R.; Sangkuhl, K.; Müller, D.J.; Ji, Y.; Leckband, S.G.; Leeder, J.S.; Graham, R.L.; Chiulli, D.L.; LLerena, A.; et al. Clinical Pharmacogenetics Implementation Consortium (CPIC) Guideline for CYP2D6 and CYP2C19 Genotypes and Dosing of Selective Serotonin Reuptake Inhibitors. *Clin. Pharmacol. Ther.* **2015**, *98*, 127–134. [CrossRef]
36. Vilches, S.; Tuson, M.; Vieta, E.; Álvarez, E.; Espadaler, J. Effectiveness of a Pharmacogenetic Tool at Improving Treatment Efficacy in Major Depressive Disorder: A Meta-Analysis of Three Clinical Studies. *Pharmaceutics* **2019**, *11*, 453. [CrossRef] [PubMed]
37. Frazer, A.; Benmansour, S. Delayed Pharmacological Effects of Antidepressants. *Mol. Psychiatry* **2002**, *7* (Suppl. 1), S23–S28. [CrossRef] [PubMed]
38. GlaxoSmithKline Inc. ZIAGEN (GlaxoSmithKline Inc): FDA Package Insert. Available online: https://druginserts.com/lib/rx/meds/ziagen-6/ (accessed on 24 August 2020).
39. Cho, S.-M.; Lee, K.-Y.; Choi, J.R.; Lee, K.-A. Development and Comparison of Warfarin Dosing Algorithms in Stroke Patients. *Yonsei Med. J.* **2016**, *57*, 635–640. [CrossRef] [PubMed]
40. Kelly, L.E.; Rieder, M.; van den Anker, J.; Malkin, B.; Ross, C.; Neely, M.N.; Carleton, B.; Hayden, M.R.; Madadi, P.; Koren, G. More Codeine Fatalities after Tonsillectomy in North American Children. *Pediatrics* **2012**, *129*, e1343–e1347. [CrossRef]
41. Thorn, C.F.; Klein, T.E.; Altman, R.B. Codeine and Morphine Pathway. *Pharm. Genom.* **2009**, *19*, 556–558. [CrossRef]
42. Crews, K.R.; Gaedigk, A.; Dunnenberger, H.M.; Klein, T.E.; Shen, D.D.; Callaghan, J.T.; Kharasch, E.D.; Skaar, T.C. Clinical Pharmacogenetics Implementation Consortium (CPIC) Guidelines for Codeine Therapy in the Context of Cytochrome P450 2D6 (CYP2D6) Genotype. *Clin. Pharmacol. Ther.* **2012**, *91*, 321–326. [CrossRef]
43. Lemke, A.A.; Hulick, P.J.; Wake, D.T.; Wang, C.; Sereika, A.W.; Yu, K.D.; Glaser, N.S.; Dunnenberger, H.M. Patient Perspectives Following Pharmacogenomics Results Disclosure in an Integrated Health System. *Pharmacogenomics* **2018**, *19*, 321–331. [CrossRef]
44. Patel, H.N.; Ursan, I.D.; Zueger, P.M.; Cavallari, L.H.; Pickard, A.S. Stakeholder Views on Pharmacogenomic Testing. *Pharmacotherapy* **2014**, *34*, 151–165. [CrossRef]
45. Haga, S.B.; Mills, R.; Moaddeb, J.; Allen Lapointe, N.; Cho, A.; Ginsburg, G.S. Patient Experiences with Pharmacogenetic Testing in a Primary Care Setting. *Pharmacogenomics* **2016**, *17*, 1629–1636. [CrossRef] [PubMed]
46. Bielinski, S.J.; St Sauver, J.L.; Olson, J.E.; Wieland, M.L.; Vitek, C.R.; Bell, E.J.; Mc Gree, M.E.; Jacobson, D.J.; McCormick, J.B.; Takahashi, P.Y.; et al. Are Patients Willing to Incur Out-of-Pocket Costs for Pharmacogenomic Testing? *Pharm. J.* **2017**, *17*, 1–3. [CrossRef] [PubMed]
47. Haga, S.B.; O'Daniel, J.M.; Tindall, G.M.; Lipkus, I.R.; Agans, R. Survey of US Public Attitudes toward Pharmacogenetic Testing. *Pharm. J.* **2012**, *12*, 197–204. [CrossRef] [PubMed]
48. Dunnenberger, H.M.; Biszewski, M.; Bell, G.C.; Sereika, A.; May, H.; Johnson, S.G.; Hulick, P.J.; Khandekar, J. Implementation of a Multidisciplinary Pharmacogenomics Clinic in a Community Health System. *Am. J. Health Syst. Pharm.* **2016**, *73*, 1956–1966. [CrossRef]
49. Wake, D.T.; Ilbawi, N.; Dunnenberger, H.M.; Hulick, P.J. Pharmacogenomics. *Med. Clin. N. Am.* **2019**, *103*, 977–990. [CrossRef]
50. Swen, J.J.; Nijenhuis, M.; de Boer, A.; Grandia, L.; Maitland-van der Zee, A.H.; Mulder, H.; Rongen, G.a.P.J.M.; van Schaik, R.H.N.; Schalekamp, T.; Touw, D.J.; et al. Pharmacogenetics: From Bench to Byte–An Update of Guidelines. *Clin. Pharmacol. Ther.* **2011**, *89*, 662–673. [CrossRef]
51. Caudle, K.E.; Klein, T.E.; Hoffman, J.M.; Muller, D.J.; Whirl-Carrillo, M.; Gong, L.; McDonagh, E.M.; Sangkuhl, K.; Thorn, C.F.; Schwab, M.; et al. Incorporation of Pharmacogenomics into Routine Clinical Practice: The Clinical Pharmacogenetics Implementation Consortium (CPIC) Guideline Development Process. *Curr. Drug Metab.* **2014**, *15*, 209–217. [CrossRef]

52. Rubinstein, W.S.; Maglott, D.R.; Lee, J.M.; Kattman, B.L.; Malheiro, A.J.; Ovetsky, M.; Hem, V.; Gorelenkov, V.; Song, G.; Wallin, C.; et al. The NIH Genetic Testing Registry: A New, Centralized Database of Genetic Tests to Enable Access to Comprehensive Information and Improve Transparency. *Nucleic Acids Res.* **2013**, *41*, D925–D935. [CrossRef]
53. Sangkuhl, K.; Berlin, D.S.; Altman, R.B.; Klein, T.E. PharmGKB: Understanding the Effects of Individual Genetic Variants. *Drug Metab. Rev.* **2008**, *40*, 539–551. [CrossRef]
54. Volpi, S.; Bult, C.J.; Chisholm, R.L.; Deverka, P.A.; Ginsburg, G.S.; Jacob, H.J.; Kasapi, M.; McLeod, H.L.; Roden, D.M.; Williams, M.S.; et al. Research Directions in the Clinical Implementation of Pharmacogenomics: An Overview of US Programs and Projects. *Clin. Pharmacol. Ther.* **2018**, *103*, 778–786. [CrossRef]
55. Caraballo, P.J.; Hodge, L.S.; Bielinski, S.J.; Stewart, A.K.; Farrugia, G.; Schultz, C.G.; Rohrer-Vitek, C.R.; Olson, J.E.; St Sauver, J.L.; Roger, V.L.; et al. Multidisciplinary Model to Implement Pharmacogenomics at the Point of Care. *Genet. Med.* **2017**, *19*, 421–429. [CrossRef] [PubMed]
56. van der Wouden, C.H.; Cambon-Thomsen, A.; Cecchin, E.; Cheung, K.C.; Dávila-Fajardo, C.L.; Deneer, V.H.; Dolžan, V.; Ingelman-Sundberg, M.; Jönsson, S.; Karlsson, M.O.; et al. Ubiquitous Pharmacogenomics Consortium. Implementing Pharmacogenomics in Europe: Design and Implementation Strategy of the Ubiquitous Pharmacogenomics Consortium. *Clin. Pharmacol. Ther.* **2017**, *101*, 341–358. [CrossRef] [PubMed]
57. Luzum, J.A.; Pakyz, R.E.; Elsey, A.R.; Haidar, C.E.; Peterson, J.F.; Whirl-Carrillo, M.; Handelman, S.K.; Palmer, K.; Pulley, J.M.; Beller, M.; et al. Pharmacogenomics Research Network Translational Pharmacogenetics Program. The Pharmacogenomics Research Network Translational Pharmacogenetics Program: Outcomes and Metrics of Pharmacogenetic Implementations Across Diverse Healthcare Systems. *Clin. Pharmacol. Ther.* **2017**, *102*, 502–510. [CrossRef] [PubMed]
58. Scott, S.A.; Sangkuhl, K.; Stein, C.M.; Hulot, J.-S.; Mega, J.L.; Roden, D.M.; Klein, T.E.; Sabatine, M.S.; Johnson, J.A.; Shuldiner, A.R. Clinical Pharmacogenetics Implementation Consortium Guidelines for CYP2C19 Genotype and Clopidogrel Therapy: 2013 Update. *Clin. Pharmacol. Ther.* **2013**, *94*, 317–323. [CrossRef]
59. Vo, T.T.; Bell, G.C.; Obeng, A.O.; Hicks, J.K.; Dunnenberger, H.M. Pharmacogenomics Implementation: Considerations for Selecting a Reference Laboratory. *Pharmacother. J. Hum. Pharmacol. Drug Ther.* **2017**, *37*, 1014–1022. [CrossRef]
60. Bousman, C.; Maruf, A.A.; Müller, D.J. Towards the Integration of Pharmacogenetics in Psychiatry: A Minimum, Evidence-Based Genetic Testing Panel. *Curr. Opin. Psychiatry* **2019**, *32*, 7–15. [CrossRef]
61. Phillips, E.J.; Sukasem, C.; Whirl-Carrillo, M.; Müller, D.J.; Dunnenberger, H.M.; Chantratita, W.; Goldspiel, B.; Chen, Y.-T.; Carleton, B.C.; George, A.L.; et al. Clinical Pharmacogenetics Implementation Consortium Guideline for HLA Genotype and Use of Carbamazepine and Oxcarbazepine: 2017 Update. *Clin. Pharmacol. Ther.* **2018**, *103*, 574–581. [CrossRef]
62. Hosono, N.; Kato, M.; Kiyotani, K.; Mushiroda, T.; Takata, S.; Sato, H.; Amitani, H.; Tsuchiya, Y.; Yamazaki, K.; Tsunoda, T.; et al. CYP2D6 Genotyping for Functional-Gene Dosage Analysis by Allele Copy Number Detection. *Clin. Chem.* **2009**, *55*, 1546–1554. [CrossRef]
63. Caudle, K.E.; Dunnenberger, H.M.; Freimuth, R.R.; Peterson, J.F.; Burlison, J.D.; Whirl-Carrillo, M.; Scott, S.A.; Rehm, H.L.; Williams, M.S.; Klein, T.E.; et al. Standardizing Terms for Clinical Pharmacogenetic Test Results: Consensus Terms from the Clinical Pharmacogenetics Implementation Consortium (CPIC). *Genet. Med.* **2017**, *19*, 215–223. [CrossRef]
64. Hershfield, M.S.; Callaghan, J.T.; Tassaneeyakul, W.; Mushiroda, T.; Thorn, C.F.; Klein, T.E.; Lee, M.T.M. Clinical Pharmacogenetics Implementation Consortium Guidelines for Human Leukocyte Antigen-B Genotype and Allopurinol Dosing. *Clin. Pharmacol. Ther.* **2013**, *93*, 153–158. [CrossRef]
65. Leckband, S.G.; Kelsoe, J.R.; Dunnenberger, H.M.; George, A.L.; Tran, E.; Berger, R.; Müller, D.J.; Whirl-Carrillo, M.; Caudle, K.E.; Pirmohamed, M. Clinical Pharmacogenetics Implementation Consortium Guidelines for HLA-B Genotype and Carbamazepine Dosing. *Clin. Pharmacol. Ther.* **2013**, *94*, 324–328. [CrossRef] [PubMed]
66. Hinderer, M.; Boeker, M.; Wagner, S.A.; Lablans, M.; Newe, S.; Hülsemann, J.L.; Neumaier, M.; Binder, H.; Renz, H.; Acker, T.; et al. Integrating Clinical Decision Support Systems for Pharmacogenomic Testing into Clinical Routine—A Scoping Review of Designs of User-System Interactions in Recent System Development. *BMC Med. Inform. Decis. Mak.* **2017**, *17*, 81. [CrossRef]

67. Blagec, K.; Koopmann, R.; Crommentuijn-van Rhenen, M.; Holsappel, I.; van der Wouden, C.H.; Konta, L.; Xu, H.; Steinberger, D.; Just, E.; Swen, J.J.; et al. Implementing Pharmacogenomics Decision Support across Seven European Countries: The Ubiquitous Pharmacogenomics (U-PGx) Project. *J. Am. Med. Inform. Assoc* **2018**, *25*, 893–898. [CrossRef] [PubMed]
68. Krebs, K.; Milani, L. Translating Pharmacogenomics into Clinical Decisions: Do Not Let the Perfect Be the Enemy of the Good. *Hum. Genom.* **2019**, *13*, 39. [CrossRef] [PubMed]
69. Plumpton, C.O.; Roberts, D.; Pirmohamed, M.; Hughes, D.A. A Systematic Review of Economic Evaluations of Pharmacogenetic Testing for Prevention of Adverse Drug Reactions. *Pharmacoeconomics* **2016**, *34*, 771–793. [CrossRef] [PubMed]
70. Cacabelos, R.; Cacabelos, N.; Carril, J.C. The Role of Pharmacogenomics in Adverse Drug Reactions. *Expert Rev. Clin. Pharmacol.* **2019**, *12*, 407–442. [CrossRef]
71. Shepherd, G.; Mohorn, P.; Yacoub, K.; May, D.W. Adverse Drug Reaction Deaths Reported in United States Vital Statistics, 1999–2006. *Ann. Pharmacother.* **2012**, *46*, 169–175. [CrossRef]
72. Ekhart, C.; van Hunsel, F.; Scholl, J.; de Vries, S.; van Puijenbroek, E. Sex Differences in Reported Adverse Drug Reactions of Selective Serotonin Reuptake Inhibitors. *Drug Saf.* **2018**, *41*, 677–683. [CrossRef]
73. Routledge, P.A.; O'Mahony, M.S.; Woodhouse, K.W. Adverse Drug Reactions in Elderly Patients. *Br. J. Clin. Pharmacol.* **2004**, *57*, 121–126. [CrossRef]
74. Wilke, R.A.; Lin, D.W.; Roden, D.M.; Watkins, P.B.; Flockhart, D.; Zineh, I.; Giacomini, K.M.; Krauss, R.M. Identifying Genetic Risk Factors for Serious Adverse Drug Reactions: Current Progress and Challenges. *Nat. Rev. Drug Discov.* **2007**, *6*, 904–916. [CrossRef]
75. Chyka, P.A. How many deaths occur annually from adverse drug reactions in the United States? *Am. J. Med.* **2000**, *109*, 122–130. [CrossRef]
76. Shrestha, S.; Shakya, R.; Shrestha, S.; Shakya, S. Adverse Drug Reaction due to Cancer Chemotherapy and its Financial Burden in Different Hospitals of Nepal. *Int. J. Pharmacovigil.* **2017**, *2*, 1–7. [CrossRef]
77. Watson, S.; Caster, O.; Rochon, P.A.; den Ruijter, H. Reported Adverse Drug Reactions in Women and Men: Aggregated Evidence from Globally Collected Individual Case Reports during Half a Century. *EClinicalMedicine* **2019**, *17*, 100188. [CrossRef] [PubMed]
78. Wilson, K. Sex-Related Differences in Drug Disposition in Man. *Clin. Pharmacokinet.* **1984**, *9*, 189–202. [CrossRef] [PubMed]
79. Mallik, S.; Palaian, S.; Ojha, P.; Mishra, P. Pattern of Adverse Drug Reactions Due to Cancer Chemotherapy in a Tertiary Care Teaching Hospital in Nepal. *Pak. J. Pharm. Sci.* **2007**, *20*, 214–218. [PubMed]
80. Jose, J.; Rao, P.G.M. Pattern of Adverse Drug Reactions Notified by Spontaneous Reporting in an Indian Tertiary Care Teaching Hospital. *Pharmacol. Res.* **2006**, *54*, 226–233. [CrossRef] [PubMed]
81. Chen, X.-W.; Liu, W.; Zhou, S.-F. Pharmacogenomics-Guided Approaches to Avoiding Adverse Drug Reactions. *Clin. Pharmacol. Biopharm.* **2012**, *1*. [CrossRef]
82. Cargnin, S.; Jommi, C.; Canonico, P.L.; Genazzani, A.A.; Terrazzino, S. Diagnostic Accuracy of HLA-B*57:01 Screening for the Prediction of Abacavir Hypersensitivity and Clinical Utility of the Test.: A Meta-Analytic Review. *Pharmacogenomics* **2014**, *15*, 963–976.
83. Mallal, S.; Phillips, E.; Carosi, G.; Molina, J.-M.; Workman, C.; Tomažič, J.; Jägel-Guedes, E.; Rugina, S.; Kozyrev, O.; Cid, J.F.; et al. HLA-B*5701 Screening for Hypersensitivity to Abacavir. *N. Engl. J. Med.* **2008**, *358*, 568–579. [CrossRef]
84. Schackman, B.R.; Scott, C.A.; Walensky, R.P.; Losina, E.; Freedberg, K.A.; Sax, P.E. The Cost-Effectiveness of HLA-B*5701 Genetic Screening to Guide Initial Antiretroviral Therapy for HIV. *AIDS* **2008**, *22*, 2025–2033. [CrossRef]
85. Hippman, C.; Nislow, C. Pharmacogenomic Testing: Clinical Evidence and Implementation Challenges. *J. Pers. Med.* **2019**, *9*, 40. [CrossRef] [PubMed]
86. Hess, G.P.; Fonseca, E.; Scott, R.; Fagerness, J. Pharmacogenomic and Pharmacogenetic-Guided Therapy as a Tool in Precision Medicine: Current State and Factors Impacting Acceptance by Stakeholders. *Genet. Res.* **2015**, *97*, e13. [CrossRef] [PubMed]
87. Botkin, J.R.; Teutsch, S.M.; Kaye, C.I.; Hayes, M.; Haddow, J.E.; Bradley, L.A.; Szegda, K.; Dotson, W.D. Outcomes of Interest in Evidence-Based Evaluations of Genetic Tests. *Genet. Med.* **2010**, *12*, 228–235. [CrossRef] [PubMed]

88. Palomaki, G.E.; Bradley, L.A.; Douglas, M.P.; Kolor, K.; Dotson, W.D. Can UGT1A1 Genotyping Reduce Morbidity and Mortality in Patients with Metastatic Colorectal Cancer Treated with Irinotecan? An Evidence-Based Review. *Genet. Med.* **2009**, *11*, 21–34. [CrossRef] [PubMed]
89. Evaluation of Genomic Applications in Practice and Prevention (EGAPP) Working Group. The EGAPP initiative: Lessons learned. *Genet. Med.* **2014**, *16*, 217–224. [CrossRef]
90. Relling, M.V.; Evans, W.E. Pharmacogenomics in the Clinic. *Nature* **2015**, *526*, 343–350. [CrossRef]
91. Sorich, M.J.; Coory, M. Interpreting the Clinical Utility of a Pharmacogenomic Marker Based on Observational Association Studies. *Pharm. J.* **2014**, *14*, 1–5. [CrossRef]
92. Dias, M.M.; Sorich, M.J.; Rowland, A.; Wiese, M.D.; McKinnon, R.A. The Routine Clinical Use of Pharmacogenetic Tests: What It Will Require? *Pharm. Res.* **2017**, *34*, 1544–1550. [CrossRef]
93. Teutsch, S.M.; Bradley, L.A.; Palomaki, G.E.; Haddow, J.E.; Piper, M.; Calonge, N.; Dotson, W.D.; Douglas, M.P.; Berg, A.O.; EGAPP Working Group. The Evaluation of Genomic Applications in Practice and Prevention (EGAPP) Initiative: Methods of the EGAPP Working Group. *Genet. Med.* **2009**, *11*, 3–14. [CrossRef]
94. Johnson, J.A.; Caudle, K.E.; Gong, L.; Whirl-Carrillo, M.; Stein, C.M.; Scott, S.A.; Lee, M.T.M.; Gage, B.F.; Kimmel, S.E.; Perera, M.A. Clinical Pharmacogenetics Implementation Consortium (CPIC) Guideline for Pharmacogenetics-Guided Warfarin dosing: 2017 Update. *Clin. Pharmacol. Ther.* **2017**, *102*, 397–404. [CrossRef]
95. Borenstein, M. (Ed.) *Introduction to Meta-Analysis*; John Wiley & Sons: Chichester, UK, 2009.
96. Liberati, A.; Altman, D.G.; Tetzlaff, J.; Mulrow, C.; Gøtzsche, P.C.; Ioannidis, J.P.A.; Clarke, M.; Devereaux, P.J.; Kleijnen, J.; Moher, D. The PRISMA Statement for Reporting Systematic Reviews and Meta-Analyses of Studies That Evaluate Health Care Interventions: Explanation and Elaboration. *PLoS Med.* **2009**, *6*, e1000100. [CrossRef] [PubMed]
97. Sorich, M.J.; Polasek, T.M.; Wiese, M.D. Challenges and Limitations in the Interpretation of Systematic Reviews: Making Sense of Clopidogrel and CYP2C19 Pharmacogenetics. *Clin. Pharmacol. Ther.* **2013**, *94*, 376–382. [CrossRef] [PubMed]
98. Genomic Epidemiology of Complex Disease: The Need for an Electronic Evidence-Based Approach to Research Synthesis. Available online: https://www.pubfacts.com/detail/16014778/Genomic-epidemiology-of-complex-disease-the-need-for-an-electronic-evidence-based-approach-to-resear (accessed on 25 August 2020).
99. Amstutz, U.; Carleton, B. Pharmacogenetic Testing: Time for Clinical Practice Guidelines. *Clin. Pharmacol. Ther.* 2011. [CrossRef] [PubMed]
100. Sorich, M.J.; Wiese, M.D.; Pekarsky, B. Cost-Effectiveness of Genotyping to Guide Treatment. *Pharmacogenomics* **2014**, *15*, 727–729. [CrossRef]
101. Tansey, K.E.; Guipponi, M.; Hu, X.; Domenici, E.; Lewis, G.; Malafosse, A.; Wendland, J.R.; Lewis, C.M.; McGuffin, P.; Uher, R. Contribution of Common Genetic Variants to Antidepressant Response. *Biol. Psychiatry* **2013**, *73*, 679–682. [CrossRef]
102. Niitsu, T.; Fabbri, C.; Bentini, F.; Serretti, A. Pharmacogenetics in Major Depression: A Comprehensive Meta-Analysis. *Prog. Neuro-Psychopharmacol. Biol. Psychiatry* **2013**, *45*, 183–194. [CrossRef]
103. Peterson, K.; Dieperink, E.; Anderson, J.; Boundy, E.; Ferguson, L.; Helfand, M. Rapid Evidence Review of the Comparative Effectiveness, Harms, and Cost-Effectiveness of Pharmacogenomics-Guided Antidepressant Treatment versus Usual Care for Major Depressive Disorder. *Psychopharmacology* **2017**, *234*, 1649–1661. [CrossRef]
104. Rosenblat, J.D.; Lee, Y.; McIntyre, R.S. Does Pharmacogenomic Testing Improve Clinical Outcomes for Major Depressive Disorder? A Systematic Review of Clinical Trials and Cost-Effectiveness Studies. *J. Clin. Psychiatry* **2017**, *78*, 720–729. [CrossRef]
105. Bousman, C.A.; Hopwood, M. Commercial Pharmacogenetic-Based Decision-Support Tools in Psychiatry. *Lancet Psychiatry* **2016**, *3*, 585–590. [CrossRef]
106. Gillis, N.K.; Innocenti, F. Evidence Required to Demonstrate Clinical Utility of Pharmacogenetic Testing: The Debate Continues. *Clin. Pharmacol. Ther.* **2014**, *96*, 655–657. [CrossRef]
107. Stanek, E.J.; Sanders, C.L.; Taber, K.A.J.; Khalid, M.; Patel, A.; Verbrugge, R.R.; Agatep, B.C.; Aubert, R.E.; Epstein, R.S.; Frueh, F.W. Adoption of Pharmacogenomic Testing by US Physicians: Results of a Nationwide Survey. *Clin. Pharmacol. Ther.* **2012**, *91*, 450–458. [CrossRef] [PubMed]

108. Conti, R.; Veenstra, D.L.; Armstrong, K.; Lesko, L.J.; Grosse, S.D. Personalized Medicine and Genomics: Challenges and Opportunities in Assessing Effectiveness, Cost-Effectiveness, and Future Research Priorities. *Med. Decis. Mak.* **2010**, *30*, 328–340. [CrossRef] [PubMed]
109. Freedman, K.J.; Bastian, A.R.; Chaiken, I.; Kim, M.J. Solid-State Nanopore Detection of Protein Complexes: Applications in Healthcare and Protein Kinetics. *Small* **2013**, *9*, 750–759. [CrossRef] [PubMed]
110. Faruki, H.; Lai-Goldman, M. Application of a Pharmacogenetic Test Adoption Model to Six Oncology Biomarkers. *Per. Med.* **2010**, *7*, 441–450. [CrossRef]
111. Dias, M.M.; Ward, H.M.; Sorich, M.J.; McKinnon, R.A. Exploration of the Perceptions, Barriers and Drivers of Pharmacogenomics Practice among Hospital Pharmacists in Adelaide, South Australia. *Pharm. J.* **2014**, *14*, 235–240. [CrossRef]
112. Klein, M.E.; Parvez, M.M.; Shin, J.-G. Clinical Implementation of Pharmacogenomics for Personalized Precision Medicine: Barriers and Solutions. *J. Pharm. Sci.* **2017**, *106*, 2368–2379. [CrossRef]
113. Becquemont, L.; Alfirevic, A.; Amstutz, U.; Brauch, H.; Jacqz-Aigrain, E.; Laurent-Puig, P.; Molina, M.A.; Niemi, M.; Schwab, M.; Somogyi, A.A.; et al. Practical Recommendations for Pharmacogenomics-Based Prescription: 2010 ESF-UB Conference on Pharmacogenetics and Pharmacogenomics. *Pharmacogenomics* **2011**, *12*, 113–124. [CrossRef]
114. Relling, M.V.; Klein, T.E. CPIC: Clinical Pharmacogenetics Implementation Consortium of the Pharmacogenomics Research Network. *Clin. Pharmacol. Ther.* **2011**, *89*, 464–467. [CrossRef]
115. Moyer, A.M.; Caraballo, P.J. The Challenges of Implementing Pharmacogenomic Testing in the Clinic. *Expert Rev. Pharm. Outcomes Res.* **2017**, *17*, 567–577. [CrossRef]

Publisher's Note: MDPI stays neutral with regard to jurisdictional claims in published maps and institutional affiliations.

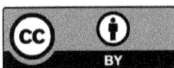

© 2020 by the authors. Licensee MDPI, Basel, Switzerland. This article is an open access article distributed under the terms and conditions of the Creative Commons Attribution (CC BY) license (http://creativecommons.org/licenses/by/4.0/).

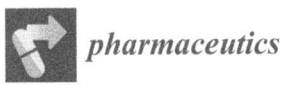

Review

Barriers to Implementing Clinical Pharmacogenetics Testing in Sub-Saharan Africa. A Critical Review

Emiliene B. Tata [1], Melvin A. Ambele [1,2] and Michael S. Pepper [1,*]

1. Institute for Cellular and Molecular Medicine, Department of Immunology, and South African Medical Research Council Extramural Unit for Stem Cell Research & Therapy, Faculty of Health Sciences, University of Pretoria, Pretoria 0084, South Africa; u19109912@tuks.co.za (E.B.T.); melvin.ambele@up.ac.za (M.A.A.)
2. Department of Oral Pathology and Oral Biology, Faculty of Health Sciences, School of Dentistry, University of Pretoria, PO BOX 1266, Pretoria 0001, South Africa
* Correspondence: michael.pepper@up.ac.za; Tel.: +27-12-319-2190

Received: 2 July 2020; Accepted: 22 August 2020; Published: 26 August 2020

Abstract: Clinical research in high-income countries is increasingly demonstrating the cost-effectiveness of clinical pharmacogenetic (PGx) testing in reducing the incidence of adverse drug reactions and improving overall patient care. Medications are prescribed based on an individual's genotype (pharmacogenes), which underlies a specific phenotypic drug response. The advent of cost-effective high-throughput genotyping techniques coupled with the existence of Clinical Pharmacogenetics Implementation Consortium (CPIC) dosing guidelines for pharmacogenetic "actionable variants" have increased the clinical applicability of PGx testing. The implementation of clinical PGx testing in sub-Saharan African (SSA) countries can significantly improve health care delivery, considering the high incidence of communicable diseases, the increasing incidence of non-communicable diseases, and the high degree of genetic diversity in these populations. However, the implementation of PGx testing has been sluggish in SSA, prompting this review, the aim of which is to document the existing barriers. These include under-resourced clinical care logistics, a paucity of pharmacogenetics clinical trials, scientific and technical barriers to genotyping pharmacogene variants, and socio-cultural as well as ethical issues regarding health-care stakeholders, among other barriers. Investing in large-scale SSA PGx research and governance, establishing biobanks/bio-databases coupled with clinical electronic health systems, and encouraging the uptake of PGx knowledge by health-care stakeholders, will ensure the successful implementation of pharmacogenetically guided treatment in SSA.

Keywords: clinical pharmacogenetics; pharmacogenetic testing; adverse drug reactions; genotype; phenotype; pharmacogene; barriers to pharmacogenetics implementation; Sub-Saharan Africa

---

1. Introduction

Pharmacogenomics is an emergent but highly actionable form of personalised genetic medicine. Pharmacogenomics studies the impact of germline and somatic genetic variations (genotype) on drug response and the incidence of adverse drug reaction (ADR) phenotypes in an individual [1]. Clinical research has demonstrated the cost-effectiveness of pharmacogenetic (PGx) testing in improving drug compliance in patients, leading to decreased hospital admissions due to ADRs, especially for psychiatric patients on anti-depressants and anti-psychotics and cardiac patients on anti-platelet medication [1,2]. Furthermore, major PGx expert organisations such as the Clinical Pharmacogenetics Implementation Consortium (CPIC) [3] and the Dutch Pharmacogenetics Working Group (DPWG) [4] provide guidelines for PGx clinical implementation of gene–drug categories, so-called "actionable variants" (gene variants with PharmGKB 1A or 1B high level of evidence) [5], with over 65 dosage recommendations in place. In addition, other expert organisations such as the EU-PIC (European Pharmacogenetics Implementation

Consortium) [6], U-PGx (Ubiquitous pharmacogenomics) [7], RELIVAF (Latin American Network for Implementation and Validation of pharmacogenomics guidelines) [8], and SEAPharm (Southeast Asian Pharmacogenomics Research Network) [9] also provide pharmacogenetically-guided dosage recommendations. Indeed, the Food and Drug Administration (FDA) has published a list of PGx biomarkers for drug labelling with pharmacogenetically guided dosing [10].

The sub-Saharan African (SSA) region accounts for 25% of the global disease burden [11], with an increasing prevalence of non-communicable diseases (NCDs) [12] and emergent infectious diseases. Distinct and complex disease patterns amongst populations in the SSA region has led to distinct ADR patterns relative to Western and Asian countries [11]. Therefore, it becomes challenging for clinicians in this region with limited knowledge on potential drug–drug, drug–gene, and drug–drug–gene interactions when prescribing multiple medications to patients. The data on ADR incidence and the efficacy of most medications in populations of African descent are relatively scarce due to inefficient or absent pharmacovigilance programs [13]. There is however increasing evidence that the integration of PGx knowledge with other clinical data that influence drug response such as gender, age, weight, co-morbidities and lifestyle, will greatly assist clinicians in prescribing safe and efficient drug regimens to patients in SSA [14].

PGx Genome-Wide Association Studies (GWAS) have uncovered several population-based genetic variants (alleles) associated with ADRs. A majority of the variants (minor allele frequencies > 0.05) are recorded in most global populations [15]. Nevertheless, a few variants are rare (minor allele frequencies < 0.005) with varying global inter-ethnic frequencies that result in unique phenotypes in some populations [16]. Global inter-ethnic variability in genetic variants and drug response will mean that selected gene–drug pairs for clinical PGx testing in one population may not be very useful in another. For instance, testing of the loss of function *CYP2D6*17* allele, associated with amitriptyline-induced adverse effects, may serve as a useful marker for African and Latin American populations relative to European populations [17,18]. However, the genomes of African populations are greatly underrepresented in global GWAS studies [19]. Unique population growth, migration and genetic drift in the SSA region has resulted in high human genetic diversity and markedly lower but diverse linkage disequilibrium patterns between genetic variants across the region [20]. Therefore, risk scores of various genetic variants in SSA populations should not be inferred from European or Asian datasets, given the peculiarity of the genomic architecture in the African populations. Varying frequencies of genetic variants across different sub-populations in SSA might suggest inter-ethnic and inter-individual variability in drug response in this region [21]. A meta-analysis of GWAS on African cohorts have revealed novel *CYP2C9* and *VKORC1* gene variants with high genome-wide association, particularly in warfarin drug response, leading to subsequent dose adjustments for these cohorts [14]. This highlights the benefit and need to identify more African PGx markers through large-scale PGx research for PGx testing in SSA.

Genomic initiatives such as the African Pharmacogenetics Consortium (APC) [22] and H3Africa [23] have been created to harmonise PGx data and to create awareness of PGx research/testing in Africa. This has led to clinical and non-clinical PGx research on African populations that has characterised some unique PGx biomarkers, thereby demonstrating the potential benefits of integrating PGx testing in clinical practice in SSA [24–29]. A classic example is the characterisation of highly prevalent *CYP2B6*6* genetic variants in African populations associated with central nervous system toxicities in HIV patients on efavirenz treatment, which has led to specific drug dosage recommendations for African cohorts, relative to European populations [30].

Priority large-scale PGx clinical research and testing in SSA should involve "actionable variants" [15] associated with drug response in diseases contributing to the greatest morbidity and mortality such as tuberculosis, HIV, malaria, filaria, cancer, diabetes, cardiovascular diseases, and mental disorders [31,32]. Notably, priority research should be on the cytochrome P450 (CYP) family, including the *CYP1*, *CYP2*, and *CYP3* sub-families of genes, which encode proteins that are involved in the metabolism of approximately 90% of commonly prescribed medications [5]. The advent of cost-effective commercial genotyping microarrays with targeted pharmacogene panels such as the Axiom Precision Medicine Diversity Research Array (Thermo Fisher Scientific, Massachusetts, USA) and other FDA-approved arrays including the Gentris Rapid Genotyping Assay—*CYP2C9* and *VKORC1* (ParagonDx, LLC)—allows for the rapid testing of thousands of pharmacogenetically relevant variants. These arrays can be customised to include unique variants of African origin together with simplified bioinformatics workflows.

PGx testing has been successfully implemented in European and North American countries, mainly through large-scale initiatives, albeit with some limitations such as the complexities in accurately genotyping pharmacogenes and lethargy by test providers [33]. However, the clinical implementation of PGx testing in SSA primary health-care settings has been slow, highlighting the need for a review of some of the challenges involved. Factors such as under-resourced clinical health-care systems, limited PGx studies, scientific and technical barriers to genotyping pharmacogene variants, and socio-cultural and ethical issues regarding patients, clinicians, and health-care stakeholders have all been identified as potential barriers to the implementation of PGx testing in SSA. This review will comprehensively address these challenges with a focus on the scientific and technical barriers, and it will propose solutions that could potentially facilitate the clinical implementation of PGx testing in SSA.

2. Under-Resourced Clinical Health-Care Systems

The implementation of clinical PGx testing in SSA will assist physicians in tailoring drug regimens and dosages [1]. A case in point is the robust evidence indicating that testing for variants in pharmacogenes (*CYP2C9/VKORC1*) affecting warfarin response significantly reduces the incidence of ADRs [2]. Randomised clinical trials (RCTs) on PGx biomarkers in a population are the gold standard for obtaining robust evidence on the clinical effectiveness of PGx tests [1]. A clinical PGx test report typically comprises the individual's genotype, predicted phenotype, and gene-guided dosing guidelines such as the CPIC guidelines. Pre-emptive testing involves genotyping an individual's pharmacogenes before a drug is prescribed. The genotypes (usually multigene and multivariant panels) and extrapolated phenotypes are stored in a clinical Electronic Health Record (EHR) coupled to a point-of-care Clinical Decision Support System (CDSS) where a physician can access the results and subsequently implement pharmacogenetically guided regimens and dosages [1]. For reactive tests, a drug is first prescribed, and where necessary, this is followed by genotyping the individual, following which drug regimen adjustments are made. However, reactive tests tend to be more expensive, have low turnaround times, and fewer gene–drug pairs are included.

Clinical EHRs typically include patients' demographic data, prescribed laboratory tests, prescribed medications, co-morbidities, and lifestyle data. Therefore, EHRs are critical in order to obtain longitudinal phenotype/genotype patient data for effective patient management, in addition to retrieving data for pre-emptive PGx testing and population-based studies. Furthermore, CDSSs, which typically contain recommended standardised PGx variant panels and automated dosage recommendations, are a prerequisite for effective pre-emptive PGx clinical testing [34]. However, the implementation of EHRs in the SSA clinical setting has been slow due to high cost, limited informatics infrastructure, lack of access and unreliable electricity supply, poor internet connection, and lethargy in the implementation of EHR by health-care stakeholders [34]. One study revealed that only 15 African countries have EHRs implemented in a few clinics, as most clinics still depend on paper-based patient health records [34].

Aquilante et al. recently demonstrated a hybrid model that facilitated the implementation of pre-emptive clinical PGx testing via the University of Colorado research biobank, coupled with efficient clinical EHRs and CDSS. This presents a unique opportunity for retrieving patient longitudinal genotype/phenotype data for dedicated PGx testing and research studies [35]. In this model, patients or healthy volunteers report to a clinic where informed consent is obtained, and a blood sample is collected. These are sent to the biobank, clinic, or research laboratory for DNA genotyping using a commercial Massarray, followed by a bioinformatic analysis. Structured PGx results are sent to a clinical EHR with patient phenotypes. Clinicians can subsequently access pharmacogenetically guided dosage recommendations based on CPIC guidelines from PGx-based CDSS tools [35]. We believe that this model could be successfully applied in in African countries with existing genetics research institutes. The feasibility of the proposed hybrid model will be made possible by engaging key stakeholders. Patients or healthy volunteers will need to be consented for DNA sample collection by clinicians and counsellors or trained community health workers. Then, clinician–geneticists will scan for evidence of PGx "actionable variants" from published literature and PGx expert guidelines to propose priority pre-emptive gene testing panels. The involvement of bioinformatics and information technology experts will be crucial in the design and setting up of a robust EHR linked to CDDS tools for easy access of PGx results by clinicians. Finally, hospitals and government leadership will need to ensure funding and logistical support, and promote the education of clinicians regarding implementing PGx testing workflows [35].

Biobanking activities are not well developed in Africa, which leads to the misrepresentation of African genetic data in global studies and databases. A biobanking and pharmacogenetics databasing initiative by African researchers at the African Institute of Biomedical Science and Technology (AiBST, Harare, Zimbabwe), catalogued 1488 DNA samples from inter-ethnic African populations, together with recorded frequencies of pharmacogene polymorphisms. Although donor clinical phenotypes were not recorded, validated clinically relevant genotype–phenotype associations could be extrapolated from the data [18]. Notably, the high frequency (14–34%) of the non-functional *CYP2D6*17* alleles recorded could have clinical relevance in anti-depressant and anti-psychotic therapy in African populations.

Recent research efforts have given rise to the establishment of more biobanks in some SSA countries such as the pan-African biobank (54gene) that has been set up in Nigeria to collect African genomic data and enforce the electronic capture of clinical data [36]. Other biobank initiatives including H3Africa, B3Africa, and the Global Emerging Pathogens Treatment Consortium [36] have curated African biospecimens and data in addition to enforcing biobanking policies in Africa. Hopefully, through these initiatives, the application of the hybrid method proposed will ensure the successful implementation of PGx testing in SSA in the near future.

3. Paucity of Clinical Pharmacogenetics Studies in SSA

Most RCTs demonstrating the clinical validity of PGx testing have been conducted on populations of European, American, African-American, and Asian descent [1]. There is a scarcity of PGx GWAS on the impact of rare genetic variants on drug response in African populations, with a few studies focusing on single gene–drug interactions. Indeed, data for pharmacogene variants for African populations are sometimes inferred from African-American populations; however, these populations have distinct ancestries and admixtures [20].

Global GWAS have commonly been employed to scan for multiple genetic variants in the human genome that are associated with drug response. Large effect sizes have been recorded for most variants linked to pharmacogenetic traits compared to other human traits. Notably large effect sizes have been established particularly for variants associated with warfarin, clopidogrel, and simvastatin therapy [16]. Candidate gene approaches have been successfully used to identify gene variants linked to drug response traits, although subsequent studies have failed to replicate previous results [37]. Therefore, drug response in humans is a complex and mostly a polygenic trait. Polygenic Risk Scores (PRS) have been developed to capture the effects of multiple combined variants across the human genome on disease risk and drug response [38]. Although the applicability of PRSs in clinical PGx testing is limited, PRSs have been applied clinically in evaluating the risk of developing diseases such as coronary artery disease and type-2 diabetes [39]. Nevertheless, few studies have demonstrated robust evidence for the utility of PRSs in statin and antidepressant drug response [40]. Importantly, the clinical utility of PRSs in PGx in African populations has not been evaluated given the scarcity of meta-analysis on African PGx data [38]. Therefore, PRS established on European and American populations have limited transferability to African populations given the disparity in population genetic architectures.

Several clinical studies on African populations (Table 1) have demonstrated the potential for PGx testing and dose adjustments in HIV patients receiving Efavirenz [26–28,30,41,42]. Other clinical studies have identified PGx biomarkers for African patients receiving rosuvastatin [43], imatinib [44], anti-retroviral (ARV) therapy, TB, and antimalarial comedication [25,45–47]. Importantly, a clinical study has demonstrated associations between genetic variants and clinical responses among Hepatitis C virus-infected patients from SSA and Europe treated with pegylated interferon-alpha/ribavirin [48]. Inter-ethnic variation in some PGx biomarkers, particularly variants in the cytochrome P450 genes, have been recorded in the SSA region. For instance, varying frequencies of some clinically relevant *CYP2B6*6* alleles in efavirenz drug response have been reported in Ugandan and Zimbabwean communities (68%) relative to South African populations (9%) [21]. Inter-ethnic variant variability could be attributable to environmental factors and differences in research designs giving rise to distinct patient cohorts. Therefore, distinctive inter-ethnic genotype–phenotype concordance should be taken into consideration in the development and clinical implementation of PGx testing.

A closer inspection reveals that most PGx research on SSA populations involves single gene–drug relationships; however, multigene–drug or gene panel testing provides a higher predictability of individual drug response. In addition, most studies have excluded pediatric populations, which is probably due to the existence of specific pediatric pharmacovigilance tools, including age-dependent drug dosage, relying on child-reported ADRs and the engagement of children and child care-givers in the research process [49]. The absence of clinical studies evaluating the economic value of implementing PGx testing in SSA health-care systems is also noteworthy, given that government and private insurers require evidence of the cost–utility of clinical tests for reimbursements. Therefore, there is an urgent need for dedicated PGx RCTs on populations of African ancestry to validate the impact of rare genetic variants on drug efficacy and ADRs while evaluating the cost-effectiveness of implementing clinical PGx testing. Although RCTs are the gold standard for providing robust evidence for clinical PGx testing, their cost-prohibitive nature calls for alternative approaches such as retrospective and prospective observational clinical studies.

The functionality of novel and rare variants uncovered in most of these studies (Table 1) have been predicted by computational algorithms. These algorithms utilise machine learning techniques based on a set of conserved variants associated with a disease; therefore, appropriate algorithms for PGx analysis need to be developed and trained on PGx variants [50]. This constitutes a challenge for the validation and subsequent inclusion of novel and rare variants in clinical testing. Experimental assays to validate the function of novel PGx variants remain the gold standard, although they are cost-prohibitive and time consuming [51]. Most experimental assays utilise knockout animal models such as mouse, Zebrafish, *Caenorhabdis elegans*, and *Drosophila*; however, the use of animal models is limited by cost together with the inaccurate extrapolation of human-specific drug disposition mechanisms. Complementary functional assays utilise transformed human cell lines, human-induced pluripotent stem cells, and organoids. For instance, stem cell-derived cardiomyocytes have been employed in identifying gene variants associated with doxorubin-induced cardiotoxicity in cancer patients. Notable advantages of employing human stem cells include the presence of human genomes that can easily be edited with tools such as CRISPR–Cas9 and the ability of these cells to differentiate into different tissues and organoids in culture [51]. The provision of more research funding and collaboration between interdisciplinary African researchers will boost robust PGx clinical research.

Co-infection and disease co-morbidity patterns are not uniform across the SSA region, which constitutes a major challenge for disease management. Co-morbidities such as malaria, neglected tropical diseases, HIV, and TB are commonly observed in Central and West Africa, while in the southern region, co-morbidities such as HIV and TB are prevalent [11]. Therefore, treatment regimens and ADR patterns for one region cannot be extrapolated to another. Furthermore, the rising incidence of NCDs such as cancer, diabetes, cardiovascular disease, and neuropsychiatric disorders [12] has complicated the burden of comorbidities, leading to multidrug regimens being prescribed to patients. Data on the frequency of ADRs and the efficacy of medications for the treatment of co-morbidities on African populations are scarce [13]. ADRs may lead to patient non-compliance and prolonged hospital stays, thereby placing a cost burden on already strained health systems.

Table 1. Clinical studies aimed at validating pharmacogenetic biomarkers on clinical outcomes on sub-Saharan African populations.

Drugs	Clinical Study Outcome	References
Efavirenz	Pharmacogenetic determinants of response to Efavirenz in Black South African HIV/AIDS patients.	[41]
	Gender, weight, and *CYP2B6* genotype influence Efavirenz HIV/AIDS and TB treatment in Zimbabwe.	[26]
	CYP2B6 variants impact plasma Efavirenz concentrations in HIV/TB patients in Tanzania.	[27]
	CYP2B6 variants correlate with Efavirenz plasma concentrations in HIV patients in Zimbabwe.	[42]
	CYP2B6 variants and pregnancy impact on Efavirenz plasma concentrations in Nigerian patients.	[28]
	Novel variants in pharmacogenes are associated with Efavirenz metabolism in HIV patients in South Africa.	[30]
	Composite *CYP2B6* alleles are significantly associated with Efavirenz-mediated central nervous system toxicity in HIV patients in Botswana.	[52]
Nevirapine	*CYP2B6* and *CYP1A2* variants impact Nevirapine plasma concentrations and HIV progression respectively in an HIV patient cohort in Zimbabwe.	[29]
PEGylated Interferon-alpha/Ribavirin	*IL28B* SNPs correlate with treatment response in Hepatitis C patients from SSA.	[48]
ARV/TB	GWAS study identified SNPs linked to drug-induced hepatotoxicity in HIV/TB patients in Ethiopia.	[47]
ARV/TB/Antimalarials	*CYP2B6*6* variant and Efavirenz concentration impact on Lumefantrine plasma levels in HIV/Malaria patients in Tanzania.	[25]
	High frequency of the *CYP2B6*6* allele is associated with poor clinical response in HIV/TB/Malaria patient cohort in Congo.	[46]
Lumefantrine	*CYP3A4*, *CYP3A5* variants impact Lumefantrine response in a cohort of pregnant women with malaria in Tanzania.	[25]
Imatinib	*CYP3A5*3* and *ABCB1 C3435T* variants influence clinical outcomes and plasma concentrations of Imatinib in Nigerian patients with chronic myeloid leukaemia.	[44]
Risperidone	*CYP2D6* variants did not significantly impact the incidence of ADRs in a South African cohort.	[53]
Amitriptyline	*CYP2D6* variants influence ADR incidence in patients with painful diabetic peripheral neuropathy in a South African cohort.	[54]
Rosuvastatin	Specific pharmacogene variants influencing rosuvastatin response in African populations.	[24]
Warfarin	*CYP2C9* and *VKORC1* variants are associated with dose–response in Warfarin-treated Sudanese patients.	[55]
	Novel *CYP2C9/VKORC1* variants influence Warfarin response in a black South African cohort.	[56]
	CYP2C9/VKORC1 variants did not correlate with Warfarin dose–response in a Ghanaian cohort.	[57]

Pharmacovigilance systems aimed at monitoring drug safety are underdeveloped or even non-existent in some SSA countries. Therefore, clinicians are not aware of the exact framework for communicating ADRs to health institutes or national health departments. Insufficient funding and lack of communication between clinicians and national health departments, as well as limited physician competency on pharmacovigilance, greatly contribute to underreporting of ADRs in SSA countries [13] (Figure 1). Most clinicians complain of a lack of time to prepare ADR reports, while some physicians in private health care might be lethargic in reporting ADRs due to fear that submitting inadequate reports may lead to legal action taken either for medical malpractice or incompetence [58]. Under-reporting of ADRs is reflected in the under-participation by SSA countries in pharmacovigilance programs where only 35 countries actively participate in the International Drug Monitoring Program run by the by the World Health Organisation [13].

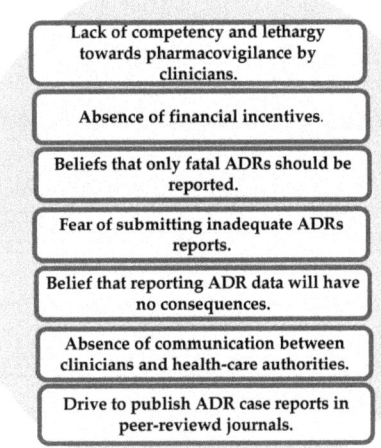

Figure 1. Main factors contributing to under-reporting of adverse drug reactions (ADRs) by clinicians in sub-Saharan African (SSA) countries.

The few studies on the impact of ADRs on affected populations and health care systems in SSA have demonstrated that ARVs contribute to 80% of ADRs and that ADRs from some antibiotics are up to 10% higher in African populations relative to other populations globally [13]. A case in point is the high frequency of ADRs such as cardiotoxicity and congestive heart failure commonly observed during anthracycline treatment in Africans relative to Caucasian populations [59]. Clinical trials on medications used to treat NCDs have mainly been carried out on populations other than African, leading to rare ADRs being recorded in Africans. Several factors could be attributable to the unique patterns of ADRs in SSA populations including host genetic factors, age, weight, polypharmacy, lifestyle, and the utilisation of counterfeit or expired medication [13]. Furthermore, there is a reported low efficacy of drugs such as beta blockers and angiotensin-converting enzyme inhibitors in African populations [60]. Therefore, large-scale PGx GWAS in African populations are needed to uncover drug–gene, drug–drug, drug–drug–gene interactions, as well as gene loci impacting ADRs and the low efficacy of some drugs.

4. Challenges in Genotyping Pharmacogene Variants

Drug response phenotypes are primarily determined by mechanisms involved in the induction or inhibition of enzymes, as well as the functionality of transporters and other proteins involved in absorption, distribution, metabolism and excretion (ADME) (pharmacokinetics). The pharmacodynamics of interactions of a drug with its target or other molecules in disease pathways also impacts drug response.

Together, polymorphisms mostly in the coding and regulatory regions of genes for these enzymes account for approximately 25% of the variability in inter-individual and inter-ethnic drug responses [61]. Other factors affecting the activities of these enzymes include epigenetic regulation, gender, age, lifestyle, and concomitant medications [62].

The Cytochrome P450 family of enzymes (including CYP1A2, CYP2D6, CYP2C9, CYP2B6, CYP2C19, CYP3A4, and CYP3A5) coded for by their respective pharmacogenes is responsible for the metabolism of almost 90% of prescribed medications [3]. Other important pharmacogenes with "actionable variants" include *SLCO1B1*, *VKORC1*, *DPYD*, *TPMT*, *NUDT15*, *HLA-A*, and *HLA-B*. Together, the "actionable variants" of pharmacogenes listed above impact the metabolism of up to 49 commonly prescribed drugs used in primary care in SSA and globally (including anti-infectives, antihypertensives, antilipidemic, antidepressants, and anticancer). The CPIC and DPGWG assigns "actionable variants" based on sufficient clinical evidence while providing gene–drug dosing guidelines [15] (Figure 2).

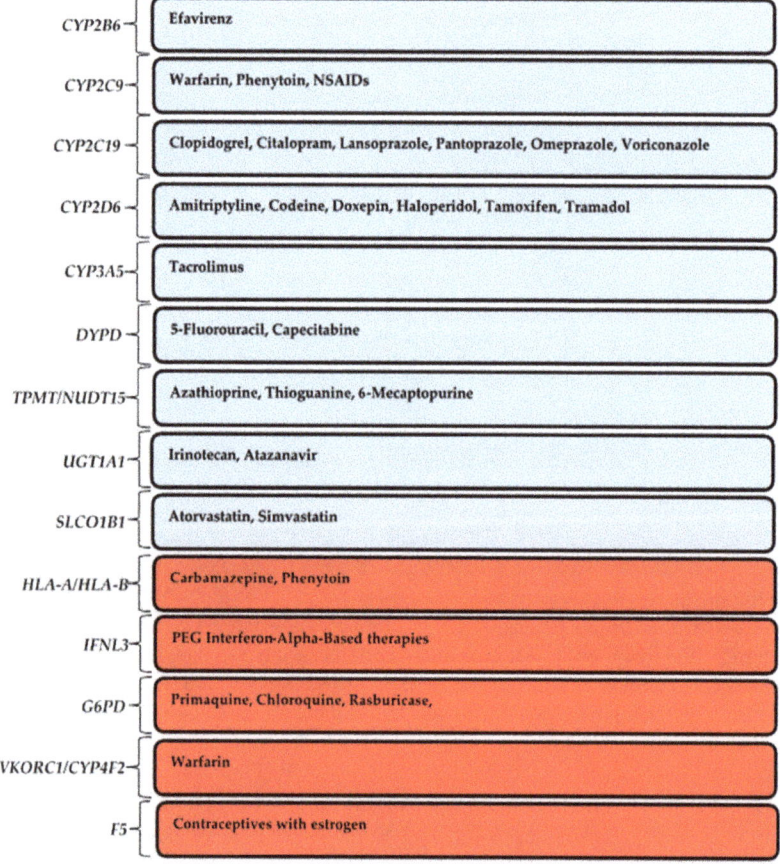

Figure 2. Pharmacokinetic (blue), pharmacodynamic (red) gene–drug pairs with Clinical Pharmacogenetics Implementation Consortium/Dutch Pharmacogenetics Working Group (CPIC/DPWG) "actionable variants" and dosage guidelines in commonly prescribed medications that will benefit patients in primary care in SSA.

Germline variants in genes coding for these enzymes (Figure 2) can be SNPs (single nucleotide polymorphisms), INDELS (insertions and deletions), and copy number variations (CNVs) including duplications, deletions, and complex structural variants (SVs) [5]. These variants result in alleles that confer different phenotypes. Specifically, phenotypes resulting from variants in the CYP2 family of enzymes are grouped into four main categories, namely (a) ultra-rapid metabolisers (UM)—carry two or more gain-of-function alleles including gene duplications; (b) normal metabolisers (NM)—carry normal-function gene alleles; (c) intermediate metabolisers (IM)—carry one non-functional allele; and (d) poor metabolisers (PM)—carry two non-functional alleles, including gene deletions [5]. PMs normally experience more ADRs in the case of the metabolism of an active drug due to high plasma levels of the active compound, while UMs will experience therapeutic failure due to the rapid metabolism and clearance of the active compound from their systems. Globally, with respect to the CYP2D6 enzyme, 0.4–5.4% of individuals are PMs, 0.4–11% are IMs, 67–90% are NMs, and 1–21% are UMs [61]. For example, the *CYP2D6*2XN* allele found in UM individuals is recorded in 1–16% of Africans, while *CYP2D6*17* found in PM individuals is recorded in 35% of African populations [21]. The high frequency of recorded PM individuals in African populations is of great clinical significance, as most of the commonly prescribed medications and food substances are metabolised by the CYP2D6 enzyme.

Global inter-ethnic variability in the frequency of PGx "actionable variants" is evident for some genes (Table 2), leading to the clustering of biogeographical populations into European, Asian, and African. The frequency of African-specific PGx biomarkers as highlighted (Table 2) reveals some population-specific variants: for instance, the high frequency of the *CYP2D6*17* allele in African populations relative to European and Asian populations. Nevertheless, the clinical relevance as well as frequencies of some "actionable variants" for specific medications have not been characterised in African populations, as is evident from the absence of frequency data on the CPIC database. Dedicated clinical PGx research with large sample sizes of African cohorts might hopefully uncover region-specific genotype–phenotype correlations.

In addition to germline variants, somatic variants have been characterised and catalogued in relation to cancer treatment responses. For instance, somatic mutations on *EGFR* and *BCR-ABL* genes are highly predictive of gefitinib and imatinib drug response respectively in non-small cell lung cancer patients of European ancestry [63]. Furthermore, few studies have demonstrated inter-ethnic variability in the frequency of some sensitising somatic variants. However, studies on somatic variant profiles in cancer patients in African populations are sparse [63]. Neoplasms are one of the leading causes of deaths from NCDs in the SSA region [12]. Therefore, it is crucial for health-care stakeholders to start prioritising PGx research and effective PGx clinical interventions in cancer patients.

Transient drug induction or the inhibition of ADME enzymes during co-medication is known as phenoconversion. The phenomenon of phenoconversion can also be a result of inflammatory processes in the body and can greatly impact the interpretation of PGx test results [64]. Very few clinical studies globally, and in Africa in particular, have demonstrated the impact of phenoconversion on PGx test result interpretation. An in vitro investigation on CYP2C19 enzyme activities in human donor liver microsomes revealed that the inclusion of phenocopying factors significantly improved phenotype prediction [65]. Phenoconversion is most likely to influence PGx results in African populations due to complex health interventions that include herbal medicines, although some enzymes such as CYP2D6 are not easily induced. Khat (*Catha edulis Forsk*), a psychoactive herb commonly used in East Africa, has been identified as a potent inhibitor of the CYP2D6 enzyme (which metabolises up to 25% of prescribed medications) [66]. Therefore, environmental factors such as regional lifestyles and co-medication should be considered in future studies and in the interpretation of clinical pharmacogenetically guided drug prescription.

Table 2. Average frequencies (%) of alleles (* star alleles) with "actionable variants" in pharmacogenes as assigned by CPIC in major global biogeographical populations. Average frequencies are based on the reported frequencies in one or multiple studies [15].

Gene	Allele	Functional Effect	Sub-Saharan Africa	African American/Afro-Caribbean	Caucasian	Central/South Asian
CYP2B6	*4	Increased function	0.0000	0.0103	0.0409	0.0990
	*5	Normal function	0.0200	0.0621	0.1155	0.0110
	*6	Decreased function	0.3749	0.3170	0.2330	0.1850
	*9	Decreased function	-	0.0465	0.0147	0.0590
	*16	Decreased function	0.0054	0.0000	0.0000	0.0000
	*18	No function	0.0577	0.0330	0.0000	0.0000
CYP2C9	*2	Decreased function	0.0131	0.0224	0.1273	0.1138
	*3	No function	0.0112	0.0301	0.0763	0.1099
	*5	Decreased function	0.0131	0.0116	0.0003	0.0000
	*11	Decreased function	0.0257	0.0139	0.0016	0.0010
CYP2C19	*2	No function	0.1568	0.1815	0.1466	0.2699
	*3	No function	0.0027	0.0028	0.0017	0.0157
	*4A/B	No function	0.0000	0.0000	0.0020	0.0000
	*5	No function	0.0000	0.0000	0.0000	0.0032
	*6	No function	0.0000	0.0000	0.0003	0.0006
	*8	No function	0.0000	0.0011	0.0034	0.0000
	*9	Decreased function	0.0270	0.0143	0.0007	0.0001
	*10	Decreased function	0.0000	0.0033	0.0000	0.0001
	*17	Increased function	0.1733	0.2072	0.2164	0.1708
CYP2D6	2XN	Increased function	0.0173	0.0188	0.0084	0.095
	*3	No function	0.0015	0.0032	0.0159	0.0011
	*4	No function	0.0338	0.0482	0.1854	0.0906
	*5	No function	0.0338	0.0482	0.1854	0.0459
	*6	No function	0.0000	0.0029	0.0111	0.0000
	*8	No function	0.0000	0.0000	0.0002	0.0000
	*9	Decreased function	0.0000	0.0044	0.0276	0.0300
	*10	Decreased function	0.0557	0.0382	0.0157	0.0867
	*14	Decreased function	-	0.0000	0.0000	-
	*17	Decreased function	0.1929	0.1688	0.0039	0.0007
	*41	Decreased function	0.1147	0.0372	0.0924	0.1230
CYP3A5	*3	No function	0.2409	0.3160	0.9249	0.6733
	*6	No function	0.1932	0.1112	0.0015	0.0000
	*7	No function	0.0864	0.1200	0.0000	-
DPYD	*2A	No function	0.0000	0.0031	0.0079	0.0051
	*13	No function	0.0000	0.0000	0.0006	0.0000
	2846A > T	Decreased function	-	0.0031	0.0037	0.0006
	1236G > A	Decreased function	0.0000	0.0031	0.0237	-
TPMT	*2	No function	0.0000	0.0053	0.0021	0.0002
	*3A	No function	0.0016	0.0080	0.0343	0.0042
	*3B	No function	0.0000	0.0000	0.0027	0.0017
	*3C	No function	0.0529	0.0240	0.0047	0.0112
NUDT15	*2*	No function	-	-	0.000	0.035
	*3	No function	-	-	0.002	0.061
	*6	Uncertain function	-	-	0.003	0.013
	*9	No function	-	-	0.002	0.000
SLCO1B1	*5	Decreased function	0.0000	0.0000	0.0083	0.0224
	*15	Decreased function	0.0297	-	0.0439	0.1214
	*17	Decreased function	-	0.1330	0.0519	-
UGT1A1	*28	Decreased function	0.4000	0.3734	0.3165	0.4142
	*6	Decreased function	0.0000	0.0040	0.0079	0.0449
	*37	Decreased function	0.0371	0.0570	0.0007	0.0000
HLA-A/HLA-B	HLA-A*31:01	High risk allele	0.52	0.98	2.84	2.20
	HLA-B*15:02	High risk allele	0.00	0.10	0.04	4.64
	HLA-B*57:01	High risk allele	0.79	0.10	3.23	4.49
	HLA-B*58:01	High risk allele	5.54	3.89	1.32	4.54
IFNL3	IL28B:CC	Increased response	26.8	15.2	36.5	1.9
	IL28B:CT	Increased response	52.4	40.62	47.6	23
	IL28B:TT	Increased response	20.8	43.75	15.9	75.1
G6PD	376A>G	Deficiency	0.312	-	0.0595	-
VKORC1	1639G>A	Decreased Warfarin dose	12.900	10.274	41.2242	15.317

The advent of improved techniques including next-generation sequencing (NGS), Sanger sequencing, and microarray genotyping techniques has completely revolutionised genotyping and GWAS, making genotyping more cost-effective, high-throughput, and accessible for clinical use [67]. Novel rare variants (including SNPs, CNVs, and complex hybrid SVs) in pharmacogenes such as the *CYP2D6* gene, with important functional effects, have recently been identified using NGS, highlighting the complexities in these genes [68]. These rare variants are thought to be differentiated amongst populations, which warrants more research on African rare variants, given the diverse genetic pool recorded in this region [20]. The high genetic diversity may result in varying efficacy and ADRs reported in African populations. South Africa in particular has a unique and complex genetic population, resulting from admixture between the native Khoisan with Bantu and European populations [20]. Recently, deep NGS of the pharmacogenes of a Bantu-speaking cohort in South Africa revealed rare novel variants with predicted functional effects that have not been recorded in other African populations [69]. This includes the identification of novel deleterious variants in the flavin-containing monooxygenase 2 gene, which is involved in the oxygenation of sulphur-containing drugs in humans [69]. Distinct and highly diverse alleles of the Cytochrome P450 family have been recorded in African populations relative to other populations, highlighting the need for further dedicated PGx and functional studies on these unique variants [21]. For instance, the loss-of-function *CYP2B6*6* allele which accounts for low efavirenz plasma levels and an increased risk of neurotoxicity, is highly prevalent in African populations relative to Europeans and Asians [30].

Novel and efficient genotyping platforms provide an opportunity for research initiatives to catalogue the structure and clinical functional effects of rare African genetic variants. Only a few private diagnostic and university research institutes in SSA are equipped with genotyping and bioinformatics technologies, while access to PGx tests is essentially limited to the private health-care sector. The cost-prohibitive nature of genetic testing and the general lack of expertise constitute barriers to setting up genetic testing laboratories. Furthermore, there are no standardised gene panels or guidelines for clinical testing between the few laboratories involved. Finally, there is lethargy in obtaining laboratory accreditation for genetic testing in countries that offer direct-to-customer testing. This stems from the absence of national guidelines for genetic testing in most SSA countries and other less developed regions [17].

Accurate genotyping and phenotype translation into actionable clinical decisions requires state-of-the-art sequencing technologies and computational platforms. Notably, the recent single-molecule real-time (SMRT) NGS platform has uncovered novel and complex SVs of the *CYP2D6* gene with predicted functional impact. Commercial genotyping arrays coupled with bioinformatics algorithms have been designed to incorporate millions of SNPs on chips, leading to high-turnaround times. SNPs (tag SNPs) incorporated in the array are selected such that they represent multiple other SNPs in the genome based on their linkage disequilibrium. Nonetheless, genomic data on most commercial arrays is based on data principally from Caucasian and Asian populations. Therefore, rare variants of African origin may not be captured using pre-designed arrays, due to differences in the linkage disequilibrium patterns between populations. This challenge is reflected in low specificities and sensitivities being recorded when these arrays are applied on African samples [67]. The challenge of genotyping novel rare variants can be overcome by using phasing and imputation software to extrapolate missing variants from whole-genome databases and subsequently customising the pre-designed array.

A H3Africa chip-based genotyping array with tag SNPs of clinically important pharmacogenes based on African genome sequences is now available for research [23]. This array will be a more accurate genotyping tool for African studies following its validation, as opposed to arrays that do not specifically include African variants. Importantly, different arrays have different sets of variants leading to the non-standardisation of variant panels tested [67]. Clinicians are faced with the challenge of selecting the most appropriate genotyping technology. There are several factors to be considered when selecting an appropriate genotyping test, including turnaround time, ability to detect/customise multiplexed variants across global ethnicities, and ease of workflow [67]. Varying sensitivities and specificities have been recorded by different genotyping platforms, leading to inconsistent variant calls. For example, inconsistent CNV and SV detection for *CYP2D6* has been recorded by different genotyping platforms, depending on their design [67,68]. Therefore, multiple genotyping platforms must be utilised for accurate phenotype prediction, which imposes a cost burden. The functional impacts of rare CNVs and SVs in *CYP2D6*, *CYP2C19*, *CYP2A6*, *SULT1A1*, and *GSTT1* have been identified with varying inter-ethnic frequencies (https://www.pharmgkb.org). These rare variants might explain the complex phenotypes unaccounted for by the "missing heritability" issue recorded in most GWAS studies. Therefore, uncovering the frequency and functional impact of pharmacogene CNVs and SVs on drug disposition in populations of African descent will greatly improve the accuracy of metaboliser status determination in clinical studies. Other challenges in genotyping include recorded allelic drop-out by different assays and the inability of some genotyping assays to determine which allele is duplicated, particularly with respect to the *CYP2D6* gene [68]. The accurate genotyping of complex PGx genes usually requires the utilisation of multiple genotyping techniques including those that are PCR-based, mass arrays, and sequencing techniques [68].

The absence of a consensus in the translation of genotyping results to actionable drug prescription presents another challenge for PGx test result interpretation. For example, the phenotypic effects of loss-of-function and gain-of-function *CYP2C19* alleles are drug-dependent [5]. Although the CPIC is continually updating guidelines for drug–gene interactions and translating "actionable variants" into phenotypes based on activity scores, clinical validity of these recommendations is still required, particularly in SSA populations. Furthermore, some guidelines for translating *CYP2D6* genotypes into actionable clinical decisions are divergent between expert organisations such as the CPIC and DPWG, although efforts are being made towards harmonising guidelines. The functional impacts of rare novel alleles are commonly predicted using computational algorithms, but experimental studies remain the gold standard. This further highlights the need for more in vivo studies on the functional impact of novel rare African gene variants. Experimental assays to validate the functionality of the novel variants could be performed by employing whole animal models, human transformed cell lines, and organoids, depending on available funding and logistics [51].

Recently, an assembled pan-African reference human genome from sequences of African individuals revealed an additional 296.6 Mb of unique sequences relative to the current reference human genome [70]. Thus, the current reference human genome is not appropriate for African PGx and genetic studies. Genomic initiatives in Africa such as H3Africa [23] and APC [22] have been supporting PGx research in Africa by sequencing and curating the genomes of African individuals, supporting genomic research capacity building and harmonising genotype and phenotype data recording. This has led to an increase in integrated capacities for PGx research as well as an increase in the utilisation of genomics and bioinformatics technologies in SSA. Other genomic initiatives such as the Southern African Human Genome Programme [71], the African Genome Variation Project [72], and the MalariaGEN project [73] have provided databases of African genome sequences. Although governments in SSA are compelled to channel their limited resources towards the fight against infectious diseases, the cataloguing of African PGx data will contribute to diagnostic and drug development pipelines tailored for African populations.

5. Socio-Cultural and Ethical Challenges vis-à-vis Clinicians

The successful implementation of PGx testing will require acceptance and adequate knowledge of PGx by health-care workers, especially physicians. Nevertheless, competency on PGx testing amongst clinicians in African populations is lacking, which has also been reported as one of the major barriers for implementing PGx in other under-resourced clinical settings such as in Latin America [17,74]. The lack of competency stems from the absence of or limited PGx training programs in health-care training institutions and universities in Africa. In addition, physicians are not aware of the available evidence and curated guidelines for PGx testing implementation [74,75]. The CPIC and PharmKGB databases are excellent resources for clinicians to acquire adequate guideline support for priority PGx testing implementation. PGx programs should be a prerequisite in health training schools and university curricula in SSA countries. The ordering, analysis, and interpretation of PGx test reports are complex, requiring access to and the incorporation of PGx data into EHRs and CDSS. Therefore, physicians require adequate knowledge concerning the logistics involved in ordering and interpreting PGx tests. Importantly, clinicians also lack confidence when counselling and/or recommending PGx tests to patients, reflecting lethargy in updating themselves regarding PGx analysis and research from peer-reviewed literature [74]. Furthermore, the absence of clear regulations for genetic testing coupled with cost-prohibitive tests in private and public laboratories in SSA greatly contributes to the non-ordering of these tests by physicians [74]. Most physicians in SSA clinics are not aware of the ethical and legal implications of returning PGx testing results to patients, stemming from the absence of national regulatory guidelines for genetic testing [74,76]. Genetic counselling of patients is required before returning PGx test results to patients. However, the absence of genetic counsellors in most public clinics in SSA places a high burden on physicians. Importantly, physicians may be wary of fatal outcomes, in the case where an inaccurate drug regimen or dosage was selected based on genotype [70]. The sharing of secondary or incidental findings of disease-related genes during PGx testing with an individual or family also poses an ethical issue. Indeed, patients need to be assured of the privacy and confidentiality of their results, especially with respect to employer and insurer decisions. Furthermore, the right to ownership of patient data and samples varies depending on the country's policies, which needs to be known and acknowledged by clinicians. The unique consenting procedure for PGx testing in SSA populations is also noteworthy. It has been suggested that informed consent for African populations needs to be modelled relative to the culture and ethics of the communities and not extrapolated from Western cultures [74,77]. A tiered informed consent involving the use of African colloquialisms to explain hereditary has been suggested for use in African cohorts [77]. Overcoming these observed social and ethical barriers will require collaboration between clinicians, genetic councillors, and research experts to provide robust institutional support for the successful implementation of PGx testing.

6. Socio-Cultural and Ethical Challenges vis-à-vis Patients

Knowledge and awareness of PGx testing by patients and caregivers in SSA populations is absent. This might lead to an unacceptability of PGx testing, as most patients from rural areas with limited education and socio-economic status will lack understanding, including misconceptions about the costs and invasiveness of the tests. Most patients do not obtain additional information on the benefits or logistics of PGx testing, and therefore, they rely more on the physician to make final decisions for them [74]. Some patients might be reluctant to perform a PGx test for psychological reasons, based on the implications of the results. This might stem from religious and cultural beliefs regarding genetic material [74]. Most African people do not have specific words in their native languages describing genetic material. Furthermore, many consider genetic material to be related to paternity and ancestry, which may affect their understanding and acceptability of PGx testing. Therefore, physicians need to implement traditional and religious symbols to facilitate patient understanding of PGx tests. Patients from rural areas in SSA countries do not have access to PGx testing services due to their cost-prohibitive nature, and only a few private laboratories offer these services to private patients in urban areas [74]. Patients and caregivers will appreciate the benefits of PGx testing in their clinical care if the tests are implemented in most clinics and are affordable.

7. Socio-Cultural and Ethical Challenges vis-à-vis Health-Care Authorities and Insurers

The implementation of clinical PGx testing in SSA poses a financial burden on already challenged public health-care systems. Health-care policy makers and government departments need robust evidence that demonstrates the cost-effectiveness of PGx testing implementation, as resources are usually directed towards urgent public health-care issues. Therefore, most researchers and clinicians rely on foreign and private funding for genetic research and testing. This highlights the need for more large-scale clinical studies in SSA populations aimed at demonstrating the cost-effectiveness and ability of PGx tests to improve the quality of life of patients. Government health departments also exhibit lethargy in engaging researchers and providing informatics support to clinics, as PGx tests are perceived to be expensive [74].

Most countries, particularly in SSA and other less developed regions [17], lack specific and clear regulatory policies for the implementation of genetic testing, and in particular PGx testing. For instance, only South Africa, Nigeria, and Malawi amongst SSA countries provide clear and specific guidelines for genetic testing and research [78]. The Academy of Science of South Africa has provided a review of ethical, legal, and social implications of genetics research and testing in South Africa [79]. Nevertheless, a final framework on data sharing and genotyping test accreditation can only be provided by the national health and science research departments. This poses a challenge for researchers and funders involved in PGx research and implementation. The implementation of PGx testing regulations in SSA countries will depend on the continued training of geneticists, setting up of national genetic testing infrastructure, and research funding from government health departments.

The non-reimbursement of PGx tests in SSA countries poses another challenge for clinical implementation. Insurers, particularly those in the private health-care sector, require standard clinical guidelines for frequent use by physicians and evidence of cost–utility for their coverage of PGx tests [74]. Given the absence of clinical studies demonstrating the cost-effectiveness and clinical utility of PGx in African populations, most insurers in this region will not provide coverage for these tests. Therefore, cost–utility analyses of implementing PGx testing in SSA populations needs to be undertaken in order to demonstrate clinical utility and provide motivation for reimbursement by health-care insurers.

8. Conclusions and Future Directives

The clinical utility and cost-effectiveness of PGx testing for improved patient health care is increasingly being demonstrated. However, the implementation of PGx testing in SSA is still lagging. This review highlights several challenges that need to be surmounted for the future implementation of routine PGx testing in SSA. These include the establishment of robust clinical health-care systems, investing in dedicated PGx studies and governance, improving scientific and technical barriers to genotyping pharmacogene variants, and PGx knowledge uptake by health-care stakeholders.

We believe the implementation of pre-emptive clinical PGx testing in SSA countries is feasible through a hybrid model that incorporates patient genetic data from research biobanks linked to other clinical data in EHS/CDDS. This will involve the input of multiple key stakeholders, including patients, clinicians, geneticists, information technology specialists, and health departments. Furthermore, this model will also provide a unique opportunity for the easy retrieval of patient phenotypic and genetic data for large-scale GWAS PGx research initiatives. Proactive strategies such as the provision of institutional support by national health departments will ensure the strengthening of health-care systems in SSA countries.

Clinical PGx research in some SSA countries has uncovered rare variants in African populations with a significant functional impact. Preliminary data from clinical studies demonstrate the benefits of implementing PGx testing in SSA for optimal patient care. Additional robust large-scale studies on populations of African ancestry will provide strong evidence for the cost-effectiveness and clinical utility of PGx testing in these populations. Robust evidence on the cost-utility of PGx testing will ensure support for clinical PGx testing implementation from health-care departments, policy makers, and health-care insurers. Furthermore, the genotypes of large populations of Africans should be catalogued by employing a combination of cost-effective high-throughput NGS and customisable massarray genotyping techniques coupled with bioinformatic analysis. Finally, the provision of additional funding and regulations for PGx research and clinical diagnostic laboratories will ensure increased expertise and accessibility to genotyping techniques in SSA.

The availability of published CPIC and PharmKGB guidelines for pharmacogenetically guided prescription provides an excellent resource for PGx testing knowledge uptake by clinicians, counsellors, and subsequently patients and caregivers in SSA. Finally, we suggest that the continual curation of clinical PGx testing evidence, the setting up and harmonisation of regulatory policies, and the education of health-care stakeholders across SSA countries by African genomic initiatives such as the H3Africa and the African Pharmacogenetics Consortium (APC) will facilitate the implementation of PGx testing in SSA.

Author Contributions: Conceptualisation, M.S.P.; Original draft writing, E.B.T.; Review and editing, E.B.T., M.A.A., M.S.P.; Supervision, M.S.P., M.A.A.; Project administration and funding, M.S.P. All authors have read and agreed to the published version of the manuscript.

Funding: M.S.P. receives funding from the South African Medical Research Council (Flagship and Extramural Unit awards), and the University of Pretoria (through the Institute for Cellular and Molecular Medicine).

Conflicts of Interest: The authors have no conflicts of interest to declare.

References

1. Cavallari, L.H.; Beitelshees, A.L.; Blake, K.V.; Dressler, L.G.; Duarte, J.D.; Elsey, A.; Eichmeyer, J.N.; Empey, P.E.; Franciosi, J.P.; Hicks, J.K.; et al. The IGNITE Pharmacogenetics Working Group: An Opportunity for Building Evidence with Pharmacogenetic Implementation in a Real-World Setting. *Clin. Transl. Sci.* **2017**, *10*, 143–146. [CrossRef] [PubMed]
2. Zhu, Y.; Swanson, K.M.; Rojas, R.L.; Wang, Z.; St Sauver, J.L.; Visscher, S.L.; Prokop, L.J.; Bielinski, S.J.; Wang, L.; Weinshilboum, R.; et al. Systematic review of the evidence on the cost-effectiveness of pharmacogenomics-guided treatment for cardiovascular diseases. *Genet. Med.* **2020**, *22*, 475–486. [CrossRef] [PubMed]
3. Relling, M.V.; Klein, T.E. CPIC: Clinical Pharmacogenetics Implementation Consortium of the Pharmacogenomics Research Network. *Clin. Pharmacol. Ther.* **2011**, *89*, 464–467. [CrossRef] [PubMed]
4. Swen, J.J.; Wilting, I.; de Goede, A.L.; Grandia, L.; Mulder, H.; Touw, D.J.; de Boer, A.; Conemans, J.M.; Egberts, T.C.; Klungel, O.H.; et al. Pharmacogenetics: From bench to byte. *Clin. Pharmacol. Ther.* **2008**, *83*, 781–787. [CrossRef]
5. PharmGKB. Available online: https://www.pharmgkb.org/ (accessed on 10 November 2019).
6. EU-PIC. Available online: https://www.eu-pic.net/ (accessed on 9 August 2020).
7. U-PGx. Available online: http://upgx.eu/ (accessed on 9 August 2020).
8. CYTED. Available online: http://www.cyted.org/es/relivaf (accessed on 9 August 2020).
9. Chumnumwat, S.; Lu, Z.H.; Sukasem, C.; Winther, M.D.; Capule, F.R.; Abdul Hamid, A.; Bhandari, B.; Chaikledkaew, U.; Chanhom, N.; Chantarangsu, S.; et al. Southeast Asian Pharmacogenomics Research Network (SEAPharm): Current Status and Perspectives. *Public Health Genom.* **2019**, *22*, 132–139. [CrossRef]
10. FDA. Available online: https://www.fda.gov/drugs/science-and-research-drugs/table-pharmacogenomic-biomarkers-drug-labeling (accessed on 10 December 2019).
11. Mhalu, F.S. Burden of diseases in poor resource countries: Meeting the challenges of combating HIV/AIDS, tuberculosis and malaria. *Tanzan. Health Res. Bull.* **2005**, *7*, 179–184. [CrossRef]
12. Gouda, H.N.; Charlson, F.; Sorsdahl, K.; Ahmadzada, S.; Ferrari, A.J.; Erskine, H.; Leung, J.; Santamauro, D.; Lund, C.; Aminde, L.N.; et al. Burden of non-communicable diseases in sub-Saharan Africa, 1990-2017: Results from the Global Burden of Disease Study 2017. *Lancet Glob. Health* **2019**, *7*, e1375–e1387. [CrossRef]
13. Ampadu, H.H.; Hoekman, J.; de Bruin, M.L.; Pal, S.N.; Olsson, S.; Sartori, D.; Leufkens, H.G.; Dodoo, A.N. Adverse Drug Reaction Reporting in Africa and a Comparison of Individual Case Safety Report Characteristics Between Africa and the Rest of the World: Analyses of Spontaneous Reports in VigiBase(R). *Drug Saf.* **2016**, *39*, 335–345. [CrossRef]
14. Asiimwe, I.G.; Zhang, E.J.; Osanlou, R.; Krause, A.; Dillon, C.; Suarez-Kurtz, G.; Zhang, H.; Perini, J.A.; Renta, J.Y.; Duconge, J.; et al. Genetic Factors Influencing Warfarin Dose in Black-African Patients: A Systematic Review and Meta-Analysis. *Clin. Pharmacol. Ther.* **2020**, *107*, 1420–1433. [CrossRef]
15. CPIC. Available online: https://cpicpgx.org/genes-drugs/ (accessed on 30 July 2020).

16. Maranville, J.C.; Cox, N.J. Pharmacogenomic variants have larger effect sizes than genetic variants associated with other dichotomous complex traits. *Pharm. J.* **2016**, *16*, 388–392. [CrossRef]
17. Quinones, L.A.; Lavanderos, M.A.; Cayun, J.P.; Garcia-Martin, E.; Agundez, J.A.; Caceres, D.D.; Roco, A.M.; Morales, J.E.; Herrera, L.; Encina, G.; et al. Perception of the usefulness of drug/gene pairs and barriers for pharmacogenomics in Latin America. *Curr. Drug Metab.* **2014**, *15*, 202–208. [CrossRef] [PubMed]
18. Matimba, A.; Oluka, M.N.; Ebeshi, B.U.; Sayi, J.; Bolaji, O.O.; Guantai, A.N.; Masimirembwa, C.M. Establishment of a biobank and pharmacogenetics database of African populations. *Eur. J. Hum. Genet.* **2008**, *16*, 780–783. [CrossRef] [PubMed]
19. Buniello, A.; MacArthur, J.A.L.; Cerezo, M.; Harris, L.W.; Hayhurst, J.; Malangone, C.; McMahon, A.; Morales, J.; Mountjoy, E.; Sollis, E.; et al. The NHGRI-EBI GWAS Catalog of published genome-wide association studies, targeted arrays and summary statistics 2019. *Nucleic Acids Res.* **2019**, *47*, D1005–D1012. [CrossRef] [PubMed]
20. Tishkoff, S.A.; Reed, F.A.; Friedlaender, F.R.; Ehret, C.; Ranciaro, A.; Froment, A.; Hirbo, J.B.; Awomoyi, A.A.; Bodo, J.M.; Doumbo, O.; et al. The genetic structure and history of Africans and African Americans. *Science* **2009**, *324*, 1035–1044. [CrossRef] [PubMed]
21. Rajman, I.; Knapp, L.; Morgan, T.; Masimirembwa, C. African Genetic Diversity: Implications for Cytochrome P450-mediated Drug Metabolism and Drug Development. *EBioMedicine* **2017**, *17*, 67–74. [CrossRef]
22. Dandara, C.; Masimirembwa, C.; Haffani, Y.Z.; Ogutu, R.; Mabuka, G.; Aklillu, E.; Bolaji, R. African Pharmacogenomics Consortium: Consolidating pharmacogenomics knowledge, capacity development and translation in Africa. *AAS Open Res.* **2019**, *2*, 19. [CrossRef]
23. H3Africa. Available online: https://h3africa.org/ (accessed on 10 November 2019).
24. Soko, N.D.; Chimusa, E.; Masimirembwa, C.; Dandara, C. An African-specific profile of pharmacogene variants for rosuvastatin plasma variability: Limited role for SLCO1B1 c.521T>C and ABCG2 c.421A>C. *Pharm. J.* **2019**, *19*, 240–248. [CrossRef]
25. Mutagonda, R.F.; Kamuhabwa, A.A.R.; Minzi, O.M.S.; Massawe, S.N.; Asghar, M.; Homann, M.V.; Farnert, A.; Aklillu, E. Effect of pharmacogenetics on plasma lumefantrine pharmacokinetics and malaria treatment outcome in pregnant women. *Malar. J.* **2017**, *16*, 267. [CrossRef]
26. Nemaura, T.; Nhachi, C.; Masimirembwa, C. Impact of gender, weight and CYP2B6 genotype on efavirenz exposure in patients on HIV/AIDS and TB treatment: Implications for individualising therapy. *Afr. J. Pharm. Pharmacol.* **2012**, *6*, 2188–2193.
27. Ngaimisi, E.; Mugusi, S.; Minzi, O.; Sasi, P.; Riedel, K.D.; Suda, A.; Ueda, N.; Janabi, M.; Mugusi, F.; Haefeli, W.E.; et al. Effect of rifampicin and CYP2B6 genotype on long-term efavirenz autoinduction and plasma exposure in HIV patients with or without tuberculosis. *Clin. Pharmacol. Ther.* **2011**, *90*, 406–413. [CrossRef]
28. Olagunju, A.; Bolaji, O.; Amara, A.; Else, L.; Okafor, O.; Adejuyigbe, E.; Oyigboja, J.; Back, D.; Khoo, S.; Owen, A. Pharmacogenetics of pregnancy-induced changes in efavirenz pharmacokinetics. *Clin. Pharmacol. Ther.* **2015**, *97*, 298–306. [CrossRef] [PubMed]
29. Mhandire, D.; Lacerda, M.; Castel, S.; Mhandire, K.; Zhou, D.; Swart, M.; Shamu, T.; Smith, P.; Musingwini, T.; Wiesner, L.; et al. Effects of CYP2B6 and CYP1A2 Genetic Variation on Nevirapine Plasma Concentration and Pharmacodynamics as Measured by CD4 Cell Count in Zimbabwean HIV-Infected Patients. *Omics* **2015**, *19*, 553–562. [CrossRef] [PubMed]
30. Decloedt, E.H.; Sinxadi, P.Z.; van Zyl, G.U.; Wiesner, L.; Khoo, S.; Joska, J.A.; Haas, D.W.; Maartens, G. Pharmacogenetics and pharmacokinetics of CNS penetration of efavirenz and its metabolites. *J. Antimicrob. Chemother.* **2019**, *74*, 699–709. [CrossRef] [PubMed]
31. WHO. Available online: https://www.who.int/bulletin/africanhealth/en/ (accessed on 25 July 2020).
32. Mpye, K.L.; Matimba, A.; Dzobo, K.; Chirikure, S.; Wonkam, A.; Dandara, C. Disease burden and the role of pharmacogenomics in African populations. *Glob. Health Epidemiol. Genom.* **2017**, *2*, e1. [CrossRef]
33. Cavallari, L.H.; Van Driest, S.L.; Prows, C.A.; Bishop, J.R.; Limdi, N.A.; Pratt, V.M.; Ramsey, L.B.; Smith, D.M.; Tuteja, S.; Duong, B.Q.; et al. Multi-site investigation of strategies for the clinical implementation of CYP2D6 genotyping to guide drug prescribing. *Genet. Med.* **2019**, *21*, 2255–2263. [CrossRef]
34. Odekunle, F.F.; Odekunle, R.O.; Shankar, S. Why sub-Saharan Africa lags in electronic health record adoption and possible strategies to increase its adoption in this region. *Int. J. Health Sci.* **2017**, *11*, 59–64.

35. Aquilante, C.L.; Kao, D.P.; Trinkley, K.E.; Lin, C.T.; Crooks, K.R.; Hearst, E.C.; Hess, S.J.; Kudron, E.L.; Lee, Y.M.; Liko, I.; et al. Clinical implementation of pharmacogenomics via a health system-wide research biobank: The University of Colorado experience. *Pharmacogenomics* **2020**, *21*, 375–386. [CrossRef]
36. Christoffels, A.; Abayomi, A. Careful governance of African biobanks. *Lancet* **2020**, *395*, 29–30. [CrossRef]
37. Border, R.; Johnson, E.C.; Evans, L.M.; Smolen, A.; Berley, N.; Sullivan, P.F.; Keller, M.C. No Support for Historical Candidate Gene or Candidate Gene-by-Interaction Hypotheses for Major Depression Across Multiple Large Samples. *Am. J. Psychiatry* **2019**, *176*, 376–387. [CrossRef]
38. Lewis, C.M.; Vassos, E. Polygenic risk scores: From research tools to clinical instruments. *Genome Med.* **2020**, *12*, 44. [CrossRef]
39. Wilson, P.W.; Meigs, J.B.; Sullivan, L.; Fox, C.S.; Nathan, D.M.; D'Agostino, R.B., Sr. Prediction of incident diabetes mellitus in middle-aged adults: The Framingham Offspring Study. *Arch. Intern. Med.* **2007**, *167*, 1068–1074. [CrossRef] [PubMed]
40. Natarajan, P.; Young, R.; Stitziel, N.O.; Padmanabhan, S.; Baber, U.; Mehran, R.; Sartori, S.; Fuster, V.; Reilly, D.F.; Butterworth, A.; et al. Polygenic Risk Score Identifies Subgroup With Higher Burden of Atherosclerosis and Greater Relative Benefit From Statin Therapy in the Primary Prevention Setting. *Circulation* **2017**, *135*, 2091–2101. [CrossRef]
41. Swart, M.; Evans, J.; Skelton, M.; Castel, S.; Wiesner, L.; Smith, P.J.; Dandara, C. An Expanded Analysis of Pharmacogenetics Determinants of Efavirenz Response that Includes 3'-UTR Single Nucleotide Polymorphisms among Black South African HIV/AIDS Patients. *Front. Genet.* **2015**, *6*, 356. [CrossRef] [PubMed]
42. Nyakutira, C.; Roshammar, D.; Chigutsa, E.; Chonzi, P.; Ashton, M.; Nhachi, C.; Masimirembwa, C. High prevalence of the CYP2B6 516G–>T(*6) variant and effect on the population pharmacokinetics of efavirenz in HIV/AIDS outpatients in Zimbabwe. *Eur. J. Clin. Pharmacol.* **2008**, *64*, 357–365. [CrossRef] [PubMed]
43. Soko, N.D.; Masimirembwa, C.; Dandara, C. Pharmacogenomics of Rosuvastatin: A Glocal (Global plus Local) African Perspective and Expert Review on a Statin Drug. *Omics* **2016**, *20*, 498–509. [CrossRef] [PubMed]
44. Adeagbo, B.A.; Bolaji, O.O.; Olugbade, T.A.; Durosinmi, M.A.; Bolarinwa, R.A.; Masimirembwa, C. Influence of CYP3A5*3 and ABCB1 C3435T on clinical outcomes and trough plasma concentrations of imatinib in Nigerians with chronic myeloid leukaemia. *J. Clin. Pharm. Ther.* **2016**, *41*, 546–551. [CrossRef]
45. Maganda, B.A.; Minzi, O.M.; Ngaimisi, E.; Kamuhabwa, A.A.; Aklillu, E. CYP2B6*6 genotype and high efavirenz plasma concentration but not nevirapine are associated with low lumefantrine plasma exposure and poor treatment response in HIV-malaria-coinfected patients. *Pharm. J.* **2016**, *16*, 88–95. [CrossRef]
46. Peko, S.M.; Gueye, N.S.G.; Vouvoungui, C.; Koukouikila-Koussounda, F.; Kobawila, S.C.; Nderu, D.; Velavan, T.P.; Ntoumi, F. Cytochrome P450 CYP2B6*6 distribution among Congolese individuals with HIV, Tuberculosis and Malaria infection. *Int. J. Infect. Dis.* **2019**, *82*, 111–116. [CrossRef]
47. Petros, Z.; Lee, M.M.; Takahashi, A.; Zhang, Y.; Yimer, G.; Habtewold, A.; Amogne, W.; Aderaye, G.; Schuppe-Koistinen, I.; Mushiroda, T.; et al. Genome-wide association and replication study of anti-tuberculosis drugs-induced liver toxicity. *BMC Genom.* **2016**, *17*, 755. [CrossRef]
48. Asselah, T.; De Muynck, S.; Broet, P.; Masliah-Planchon, J.; Blanluet, M.; Bieche, I.; Lapalus, M.; Martinot-Peignoux, M.; Lada, O.; Estrabaud, E.; et al. IL28B polymorphism is associated with treatment response in patients with genotype 4 chronic hepatitis C. *J. Hepatol.* **2012**, *56*, 527–532. [CrossRef]
49. Carpenter, D.; Gonzalez, D.; Retsch-Bogart, G.; Sleath, B.; Wilfond, B. Methodological and Ethical Issues in Pediatric Medication Safety Research. *Pediatrics* **2017**, *140*, e20170195. [CrossRef] [PubMed]
50. Zhou, Y.; Mkrtchian, S.; Kumondai, M.; Hiratsuka, M.; Lauschke, V.M. An optimized prediction framework to assess the functional impact of pharmacogenetic variants. *Pharm. J.* **2019**, *19*, 115–126. [CrossRef] [PubMed]
51. Musunuru, K.; Bernstein, D.; Cole, F.S.; Khokha, M.K.; Lee, F.S.; Lin, S.; McDonald, T.V.; Moskowitz, I.P.; Quertermous, T.; Sankaran, V.G.; et al. Functional Assays to Screen and Dissect Genomic Hits: Doubling Down on the National Investment in Genomic Research. *Circ. Genom. Precis. Med.* **2018**, *11*, e002178. [CrossRef] [PubMed]
52. Vujkovic, M.; Bellamy, S.L.; Zuppa, A.F.; Gastonguay, M.R.; Moorthy, G.S.; Ratshaa, B.; Han, X.; Steenhoff, A.P.; Mosepele, M.; Strom, B.L.; et al. Polymorphisms in cytochrome P450 are associated with extensive efavirenz pharmacokinetics and CNS toxicities in an HIV cohort in Botswana. *Pharm. J.* **2018**, *18*, 678–688.

53. Dodgen, T.M.; Eloff, A.; Mataboge, C.; Roos, L.J.; van Staden, W.C.; Pepper, M.S. Risperidone-associated adverse drug reactions and CYP2D6 polymorphisms in a South African cohort. *Appl. Transl. Genom.* **2015**, *5*, 40–46. [CrossRef] [PubMed]
54. Chaudhry, M.; Alessandrini, M.; Rademan, J.; Dodgen, T.M.; Steffens, F.E.; van Zyl, D.G.; Gaedigk, A.; Pepper, M.S. Impact of CYP2D6 genotype on amitriptyline efficacy for the treatment of diabetic peripheral neuropathy: A pilot study. *Pharmacogenomics* **2017**, *18*, 433–443. [CrossRef]
55. Shrif, N.E.; Won, H.H.; Lee, S.T.; Park, J.H.; Kim, K.K.; Kim, M.J.; Kim, S.; Lee, S.Y.; Ki, C.S.; Osman, I.M.; et al. Evaluation of the effects of VKORC1 polymorphisms and haplotypes, CYP2C9 genotypes, and clinical factors on warfarin response in Sudanese patients. *Eur. J. Clin. Pharmacol.* **2011**, *67*, 1119–1130. [CrossRef]
56. Mitchell, C.; Gregersen, N.; Krause, A. Novel CYP2C9 and VKORC1 gene variants associated with warfarin dosage variability in the South African black population. *Pharmacogenomics* **2011**, *12*, 953–963. [CrossRef]
57. Kudzi, W.A.S.; Dzudzor, B.; Olayemi, E.; Nartey, E.T.; Asmah, R.H. Genetic polymorphisms of patients on stable warfarin maintenance therapy in a Ghanaian population. *BMC Res. Notes* **2019**, *9*, 507. [CrossRef]
58. Maigetter, K.; Pollock, A.M.; Kadam, A.; Ward, K.; Weiss, M.G. Pharmacovigilance in India, Uganda and South Africa with reference to WHO's minimum requirements. *Int. J. Health Policy Manag.* **2015**, *4*, 295–305. [CrossRef]
59. Hershman, D.; McBride, R.; Jacobson, J.S.; Lamerato, L.; Roberts, K.; Grann, V.R.; Neugut, A.I. Racial disparities in treatment and survival among women with early-stage breast cancer. *J. Clin. Oncol.* **2005**, *23*, 6639–6646. [CrossRef] [PubMed]
60. Ramamoorthy, A.; Pacanowski, M.A.; Bull, J.; Zhang, L. Racial/ethnic differences in drug disposition and response: Review of recently approved drugs. *Clin. Pharmacol. Ther.* **2015**, *97*, 263–273. [CrossRef] [PubMed]
61. Gaedigk, A.; Sangkuhl, K.; Whirl-Carrillo, M.; Klein, T.; Leeder, J.S. Prediction of CYP2D6 phenotype from genotype across world populations. *Genet. Med.* **2017**, *19*, 69–76. [CrossRef] [PubMed]
62. Thummel, K.E.; Lin, Y.S. Sources of interindividual variability. *Methods Mol. Biol.* **2014**, *1113*, 363–415.
63. Wang, S.; Pitt, J.J.; Zheng, Y.; Yoshimatsu, T.F.; Gao, G.; Sanni, A.; Oluwasola, O.; Ajani, M.; Fitzgerald, D.; Odetunde, A.; et al. Germline variants and somatic mutation signatures of breast cancer across populations of African and European ancestry in the US and Nigeria. *Int. J. Cancer* **2019**, *145*, 3321–3333. [CrossRef]
64. Shah, R.R.; Smith, R.L. Inflammation-induced phenoconversion of polymorphic drug metabolizing enzymes: Hypothesis with implications for personalized medicine. *Drug Metab. Dispos.* **2015**, *43*, 400–410. [CrossRef]
65. Kiss, A.F.; Vasko, D.; Deri, M.T.; Toth, K.; Monostory, K. Combination of CYP2C19 genotype with non-genetic factors evoking phenoconversion improves phenotype prediction. *Pharmacol. Rep.* **2018**, *70*, 525–532. [CrossRef]
66. Bedada, W.; de Andres, F.; Engidawork, E.; Hussein, J.; LLerena, A.; Aklillu, E. Effects of Khat (Catha edulis) use on catalytic activities of major drug-metabolizing cytochrome P450 enzymes and implication of pharmacogenetic variations. *Sci. Rep.* **2018**, *8*, 12726. [CrossRef]
67. Bousman, C.A.; Jaksa, P.; Pantelis, C. Systematic evaluation of commercial pharmacogenetic testing in psychiatry: A focus on CYP2D6 and CYP2C19 allele coverage and results reporting. *Pharm. Genom.* **2017**, *27*, 387–393. [CrossRef]
68. Nofziger, C.; Paulmichl, M. Accurately genotyping CYP2D6: Not for the faint of heart. *Pharmacogenomics* **2018**, *19*, 999–1002. [CrossRef]
69. Tshabalala, S.; Choudhury, A.; Beeton-Kempen, N.; Martinson, N.; Ramsay, M.; Mancama, D. Targeted ultra-deep sequencing of a South African Bantu-speaking cohort to comprehensively map and characterize common and novel variants in 65 pharmacologically-related genes. *Pharm. Genom.* **2019**, *29*, 167–178. [CrossRef] [PubMed]
70. Rusk, N. Pan-African genome. *Nat. Methods* **2019**, *16*, 143. [CrossRef] [PubMed]
71. Choudhury, A.; Ramsay, M.; Hazelhurst, S.; Aron, S.; Bardien, S.; Botha, G.; Chimusa, E.R.; Christoffels, A.; Gamieldien, J.; Sefid-Dashti, M.J.; et al. Whole-genome sequencing for an enhanced understanding of genetic variation among South Africans. *Nat. Commun.* **2017**, *8*, 2062. [CrossRef] [PubMed]
72. Gurdasani, D.; Carstensen, T.; Tekola-Ayele, F.; Pagani, L.; Tachmazidou, I.; Hatzikotoulas, K.; Karthikeyan, S.; Iles, L.; Pollard, M.O.; Choudhury, A.; et al. The African Genome Variation Project shapes medical genetics in Africa. *Nature* **2015**, *517*, 327–332. [CrossRef]
73. MalariaGEN. Available online: https://www.malariagen.net/ (accessed on 23 July 2019).

74. Zhong, A.; Darren, B.; Loiseau, B.; He, L.Q.B.; Chang, T.; Hill, J.; Dimaras, H. Ethical, social, and cultural issues related to clinical genetic testing and counseling in low- and middle-income countries: A systematic review. *Genet. Med.* **2018**. [CrossRef]
75. Carroll, J.C.; Rideout, A.L.; Wilson, B.J.; Allanson, J.M.; Blaine, S.M.; Esplen, M.J.; Farrell, S.A.; Graham, G.E.; MacKenzie, J.; Meschino, W.; et al. Genetic education for primary care providers: Improving attitudes, knowledge, and confidence. *Can. Fam. Physician* **2009**, *55*, e92–e99.
76. Jegede, A.S. Culture and genetic screening in Africa. *Dev. World Bioeth.* **2009**, *9*, 128–137. [CrossRef]
77. Nembaware, V.; Johnston, K.; Diallo, A.A.; Kotze, M.J.; Matimba, A.; Moodley, K.; Tangwa, G.B.; Torrorey-Sawe, R.; Tiffin, N. A framework for tiered informed consent for health genomic research in Africa. *Nat. Genet.* **2019**, *51*, 1566–1571. [CrossRef]
78. De Vries, J.; Munung, S.N.; Matimba, A.; McCurdy, S.; Ouwe Missi Oukem-Boyer, O.; Staunton, C.; Yakubu, A.; Tindana, P.; Consortium, H.A. Regulation of genomic and biobanking research in Africa: A content analysis of ethics guidelines, policies and procedures from 22 African countries. *BMC Med. Ethics* **2017**, *18*, 8. [CrossRef]
79. Academy of Science of South Africa (ASSAf). Available online: http://hdl.handle.net/20.500.11911/106 (accessed on 25 July 2020).

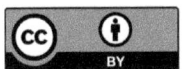

© 2020 by the authors. Licensee MDPI, Basel, Switzerland. This article is an open access article distributed under the terms and conditions of the Creative Commons Attribution (CC BY) license (http://creativecommons.org/licenses/by/4.0/).

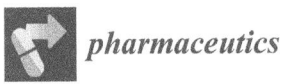

Article

Linking Pharmacogenomic Information on Drug Safety and Efficacy with Ethnic Minority Populations

Dan Li [1], April Hui Xie [1,2], Zhichao Liu [1], Dongying Li [1], Baitang Ning [1], Shraddha Thakkar [1,3], Weida Tong [1] and Joshua Xu [1,*]

1. Division of Bioinformatics and Biostatistics, National Center for Toxicological Research, U.S. Food and Drug Administration, Jefferson, AR 72079, USA; dan.li@fda.hhs.gov (D.L.); april.xie@gmail.com (A.H.X.); zhichao.liu@fda.hhs.gov (Z.L.); Dongying.Li@fda.hhs.gov (D.L.); Baitang.Ning@fda.hhs.gov (B.N.); Shraddha.Thakkar@fda.hhs.gov (S.T.); Weida.Tong@fda.hhs.gov (W.T.)
2. School of Pharmacy, Virginia Commonwealth University, Richmond, VA 23298, USA
3. Office of Computational Sciences, Office of Translational Sciences, Center for Drug Evaluation and Research, U.S. Food and Drug Administration, Silver Spring, MD 20993, USA
* Correspondence: Joshua.xu@fda.hhs.gov

Received: 8 October 2020; Accepted: 23 October 2020; Published: 25 October 2020

Abstract: Numerous prescription drugs' labeling contains pharmacogenomic (PGx) information to aid health providers and patients in the safe and effective use of drugs. However, clinical studies for such PGx biomarkers and related drug doses are generally not conducted in diverse ethnic populations. Thus, it is urgently important to incorporate PGx information with genetic characteristics of racial and ethnic minority populations and utilize it to promote minority health. In this project a bioinformatics approach was developed to enhance the collection of PGx information related to ethnic minorities to pave the way toward understanding the population-wide utility of PGx information. To address this challenge, we first gathered PGx information from drug labels. Second, we extracted data on the allele frequency information of genetic variants in ethnic minority groups from public resources. Then, we collected published research articles on PGx biomarkers and related drugs for reference. Finally, the data were integrated and formatted to build a new PGx database containing information on known drugs and biomarkers for ethnic minority groups. This database provides scientific information needed to evaluate available PGx information to enhance drug dose selection and drug safety for ethnic minority populations.

Keywords: pharmacogenomic; minority; data collection; drug; biomarker

1. Introduction

Pharmacogenomic (PGx) information can be utilized to improve the medical decision-making process and avoid severe adverse drug reactions. Drug labeling with PGx information can be used to promote drug safety and drug efficacy. In general, PGx studies include evaluation of genetic or genomic variations that serve as predictive PGx biomarkers to distinguish between responders and non-responders to specific drugs [1]. Knowing whether a patient carries a specific genetic variation or has altered expression levels of genes can help prescribers to individualize drug therapy, mitigate the chance of adverse events, and optimize the effectiveness of the drug with a proper dose [2–5]. Tools such as genotyping technologies and databases have been developed to incorporate the genetic information of patients into routine clinical practice to carefully identify and prescribe a drug to the appropriate ethnic group of patients [6,7]. However, a genetic variant associated with drug responses may show a widely diverse prevalence among populations, affecting drug efficiency and drug safety for different ethnic groups. Diverse ethnicities usually harbor variability in drug dose requirements, and genotyping of clinically relevant PGx biomarkers has been advocated to guide drug dosing/indication optimization for different patient populations [8]. Therefore, a reliable collection of PGx information with biomarkers/drugs and their behaviors in various minority groups is needed to provide guidance for effective and safe medication to treat ethnic minority populations. Unfortunately, clinical studies to characterize PGx biomarkers generally have not been conducted for diverse ethnic populations. Although some studies have considered the allele frequencies of genetic variants in different ethnic groups and have utilized genotype-guided algorithms for dose selection in the prescription of some drugs such as warfarin, acenocoumarol, and phencopromon to benefit certain ethnic populations [9,10], it remains challenging to improve the health of such groups with the current level of PGx information. Further systematic collection and evaluation of PGx biomarkers and related drugs for diverse ethnic groups is needed.

In this manuscript we describe the development and implementation of a bioinformatics workflow aimed to enhance the collection and utilization of PGx information related to ethnic minority groups (Figure 1). Labeling of a number of drugs and biologics approved by the United States Food and Drug Administration (FDA) include PGx information [11,12]; we utilized the information in the FDA Table of Pharmacogenomic Biomarkers in Drug Labeling (TPGxBMDL) from the FDA website (https://www.fda.gov/drugs/science-and-research-drugs/table-pharmacogenomic-biomarkers-drug-labeling). We also searched for PGx information containing relationships between drugs and their associated genetic variants from public resources such as DrugBank [13], Pharmacogenomics Knowledge Base (PharmGKB) [14], Clinical Interpretation of Variants in Cancer (CIViC) [15], and Gene Drug Knowledge Database (GDKD) [16]. Then, we filtered the collected data to focus on single nucleotide polymorphisms (SNPs) in the reported biomarkers that interact with non-oncology drugs. The allele frequency (AF) information of SNPs for different ethnicities were collected from the Allele Frequency Aggregator (ALFA) project [17], which provides a great opportunity to collect population-specific information for genetic variants. In total, allele frequency information of 67 SNPs associated with specific drug–biomarker pairs was collected. PGx drug and biomarker pairs were further explored in the PubMed database, and related articles with their PubMed IDs (PMIDs) were collected. Finally, all data were integrated into a database to provide researchers with information regarding drugs, paired PGx biomarkers, and associated AFs of SNPs for minority ethnic groups and to adjust drug doses and indications during drug development and drug application.

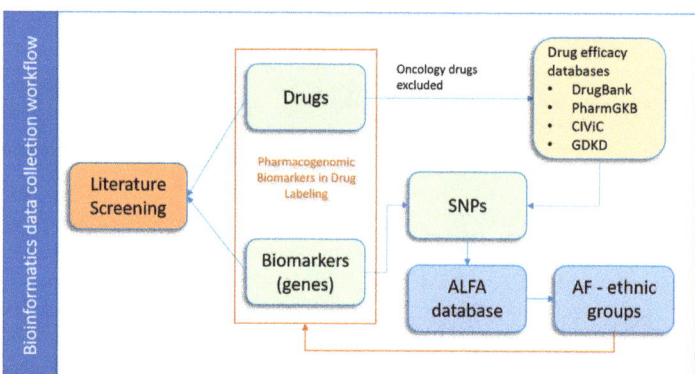

Figure 1. Overall data collection workflow. The paired PGx biomarkers and drugs were first downloaded from TPGxBMDL. The oncology drugs were excluded based on the therapeutic area information within TPGxBMDL. Then, SNPs that potentially interacted with the remaining drugs were collected from public drug efficacy databases. These SNPs thus linked the drugs and the PGx biomarkers (genes) in which they are located. Next, the AF information of the SNPs across ethnic groups were collected from the ALFA database. Additionally, PubMed literatures were searched for potential information on ethnic minority groups regarding the PGx biomarker and drug pairs.

2. Methods

2.1. Data Collection and Processing

The therapeutic area for each drug along with its associated pharmacogenomic biomarkers was archived from TPGxBMDL. Drugs in the oncology therapeutic area were excluded from this study. Remaining non-oncology drugs were searched in four drug databases (DrugBank, PharmGKB, CIViC, and GDKD) to obtain drug–SNP interactions. We then normalized results by removing redundant information and built unique drug variant–gene interaction relationships.

The SNP allele frequency data was downloaded from ALFA. Only six ethnicities were investigated in this study due to an insufficient number of subjects from other ethnic groups (Table S1). We focused on nonsynonymous SNPs in the coding region, and a further SNP filter was applied to restrict the SNPs to NSF, NSM, and NSN only. NSF, NSM, and NSN are explained below. Annotation for the SNPs was downloaded from the Single Nucleotide Polymorphism Database (dbSNP) developed and hosted by the National Center for Biotechnology Information (NCBI) (dbSNP human build 154: https://ftp.ncbi.nih.gov/snp/archive/b154/VCF/). Allele frequency was calculated as alternative allele counts divided by total allele counts.

- NSF: Nonsynonymous frameshift. A coding region variation where one allele in the set changes all downstream amino acids.
- NSM: Nonsynonymous missense. A coding region variation where one allele in the set changes a protein peptide.
- NSN: Nonsynonymous nonsense. A coding region variation where one allele in the set changes to a stop codon, i.e., a termination codon.

2.2. Allele Frequency Thresholds Based on the European Population

The allele frequency of a SNP in the European group (AF_e) was used as the baseline for the evaluation of the SNP's allele frequencies among other ethnicities. A threshold was configured to identify the substantial changes in SNP allele frequency between the European group and another group. Specifically, when $AF_e < 0.05$ the threshold is $AF_e + 0.05$, which indicates, if the SNP AF in another group is greater than AF_e by 0.05, the change is considered substantial. When $AF_e \geq 0.4$, the threshold was $AF_e \pm 0.2$. For higher AF_e values, 0.2 was high enough to be considered substantially different between ethnic groups.

For $0.05 < AF_e < 0.4$, we fitted a formula that restricted the AF threshold depending on AF_e. The threshold increased along with the AF_e and had a maximum value of 0.2.

$$AF_{Threshold} = AF_e \pm AF_{diff}$$

$$AF_{diff} = \frac{0.4}{(1 + 0.4/(AF_e + 0.01))}$$

2.3. Literature Screening Process

We used the R package easyPubMed [18] to search and download abstracts of interest from PubMed. We tracked each article published after the year 2000 that contained a given drug name and then downloaded the Year, PMID, ArticleTitle, and AbstractText. Next, abstracts containing paired biomarkers associated with a drug were retained. Finally, to narrow the PubMed articles down to ethnic minority-associated studies, we selected nine secondary keywords (African, Asian, Latin, European, Chinese, American, pharmacogenomic, metabolizer, minority, metabolism, dose, hypersensitivity, adverse reaction) to compile the final literature candidates. PMIDs were then listed for each of the drugs.

3. Results

3.1. Data Collection by Drugs

The 2 February 2020 version of TPGxBMDL was downloaded from https://www.fda.gov/drugs/science-and-research-drugs/table-pharmacogenomic-biomarkers-drug-labeling. Therapeutic products from Drugs@FDA with drug labels containing PGx information are listed in this table. In total, 404 PGx drug–biomarker pairs were constructed with 283 unique drugs and 86 predetermined biomarkers (genes), excluding three fusion genes (PML-RARA, BCR-ABL1, and FIP1L1-PDGFRA). The therapeutic area and labeling sections of a given drug were included as well. As shown in Figure 2a, most of these drugs are in the therapeutic areas of Oncology (94), Psychiatry (34), and Infectious Diseases (31). In general, the biomarkers for oncology drugs are not related to germline variants. In most cases somatic mutations of cancer patients are investigated to select oncology drugs guided by the somatic mutation biomarkers. Therefore, we excluded the oncology drugs from our study to focus on other drugs to which ethnic minority populations may show a varied response.

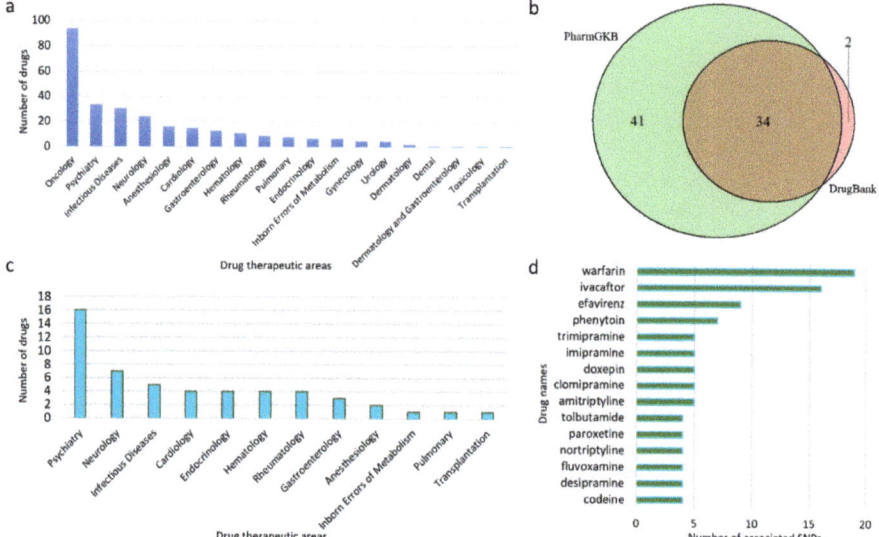

Figure 2. Summary of data collection by drugs. (**a**) The distribution of all drugs with PGx information in drug labels across therapeutic areas. (**b**) The numbers of non-oncology drugs with PGx information that were from PharmGKB and DrugBank. PharmGKB and DrugBank shared a great portion of drugs from our selection. (**c**) The distribution of therapeutic areas for non-oncology drugs with information on SNP allele frequency in six ethnic groups. (**d**) Top drugs that interact with the greatest number of SNPs with reported allele frequency information.

To better present PGx information for various ethnic populations, we collected and investigated the allele frequency distribution of genetic variants associated with drugs and related genes across ethnic groups. We focused on six groups: African, South Asian, African American, Latin American, European, and Other, excluding groups in which studies contained fewer than 400 subjects per group (Table S1). Drugs in FDA labels were searched and data on clinically actionable drug–gene interaction were collected from drug knowledge databases. Seventy-seven non-oncology drugs listed in TPGxBMDL were found in PharmGKB (75 drugs) and DrugBank (36 drugs). Most (34 of 36) of the drugs found in DrugBank were also included in PharmGKB (Figure 2b).

These 77 drugs were associated with 839 SNPs, as reported by PharmGKB and DrugBank. However, only 168 of these SNPs are located in 19 genes which are also listed as PGx biomarkers in TPGxBMDL. Allele frequency data for different ethnicities were then collected from the ALFA project, which contains approximately 447 million SNPs from more than 100,000 subjects of different ethnicities according to the newly released version 20200227123210. The ALFA dataset is updated quarterly with 100,000–200,000 new subjects of genotype and phenotype data, serving as a comprehensive and relevant reference [17]. Nonsynonymous SNPs that cause frameshift, missense, or nonsense, with ethnicity-specific allele frequency information were further selected (see Methods for details). As a result, only 67 SNPs with allele frequency demographic information were collected, which were related to 148 drug–SNP pairs made from 42 non-oncology drugs and 16 (out of 86) PGx biomarkers.

Figure 2c shows the therapeutic area distribution of these 42 drugs with data on related SNP allele frequencies. Some of the drugs interact with multiple SNPs. For example, warfarin interacts with 19 SNPs (Figure 2d). As warfarin is the most commonly prescribed oral anticoagulant used to treat thromboembolic disease, its narrow therapeutic index requires close attention to the individual variability in patient response. Studies have shown the importance of predicting or optimizing dose requirements among different ethnicities [9,19,20].

After removing rare SNPs (sum $AF < 0.01$), allele frequencies of the remaining 33 SNPs were evaluated. A two-way classification of allele frequencies was applied to group ethnicities and SNPs together (Figure 3a). Even though African and African American ethnicities were listed as two independent groups by the ALFA project, their allele frequencies for the SNPs were similar to each other and were, thus, grouped together. Meanwhile, the Other group was classified together with the European group, indicating this group may be a population or a mixed population genetically close to the European group. Allele frequencies of these SNPs for South Asian and Latin American groups were different from the other four groups, highlighting the genotype variability among diverse ethnic groups. It is apparent that rs1135840 exhibits high allele frequencies close to 0.6 in the African group and the other three groups compared to below 0.2 in the South Asian and Latin American groups. Located in CYP2D6, this SNP is associated with clozapine that is a widely used drug for schizophrenia treatment. Some other SNPs such as rs8103142 showed the highest allele frequency in the South Asian group (Figure 3a), indicating that South Asian and Latin American groups may require dose justification for certain drugs in comparison to other ethnic populations.

SNP allele frequencies were usually different from one ethnic group to another. Taking the European group that has a large number of subjects as the baseline, we compared the allele frequency of each SNP across ethnic groups (Figure 3b). Thresholds for substantial allele frequency difference were chosen according to the corresponding baseline values in the European group (see Methods for details). Any allele frequency value above or below the thresholds is marked in purple on the plot. Because African and African American groups were genetically close, the African group was not assessed in Figure 3b. As a result, 4, 0, 5, and 8 SNPs were identified with considerably different allele frequencies in the African American, Other, South Asian, and Latin American groups, respectively. Given that a total of 33 SNPs was assessed, 24.2% (8/33) of them exhibited substantially different allele frequencies in the Latin American group than in the European group. Moreover, 79% of these SNPs (26 of 33) showed a coefficient of variation over 0.5 (Figure 3c), indicating considerable diversity in allele frequency among ethnic groups, which health care providers should regard as significant for determination of patient treatment.

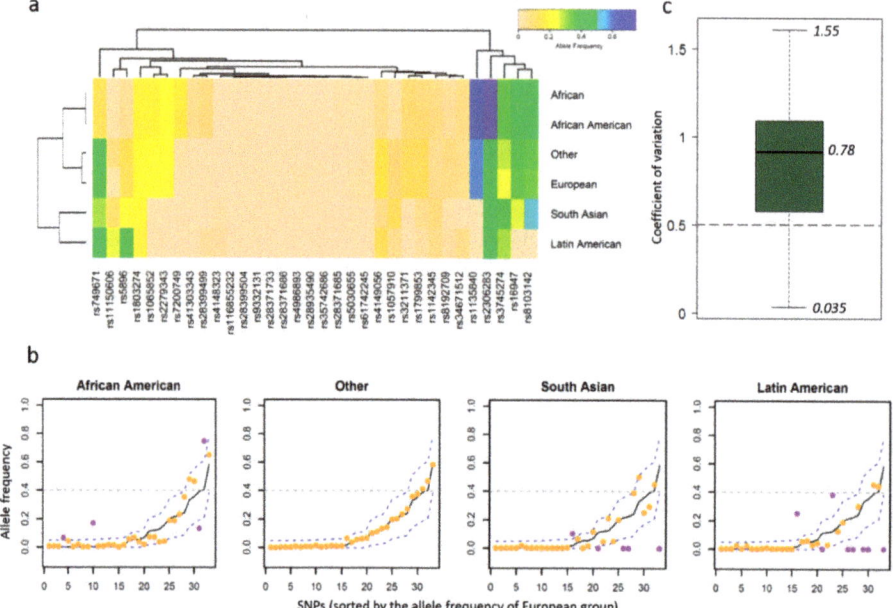

Figure 3. Analysis of the SNP allele frequency in diverse ethnic groups. (**a**) The heatmap of allele frequencies across ethnic groups (rows) and SNPs (columns). A two-way classification was performed on the allele frequency matrix. (**b**) The allele frequencies of the other four groups were plotted with those of the European population as baseline (middle black line). Any value beyond the thresholds (blue dash lines) is marked in purple, highlighting the substantial variability between ethnic groups. (**c**) The coefficient of variation distribution of SNP allele frequencies in six groups. The median coefficient of variation was 0.78, and 26 of 33 SNPs were with CVs over 0.5.

3.2. PGx Information of Biomarkers

According to the information provided in TPGxBMDL, 52 biomarkers interacted with non-oncology drugs. In 23 of these biomarkers we then identified 231 and 21 SNPs from PharmGKB and DrugBank, respectively. Fifteen SNPs were included in both resources, leaving 29 PGx biomarkers. These results suggest that the functions of SNPs in those 29 remaining PGx biomarkers may interact with non-oncology drugs.

Some genes, especially those from the Cytochrome P450 family, contained more drug-related SNPs than others, which have attracted more attention for PGx research (Figure 4a). However, when counting drugs that interact with these SNPs, many of them were not included in TPGxBMDL (Figure 4b), suggesting that the potential PGx information for these drugs has not been included in drug labels. For example, there are only 12 SNPs in the gene CYP2D6 (Figure 4a) that is one of the most important enzymes for the metabolism of xenobiotics. These 12 SNPs were found to be associated with 46 different drugs reported by PharmGKB and DrugBank, and only 16 (Figure 4b) were paired with CYP2D6 according to TPGxBMDL.

Next, we collected SNPs with allele frequency data in different ethnic groups reported by the current version of the ALFA database. As a result, 62 SNPs with allele frequencies in 15 PGx biomarkers were found to be associated with the non-oncology drugs in TPGxBMDL (Figure S1). Results showed that SNP information for many drugs is not available for diverse populations. Some biomarkers were not studied extensively, and inter-ethnicity variability was not addressed, which was likely due to a lack of enrollment of ethnic minorities in these clinical studies.

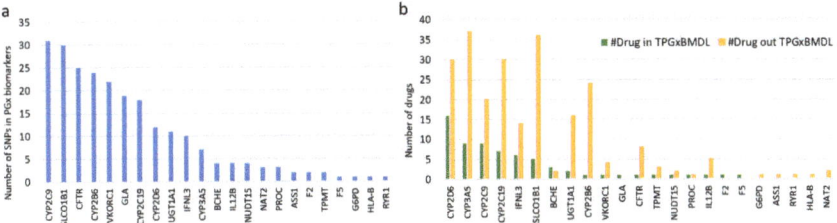

Figure 4. Numbers of SNPs and drugs related to biomarkers in TPGxBMDL. (**a**) The number of SNPs reported by public databases that are contained by biomarkers associated with drugs. (**b**) The number of drugs associated with SNPs in the biomarkers. Green bars represent the number of drugs listed in TPGxBMDL.

3.3. Literature Screening to Provide PGx PubMed IDs

We queried the drugs in labeling data to collect information related to ethnicity. Ethnicity-specific information such as metabolizer status (poor metabolizer, intermediate metabolizer, and ultrarapid metabolizer) for 40 drugs were identified in South Asian and African American ethnic groups; only 20 of these drugs were found to be associated with SNPs from the ALFA project, suggesting that more ethnicity-involved pharmacogenomics studies are needed for a larger number of drugs.

To further interpret the PGx data for diverse ethnicities and to provide additional PGx information for ethnic minorities, we searched PubMed to identify potential articles related to PGx in ethnic populations. Specifically, we searched and downloaded abstracts from studies that focused on drugs in TPGxBMDL. If an abstract contained a paired biomarker with a given drug and at least one of the keywords focused on ethnic groups (see Methods for details), the PMID of the abstract was added to the database as a potentially relevant article. Currently, 1329 articles covering 120 unique PGx drug–biomarker pairs have been identified and stored in the database (Figure S2, Methods).

Abacavir, a nucleoside analog that works as a reverse transcriptase inhibitor, is widely used to treat HIV infection. Per our screening, the PGx pair abacavir/HLA-B was mentioned in a great number of articles (19) that contained at least one keyword in the abstracts. However, no SNP with allele frequency information was reported by the ALFA project that links abacavir and HLA-B. We then reviewed the full articles for additional information on the diversity of ethnic samples involved in the studies. For example, the article PMID 29921043 reported an association between abacavir and biomarker HLA-B*57:01, where the authors demonstrated an ethnicity-specific association between the SNP and carbamazepine hypersensitivity via a comparison of risks among different ethnic populations of Asians in Hong Kong, Thailand, Malaysia, India, Korea, and Japan [21]. The PMIDs linked to articles that contain potential drugs and associated risk alleles with ethnicity-specific information were also stored in the database. The literature research potentially provided additional PGx information relevant to ethnic minorities. Unfortunately, most of these studies used a small number of subjects from ethnic minority populations, again indicating the lack of clinical PGx studies with sufficient numbers of ethnic minority subjects.

3.4. Database Development

Finally, using Microsoft Access, we developed a database of PGx information related to ethnic minorities. The main data table was built using each drug as a key basis of information. Each drug was listed in the first column, followed by columns listing SNPs and drug-interacting biomarkers. Allele frequencies of SNPs in six ethnic groups and in the total population were also listed, along with therapeutic area, and public databases that provided resources of drug SNP interaction information. Hyperlinks to public databases for each individual drug were also provided in the data table. Literature screening results were provided in a separate data table where related PMIDs were listed for each drug. The Access database is published as Supplementary File 1 and future updated versions will be shared upon request.

4. Discussion

We extracted PGx information from the ALFA database and four pharmacological databases. Although other public resources, such as 1000 Genomes [22] and gnomAD [23], could be used to acquire information on allele frequencies, the ALFA database contains SNP information for more ethnicities, and the SNP information in the ALFA database was derived from a larger sample size. Meanwhile, the ALFA database is evolving and SNP information from over 100,000 subjects is added quarterly. In our opinion, using the ALFA database will keep the information collection consistent and will benefit our database with continuous updates.

To demonstrate the utility of our database, here, we briefly describe the following case study. SNP rs3892097 *(CYP2D6*4)* is one of the most common variant alleles (allele frequency of 20%) in Caucasian populations [24]. It is a common nonfunctional allele leading to poor drug metabolism, accounting for over 75% of poor metabolizer patients [25]. We found seven antidepressant drugs that were impacted by this SNP from Clinvar, which is a public archive that aggregates information about genomic variation and its relationship to human health [26]: Amitriptyline, clomipramine, trimipramine, nortriptyline, imipramine, desipramine, and doxepin [27]. All drugs were included in TPGxBMDL. However, only nortriptyline and desipramine have polymorphism information in their drug labels. Since the ALFA project currently reports few and biased samples for this SNP among minority groups (10,434 of 11,174 were in the European and Other groups), we instead used gnomAD data that have slightly different ethnic groups than ALFA and contains 178,714 samples to compare the allele frequency of rs3892097 among various population groups: European—0.176, African—0.076, East Asian—0.0039, Latin American—0.114, and Other—0.151. It is estimated in drug labels that approximately 7–10% of Caucasians were poor metabolizers of P450 2D6 drugs. In light of the frequencies seen with this SNP, there is possibly an underestimation of poor metabolizer prevalence in the labeling among the European group. Substantially lower allele frequencies were found in African and South Asian populations compared to European populations, highlighting inter-population variability and the need for more data to confirm allele frequencies among the East Asian population. Our results indicate that more research is needed to enhance the collection of PGx information to further improve our understanding and practice of drug safety and efficacy for minorities.

Through our literature research we found over 40 PGx studies that tested non-oncology drugs for diverse ethnicities. Only 15 of these studies enrolled more than 100 patients, and numbers of ethnic minority patients were usually limited, accounting for about 5–20% of total participants. Literature research resulted in a small increase in the number of drugs with SNP information for ethnic minorities. Apparently, there is a lack of clinical studies on PGx biomarkers for these minority groups. Further, details of the analytical validation of methods used to detect and measure the biomarkers may not be available. Therefore, it is challenging to integrate all findings to further enhance our understanding of PGx information for ethnic minority groups.

5. Conclusions

We report here the development of a PGx knowledge database focusing on drugs and biomarkers in FDA drug labels to provide essential PGx information related to ethnic minorities. Such information is urgently needed for the promotion of drug safety and efficacy for diverse ethnic groups. Information on allele frequencies of SNPs related to drugs and PGx biomarkers in different ethnic populations provided an informative resource for improved clinical practice, by which appropriate drug selection and dose optimization can be conducted for diverse patient groups. By comparing multiple populations with the European population, which represents the largest sample size in the ALFA project, several SNPs were identified to exhibit distinct allele frequencies for other ethnicities, suggesting that closer attention should be paid when the same drug is prescribed for different ethnicities in the practice of personalized treatment. A literature research focusing on ethnic minority groups provided additional PGx information and highlighted the lack of studies on PGx biomarkers for ethnic minorities. The database developed in this study provides scientific support for drug reviewers and researchers to assess available PGx information for different ethnicities, which could promote the practice of personalized medicine in ethnic minority groups.

Supplementary Materials: The following are available online at http://www.mdpi.com/1999-4923/12/11/1021/s1. Figure S1: The number of SNPs in each biomarker that were associated with drugs in TPGxBMDL. Figure S2: The number of PubMed articles mentioning drug–biomarker pairs and ethnic group keywords in their abstracts. In total, 94 drug–biomarker pairs covered by 463 articles were obtained and only the pairs with more than 10 articles are shown here. Table S1: Ethnic group and subject information of the ALFA project. Supplementary File 1: The Microsoft Access database of PGx information related to ethnic minorities.

Author Contributions: Conceptualization, J.X., Z.L. and W.T.; methodology, D.L. (Dan Li), A.H.X. and J.X.; software, D.L. (Dan Li) and A.H.X.; validation, D.L. (Dongying Li), S.T., B.N. and Z.L.; formal analysis, D.L. (Dan Li) and J.X.; writing—original draft preparation, D.L. (Dan Li) and J.X.; writing—review and editing, D.L. (Dongying Li), S.T., B.N. and Z.L.; supervision, J.X.; project administration, J.X. and W.T. All authors have read and agreed to the published version of the manuscript.

Funding: This research received no external funding.

Acknowledgments: This project was partially funded by the FDA Office of Minority Health & Health Equity. April Hui Xie is grateful to the FDA's National Center for Toxicological Research (NCTR) for the financial support provided through the Summer Student Research Program administered by the Oak Ridge Institute for Science and Education (ORISE) through an interagency agreement between the U.S. Department of Energy (DOE) and the FDA.

Conflicts of Interest: The authors declare no conflict of interest.

Disclaimer: The views presented in this article do not necessarily reflect those of the U.S. Food and Drug Administration. Any mention of commercial products is for clarification and is not intended as an endorsement.

References

1. Karczewski, J.K.; Daneshjou, R.; Altman, R.B. Pharmacogenomics. *PLoS Comput. Biol.* **2012**, *8*, e1002817. [CrossRef] [PubMed]
2. Carr, D.F.; Alfirevic, A.; Pirmohamed, M. Pharmacogenomics: Current state-of-the-art. *Genes* **2014**, *5*, 430–443. [CrossRef] [PubMed]
3. Lee, J.W.; Aminkeng, F.; Bhavsar, A.P.; Shaw, K.; Carleton, B.C.; Hayden, M.R.; Ross, C.J.D. The emerging era of pharmacogenomics: Current successes, future potential, and challenges. *Clin. Genet.* **2014**, *86*, 21–28. [CrossRef] [PubMed]
4. Daly, A.K. Pharmacogenomics of adverse drug reactions. *Genom. Med.* **2013**, *5*, 5. [CrossRef] [PubMed]
5. Weng, L.; Zhang, L.; Peng, Y.; Huang, R.S. Pharmacogenetics and pharmacogenomics: A bridge to individualized cancer therapy. *Pharmacogenomics* **2013**, *14*, 315–324. [CrossRef] [PubMed]
6. Hicks, J.K.; Stowe, D.; Willner, M.A.; Wai, M.; Daly, T.; Gordon, S.M.; Moss, T. Implementation of clinical pharmacogenomics within a large health system: From electronic health record decision support to consultation services. *Pharmacother. J. Hum. Pharmacol. Drug Ther.* **2016**, *36*, 940–948. [CrossRef]
7. Bell, G.C.; Crews, K.R.; Wilkinson, M.R.; Haidar, C.E.; Hicks, J.K.; Baker, D.K.; Freimuth, R.R. Development and use of active clinical decision support for preemptive pharmacogenomics. *J. Am. Med. Inform. Assn.* **2014**, *21*, e93–e99. [CrossRef]
8. Van der Wouden, C.H.; Cambon-Thomsen, A.; Cecchin, E.; Cheung, K.C.; Dávila-Fajardo, C.L.; Deneer, V.H.; Kriek, M. Implementing pharmacogenomics in Europe: Design and implementation strategy of the ubiquitous pharmacogenomics consortium. *Clin. Pharmacol. Ther.* **2017**, *101*, 341–358. [CrossRef]
9. Kaye, J.B.; Veenstra, D.L. Warfarin pharmacogenomics in diverse populations. *Pharmacother. J. Hum. Pharmacol. Drug Ther.* **2017**, *37*, 1150–1163. [CrossRef]
10. Verhoef TIRagia, G.; de Boer, A.; Barallon, R.; Kolovou, G.; Kolovou, V.; Redekop, W.K. A randomized trial of genotype-guided dosing of acenocoumarol and phenprocoumon. *N. Engl. J. Med.* **2013**, *369*, 2304–2312. [CrossRef]

11. Frueh, F.W.; Amur, S.; Mummaneni, P.; Epstein, R.S.; Aubert, R.E.; DeLuca, T.M.; Lesko, L.J. Pharmacogenomic biomarker information in drug labels approved by the United States food and drug administration: Prevalence of related drug use. *Pharmacother. J. Hum. Pharmacol. Drug Ther.* **2008**, *28*, 992–998. [CrossRef] [PubMed]
12. Tutton, R. Pharmacogenomic biomarkers in drug labels: What do they tell us? *Pharmacogenomics* **2014**, *15*, 297–304. [CrossRef] [PubMed]
13. Wishart, D.S.; Feunang, Y.D.; Guo, A.C.; Lo, E.J.; Marcu, A.; Grant, J.R.; Assempour, N. DrugBank 5.0: A major update to the DrugBank database for 2018. *Nucleic Acids Res.* **2018**, *46*, D1074–D1082. [CrossRef] [PubMed]
14. Whirl-Carrillo MMcDonagh, E.M.; Hebert, J.M.; Gong, L.; Sangkuhl, K.; Thorn, C.F.; Klein, T.E. Pharmacogenomics knowledge for personalized medicine. *Clin. Pharmacol. Ther.* **2012**, *92*, 414–417. [CrossRef]
15. Griffith, M.; Spies, N.C.; Krysiak, K.; McMichael, J.F.; Coffman, A.C.; Danos, A.M.; Barnell, E.K. CIViC is a community knowledgebase for expert crowdsourcing the clinical interpretation of variants in cancer. *Nat. Genet.* **2017**, *49*, 170–174. [CrossRef]
16. Dienstmann, R.; Jang, I.S.; Bot, B.; Friend, S.; Guinney, J. Database of genomic biomarkers for cancer drugs and clinical targetability in solid tumors. *Cancer Discov.* **2015**, *5*, 118–123. [CrossRef]
17. Phan, L.; Jin, Y.; Zhang, H.; Qiang, W.; Shekhtman, E.; Shao, D.; Kimura, M. ALFA: Allele Frequency Aggregator. National Center for Biotechnology Information, US National Library of Medicine. Available online: www.ncbi.nlm.nih.gov/snp/docs/gsr/alfa/ (accessed on 10 March 2020).
18. Cavallari, L.H.; Limdi, N.A. Warfarin pharmacogenomics. *Curr. Opin. Mol. Ther.* **2009**, *11*, 243.
19. Johnson, J.A.; Cavallari, L.H. Warfarin pharmacogenetics. *Trends Cardiovas. Med.* **2015**, *25*, 33–41. [CrossRef]
20. Jung, J.-W.; Kim, J.Y.; Park, I.W.; Choi, B.W.; Kang, H.R. Genetic markers of severe cutaneous adverse reactions. *Korean J. Intern. Med.* **2018**, *33*, 867. [CrossRef]
21. Fantini, D. easyPubMed: *Search and Retrieve Scientific Publication Records from PubMed*; PubMed Help: Bethesda, MD, USA, 2019. Available online: https://cran.r-project.org/web/packages/easyPubMed/vignettes/getting_started_with_easyPubMed.html (accessed on 15 October 2020).
22. Purcell, S.; Neale, B.; Todd-Brown, K.; Thomas, L.; Ferreira, M.A.; Bender, D.; Sham, P.C. PLINK: A tool set for whole-genome association and population-based linkage analyses. *Am. J. Hum. Genet.* **2007**, *81*, 559–575. [CrossRef]
23. Karczewski, K.J.; Francioli, L.C.; Tiao, G.; Cummings, B.B.; Alföldi, J.; Wang, Q.; Collins, R.L.; Laricchia, K.M.; Ganna, A.; Gauthier, L.D.; et al. The mutational constraint spectrum quantified from variation in 141,456 humans. *Nature* **2020**, *581*, 434–443. [CrossRef] [PubMed]
24. Bradford, L.D. CYP2D6 allele frequency in European Caucasians, Asians, Africans and their descendants. *Pharmacogenomics* **2002**, *3*, 229–243. [CrossRef] [PubMed]
25. Bijl, M.J.; Visser, L.E.; Hofman, A.; Vulto, A.G.; Van Gelder, T.; Stricker, B.H.C.; Van Schaik, R.H. Influence of the CYP2D6*4 polymorphism on dose, switching and discontinuation of antidepressants. *Br. J. Clin. Pharmacol.* **2008**, *65*, 558–564. [CrossRef] [PubMed]
26. Landrum, M.J.; Lee, J.M.; Benson, M.; Brown, G.; Chao, C.; Chitipiralla, S.; Jang, W. ClinVar: Public archive of interpretations of clinically relevant variants. *Nucleic Acids Res.* **2015**, *44*, D862–D868. [CrossRef]
27. Landrum, M.J.; Lee, J.M.; Benson, M.; Brown, G.R.; Chao, C.; Chitipiralla, S.; Karapetyan, K. ClinVar: Improving access to variant interpretations and supporting evidence. *Nucleic Acids Res.* **2018**, *46*, D1062–D1067. [CrossRef] [PubMed]

Publisher's Note: MDPI stays neutral with regard to jurisdictional claims in published maps and institutional affiliations.

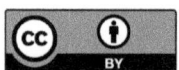

© 2020 by the authors. Licensee MDPI, Basel, Switzerland. This article is an open access article distributed under the terms and conditions of the Creative Commons Attribution (CC BY) license (http://creativecommons.org/licenses/by/4.0/).

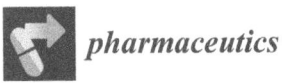

Communication

Impact of Polypharmacy on Candidate Biomarker miRNomes for the Diagnosis of Fibromyalgia and Myalgic Encephalomyelitis/Chronic Fatigue Syndrome: Striking Back on Treatments

Eloy Almenar-Pérez [1], Teresa Sánchez-Fito [1], Tamara Ovejero [2], Lubov Nathanson [3,4] and Elisa Oltra [2,5,*]

[1] Escuela de Doctorado, Universidad Católica de Valencia San Vicente Mártir, 46001 Valencia, Spain; eloy.almenar@ucv.es (E.A.-P.); mt.sanchez@ucv.es (T.S.-F.)
[2] School of Medicine, Universidad Católica de Valencia San Vicente Mártir, 46001 Valencia, Spain; tamara.ovejero@ucv.es
[3] Kiran C Patel College of Osteopathic Medicine, Nova Southeastern University, Ft Lauderdale, FL 33314, USA; lnathanson@nova.edu
[4] Institute for Neuro Immune Medicine, Nova Southeastern University, Ft Lauderdale, FL 33314, USA
[5] Unidad Mixta CIPF-UCV, Centro de Investigación Príncipe Felipe, 46012 Valencia, Spain
* Correspondence: elisa.oltra@ucv.es; Tel.: +34-963-637-412

Received: 15 January 2019; Accepted: 5 March 2019; Published: 18 March 2019

Abstract: Fibromyalgia (FM) and myalgic encephalomyelitis/chronic fatigue syndrome (ME/CFS) are diseases of unknown etiology presenting complex and often overlapping symptomatology. Despite promising advances on the study of miRNomes of these diseases, no validated molecular diagnostic biomarker yet exists. Since FM and ME/CFS patient treatments commonly include polypharmacy, it is of concern that biomarker miRNAs are masked by drug interactions. Aiming at discriminating between drug-effects and true disease-associated differential miRNA expression, we evaluated the potential impact of commonly prescribed drugs on disease miRNomes, as reported by the literature. By using the web search tools SM2miR, Pharmaco-miR, and repoDB, we found a list of commonly prescribed drugs that impact FM and ME/CFS miRNomes and therefore could be interfering in the process of biomarker discovery. On another end, disease-associated miRNomes may incline a patient's response to treatment and toxicity. Here, we explored treatments for diseases in general that could be affected by FM and ME/CFS miRNomes, finding a long list of them, including treatments for lymphoma, a type of cancer affecting ME/CFS patients at a higher rate than healthy population. We conclude that FM and ME/CFS miRNomes could help refine pharmacogenomic/pharmacoepigenomic analysis to elevate future personalized medicine and precision medicine programs in the clinic.

Keywords: fibromyalgia (FM); myalgic encephalomyelitis/chronic fatigue syndrome (ME/CFS); microRNA; miRNome; pharmacogenomics; pharmacoepigenomics; SM2miR; Pharmaco-miR; repoDB; ME/CFS Common Data Elements (CDEs)

---

1. Introduction

Fibromyalgia (FM) is a debilitating disorder characterized by a low pain threshold and muscle tenderness accompanied by bowel abnormalities, sleep disturbances, depressive episodes, cognitive problems, and chronic pain [1–4]. Though commonly comorbid with myalgic encephalomyelitis/chronic fatigue syndrome (ME/CFS), a disease also showing a complex clinical pathophysiology [5–11], these syndromes have been classified by the International Classification of Diseases, Tenth Revision,

Clinical Modification (ICD-10-CM), with separate codes (M79.7 and R53.82 or G93.3 if post-viral, for FM and ME/CFS, respectively) [12]. However, disease distinctions remain under debate [5].

Although possibly underestimated, the global prevalence for FM has been set at 2–8% and at 0.23–0.41 for ME/CFS with predominant ratios of females over males [13–17]. In addition, increasing numbers of patients being affected at early ages [18] highlights the considerable and raising needs for appropriate healthcare programs and the stepping demands for the alleviation of associated economic/social burdens.

Post-exertional malaise (PEM), a clinical hallmark of ME/CFS, together with additional clinical and biological parameters differing between these two diseases [19–24] seem to support a distinct underlying pathophysiology and possibly etiology for FM and ME/CFS. Aimed at clarifying this diagnostic conflict through an improved understanding of the biology of disease onset and evolution, some research groups, ours included, have set out to identify molecular biomarkers of these illnesses [25].

MicroRNAs or miRs constitute attractive candidates for the diagnosis of FM and ME/CFS, as they have been found to associate with the disease state of other complex chronic diseases [26,27] and may even be used to measure disease stage and response to treatments [28]. In their mature form (20–22 nts), they epigenetically control gene expression by directing particular sets of mRNAs, presenting partial complementation in their 3′UTRs, to degradation [29]. Other regulatory mechanisms have also been linked to the activity of these small molecules [30].

In addition to their biomarker value, miRNAs could potentially be targeted by small drugs, either directly through the binding of chemical compounds to particular grooves or pockets of their secondary structures, in their mature or precursor forms, as isolated or complexed molecules, or indirectly by interfering with proteins involved in their biogenesis or recycling, including regulation of transcription factors driving miRNA synthesis [31–34]. Therefore, directional FM and ME/CFS treatments based on miRNA targeting strategies are envisioned as potential curative therapies by themselves or as co-adjuvants in the near future.

MiRNA capacity to sense and respond to environmental cues [35–37], however, makes the establishment of correlations between particular disease states and miRNA profile changes challenging. To minimize potential environmental confounding factors, healthy participants are often population-matched by sex, age, and quite frequently BMI (body mass index) with the participating patient group. Careful selection of participants and proper study design are key factors in identifying miRNA disease-associated profiles (disease miRNomes), as miRNA levels also change in response to hormone challenges, during aging and metabolic states [38–41], including the post-prandial estate [42]. In the context of FM and ME/CFS, since miRNomes change with exercise [43], inclusion of sedentary control groups would be desirable.

Current treatments of both FM and ME/CFS diseases are symptom-palliative only [44–48]. Due to multi-symptomatology, patient prescriptions frequently involve polypharmacy, which may significantly impact downstream molecular analysis of the disease. With this perspective, a recent joint initiative worked out by the NINDS (National Institute of Neurological Disorders and Stroke) at the NIH (National Institute of Health) in Bethesda, MD (USA) and other federal agencies has made available case report forms (CRFs) and guidelines to register drug use in ME/CFS studies [49]. The ME/CFS Common Data Elements initiative or CDE Project aimed at standardizing clinical relevant variables for the study of ME/CFS covers various areas organized by domains and sub-domains. Information is publicly available at the NINDS Common Data Elements web page [49].

A recently observed feature of miRNAs is their role in determining drug efficacy [50,51]. The traditional field of pharmacogenomics dealing with how individual genomic features, including SNPs (single nucleotide polymorphisms) and CNVs (copy number variants), influence a patient's response to drug-based treatments and sensitivity to toxic effects is becoming complemented by individual epigenetic profiles including alternative splicing events and miRNomes (pharmacoepigenomics), with the aim of elevating predictions of the most effective and safest options towards improved personalized treatments in the clinic [52–55]. In addition to epigenetic regulation of drug targets, regulation of genes related to drug absorption, distribution, metabolism, and excretion (ADME) may translate into significant inter-individual differences to drug response [56]. In this context, it should be of relevance to take into account a patient's FM or/and ME/CFS condition when standardized treatments for diseases other than FM and ME/CFS are in need. In particular, FM and ME/CFS associated miRNA profiles might promote drug efficacy or inhibit drug function when compared to non-FM and non-ME/CFS patients and consequently impact or influence an FM and ME/CFS patient's response to pharmacological treatments or sensitivity to adverse reactions. Interestingly, and in line with this, FM and ME/CFS patients report suffering from multiple chemical sensitivity [57].

In this paper, we have interrogated the potential impact of commonly prescribed drugs to treat FM and ME/CFS on miRNA profiles in an effort to discern between miRNAs potentially linked to disease from those that might be a consequence of drug intake. We have also evaluated miRNA–target gene–drug interactions of differentially expressed (DE) miRNAs in FM and ME/CFS as an approach to determine the ability or predisposition of these patients to respond to common clinical treatments for diseases in general, including diseases other than FM and ME/CFS, which may appear comorbid at some point in FM and ME/CFS patients' lives.

2. Materials and Methods

2.1. Study Search

To locate experimental work aimed at studying miRNA profiles in FM or ME/CFS, a bibliographic search following the Preferred Reporting Items for Systematic Reviews and Meta-Analyses (PRISMA) criteria [58] was performed using Pubmed and Web of Science databases [59,60] up to January 2019. The search terms used in "all fields" included: "fibromyalgia" AND "microRNA" OR "miR" on one search, and "chronic fatigue syndrome" AND "CFS" in combination with "microRNA" OR "miR" in another. The use of the term "myalgic encephalomyelitis" to describe the disease in other searches did not yield any additional experimental publications in the field. The trial Pubmed Labs tool, including article snippets and other improvements was also used in the search [61]. Manual curation to filter out non-experimental or unrelated hits was applied.

For compounds commonly prescribed to treat symptoms in FM and ME/CFS, a search in the Cochrane library and Pubmed databases [59,62] was performed using as search terms either "fibromyalgia systematic review" AND "drug," "chronic fatigue syndrome" AND "CFS systematic review" AND "drug," or "myalgic encephalomyelitis systematic review" AND "drug." Most recently updated reviews were adopted as reference manuscripts.

2.2. Identification of miRNA–Drug–Disease Interactions

Features of miRNA and drug understudies, International Union of Pure and Applied Chemistry (IUPAC) names included, were found in miRBase and Drugbank databases, respectively [63,64]. FM and ME/CFS miRNomes were evaluated for miRNA–drug interactions using either SM2miR or Pharmaco-miR web search tools [50,65]. To find potential miRNomes derived from patient polypharmacy, SM2miR output was filtered using as criteria "drugs commonly prescribed to treat FM and ME/CFS symptoms," as described in the previous Section 2.1. Treatments to disease to which FM and ME/CFS patients may respond differently from non-FM and non-ME/CFS populations were spotted by searching the repoDB database [66] with the Pharmaco-miR drug hits obtained with FM or ME/CFS miRNome searches.

3. Results

3.1. miRNomes Associating with the Studied Diseases

3.1.1. miRNomes of FM

By reviewing the literature, as described in Methods, we found five studies reporting differential expression (DE) of particular miRNAs in FM patients with respect to healthy populations using multiplex approaches, either microarrays or RT-qPCR panels (Table 1 and Table S1). One of them measured miRNA levels in cerebrospinal fluid (CSF) [67], while the rest evaluated them in blood fractions [68–71]—two used white blood cells [69,71] and two analyzed serum [68,70].

According to these reports, a total of 85 FM patients and 86 healthy participants were screened for differential miRNA expression, and little coincidence was found (only 9 miRNAs reported by more than one study) (Table 1, miRNAs in bold) even within the same blood fraction type and in spite of using common diagnostic criteria (ACR 1990). Gene Ontology (GO) analysis, however, more commonly showed metabolic and neural pathways associating to DE miRNAs, indicating common cellular pathways affected by different FM miRNomes.

3.1.2. miRNomes of ME/CFS

A similar bibliographic search to the one performed in FM (Section 3.1.1 of this manuscript) yielded, after filtering out unrelated, gene-focused studies, only three studies showing DE of miRNAs in ME/CFS at basal levels, yet, they included a similar total number of patients and controls (83 and 47, respectively) (Table 2) [72–74]. It should be noted that an additional multiplex miRNA study evaluating the DE of miRNAs in ME/CFS upon an exercise challenge was excluded on the basis of reporting no basal disease miRNomes [75]. Again, as in FM studies, little overlap of DE miRNAs could be found across ME/CFS studies (only 4 miRNAs were reported by more than one ME/CFS study, bold miRNAs in Table 2). In this case, this could be somehow expected as blood fractions and diagnostic criteria varied across studies. In fact, only the most recent study by Petty et al. included the more restrictive Canadian criteria for patient selection [74]. Nevertheless, once more, a coincidence of mainly affected GO terms was found, indicating major immune defects in ME/CFS through different miRNomes.

Table 1. Summary of studies evaluating fibromyalgia (FM) miRNomes by multiplex approaches.

Source of RNA	Diagnostic Criteria /Clinical Parameters	Cohorts	Technical Approach	Over-Expressed microRNAs	Under-Expressed microRNAs	RT-qPCR Validated miRNAs	GO Terms Mainly Affected	References
Cerebrospinal fluid (CSF)	ACR 1990, FIQ & MFI-20 *	10 FM 8 HC	microRNA Ready-to-Use PCR microchip (Exiqon, Denmark Cat No 203608)		miR-21-5p, **miR-145-5p**, miR-29a-3p, **miR-99b-5p**, miR-125b-5p, **miR-23a-3p**, miR-23b-3p, miR-195-5p, **miR-223-3p**	N/A	Glial and neuronal response, insulin-like growth factor pathway, Alzheimer's and Parkinson's, autoimmunity and energy metabolism	Bjersing et al., 2013 [67]
Serum	ACR 1990, FIQ & MFI-20 *	20 FM 20 HC	microRNA Ready-to-Use PCR microchip (Exiqon, Denmark Cat No 203608)	miR-320a	**miR-103a-3p**, **miR-107**, let-7a-5p, miR-30b-5p, **miR-151a-5p**, miR-142-3p, miR-374b-5p.	N/A	Neuronal regeneration, opioid tolerance, dopamine neurotransmitter receptor activity, cell division, stress response, energy metabolism, lipid metabolism, Alzheimer's	Bjersing et al., 2014 [68]
PBMCs	ACR 1990, FIQ & MFI-20 *	11 FM 10 HC	3D-Gene Human miRNA Oligo chips (version 16.0; Toray Industries)		**miR-223-3p**, miR-451a, miR-338-3p, **miR-143-3p**, **miR-145-5p**, **miR-21-5p**	miR-223-3p, miR-451a, miR-338-3p, miR-143-3p, miR-145-5p	Nervous system, inflammation, diabetes, major depressive disorder	Cerdá-Olmedo et al., 2015 [69]
Serum	ACR 1990/2010, FIQ, FAS, HAQ & ZSAS/ZSDS *	14 FM 14 HC	Serum/Plasma Focus miRNA PCR Panel I+II (96-wells Exiqon)	Pooled Sera: miR-10a-5p, **miR-320b**, miR-424-5p	Pooled Sera: miR-20a-3p, miR-139-5p Individual Sera: **miR-23a-3p**, miR-1, miR-133a, miR-346, miR-139-5p, **miR-320b**	N/A	Brain development, immune response, osteogenesis, myoblast differentiation, autism, epilepsy, cellular proliferation and differentiation, muscular atrophy, complex regional pain syndrome, among others	Masotti et al., 2016 [70]
White blood cell (WBC)	ACR 1990, FIQ, NPSI-G, GCPS & ADS *	30 FM 34 HC	miRCURY LNA miRNA array (Exiqon, Vedbaek, version 19.0, with 2042 analyzed microRNAs)	miR-136-5p, miR-4306, miR-744-5p, miR-4301, miR-151a-3p, miR-584-5p, miR-4288, miR-221-3p, **miR-151a-5p**, miR-199a-5p, miR-126-3p, miR-126-5p, miR-130a-3p, miR-146a-5p, miR-125a-5p, miR-4429, **miR-320b**, **miR-320a**, miR-320c, miR-17-3p, miR-423-3p, miR-425-5p, miR-4291, miR-652-3p, miR-103b-3p, miR-199a-3p, miR-335-5p, miR-331-3p, miR-339-5p, miR-92a-3p, let-7b-5p, miR-222-3p, miR-33a, let-7c-5p, miR-185-5p, miR-22-3p, miR-148b-3p, **miR-103a-3p**, let-7d-5p, miR-4289, **miR-107**, miR-30d-5p, miR-301a-3p, miR-374c-5p, miR-17-5p, miR-188-5p, miR-1	miR-4639-3p, miR-3685, miR-943, miR-877-3p	miR-199a, miR-151, miR-103, Let-7d, miR-146a	Cell proliferation, differentiation, brain development, opioid tolerance	Leinders et al., 2016 [71]

* ACR: American College of Rheumatology 1990/2010 criteria; FIQ: Fibromyalgia Impact Questionnaire; FAS: Fibromyalgia Assessment Status; HAQ: Health Assessment Questionnaire; ZSAS, ZSDS: Zung Self-Rating Anxiety and Zung Self-Rating Depression Scale; NPSI-G: Neuropathic Pain Symptom Inventory; GCPS: Graded Chronic Pain Scale; ADS: Allgemeine Depressions-Skala. Bolded miRs correspond to miRs differentially expressed (DE) according to more than one FM study. Underlined miRs correspond to miRs DE in FM and myalgic encephalomyelitis/chronic fatigue syndrome (ME/CFS) studies.

Table 2. Summary of studies evaluating ME/CFS miRNomes by multiplex approaches.

Source of RNA	Diagnostic Criteria	Cohorts	Technical Approach	Over-Expressed microRNAs	Under-Expressed microRNAs	RT-qPCR Validated microRNAs	GO Terms Mainly Affected	References
NK & CD8+ cells	Fukuda	28 ME/CFS 28 HC	Analyzed by RT-qPCR 19 microRNAs: miR-10a, miR-16, miR-15b, miR-107, miR-128b, miR-146a, miR-191, miR-21, miR-223, miR-17-5p, miR-191, miR-150, miR-103, miR-106b, miR-126, miR-142-3p, miR-146-5p, miR-152, miR-181, let-7a.		NK: miR-10a, miR-146a, miR-191, miR-223, miR-17-5p, miR-21, miR-106, miR-152, miR-103 CD8+: miR-21	N/A	Cytotoxicity of NK and CD8+ cells, cytokine expression, cell proliferation, apoptosis, development and differentiation of effector CD8+	Brenu et al., 2012 [72]
Plasma	Fukuda	20 ME/CFS 20 HC	MicroRNA profiling by HiSeq2000 sequencing (Illumina HiSeq2000)	miR-548j, miR-548ax, miR-127-3p, miR-381-3p, **miR-331-3p**, miR-136-3p, miR-142-5p, miR-493-5p, miR-143-3p, miR-370, miR-4532	**miR-126**, miR-450b-5p, miR-641, miR-26a-1-3p, miR-3065-3p, miR-5187-3p, miR-16-2-3p, let-7g-3p	miR-127-3p, miR-142-5p, miR-143-3p	Autoimmunity, T cell development, cytokine production, inflammatory responses, apoptosis	Brenu et al., 2014 [73]
PBMCs	Fukuda & Canadian	35 ME/CFS 50 HC	Ambion Bioarray microarrays (version 1 targeting 385 miRNA sequences)	let-7b, **miR-103**, **miR-126**, miR-145, miR-151, miR-181a, miR-185, **miR-191**, miR-197, miR-199a, miR-19b, miR-210, miR-22-5p, miR-24, miR-27a, miR-27b, miR-30c, miR-30d, miR-320, miR-324-3p, miR-324-5p, miR-326, miR-330, **miR-331-3p**, miR-339, miR-422b, miR-423, miR-92, miR-99b		miR-99b, miR-30c, miR-126, miR-330-3p	Angiogenesis, invasion, migration and proliferation in dendritic cells, proliferative, cytotoxic and cytokine effector function in NK cells	Petty, et al., 2016 [74]

Bolded miRs correspond to miRs DE according to more than one ME/CFS study. Underlined miRs correspond to miRs DE in FM and ME/CFS studies. This table has been adapted from Almenar-Perez, E.; Ovejero, T.; Sánchez-Fito, T.; Espejo, J.A.; Nathanson, L.; Oltra, E. Epigenetic components of Myalgic Encephalomyelitis/Chronic Fatigue Syndrome (ME/CFS) uncover potential transposable element activation (Clin Ther, accepted, special issue: "Immunology Specialty Update on CFS/ME.", Elsevier 2019).

Surprisingly as many as 19 miRNAs were found to be commonly reported as DE by FM and ME/CFS studies, the significance of which is unknown at present (miRNAs underlined in Tables 1 and 2).

3.2. Polypharmacy Potentially Impacting miRNA Profiles

As mentioned above, our general aims included determining drug–miRNA and drug–disease interactions in the context of FM, or ME/CFS miRNomes, for the purpose of identifying potential interference of drugs in miRNA profiling, which could bias research outcomes on one hand and, on the other, determine whether disease miRNA profiles could influence drug response in these patients. This section focuses on selecting drugs commonly prescribed to FM and ME/CFS patients to evaluate the effect that polypharmacy might have on miRNomes of these diseases.

3.2.1. Polypharmacy in FM

Based on the recent Cochrane report by Häuser et al. [44], drugs that have been commonly used to treat FM in the clinical practice can be classified into the following six classes: antidepressants, antiepileptics, antipsychotics, cannabinoids, nonsteroidal anti-inflammatory drugs (NSAIDs), and opioids. Rather than analyzing the quality of evidence of clinical trials using these substances, we were interested in assigning the active principle and IUPAC names to the reported compounds, to facilitate our downstream analysis (Table 3). Additional literature supporting the use of compounds for each of the six classes described by Häuser et al. to treat FM patients is provided in Table 3 [76–93].

3.2.2. Polypharmacy in ME/CFS

Opposite to FM, no drug-based Cochrane review for the treatment of ME/CFS could be found. The three hits obtained by using the MeSH search terms "chronic fatigue syndrome" were reviews on exercise, CBT (cognitive behaviour therapy) and Chinese herbs [94–96]. Therefore, we decided to use the recent reviews by Collatz et al. and Smith et al. as reference papers to evaluate common drug-based ME/CFS therapies [46,47]. Additional bibliography supporting the use of polypharmacy in ME/CFS was also included [46,48,97–105]. Similar to what has been described in Section 3.2.1, a documented summary of drugs commonly prescribed to ME/CFS patients that could impact miRNA screenings is shown in Table 4 together with active principles and IUPAC names.

Although possibly not complete, Tables 3 and 4 include the most representative compounds to treat FM and ME/CFS according to the consulted authors [44,48,76–93,97–105]. Unexpectedly, a single IUPAC overlap, corresponding to the selective serotonin reuptake inhibitor (SSRI) fluoxetine, was found for drugs commonly prescribed for FM and ME/CFS (in bold in Tables 3 and 4), indicating little prescription overlap at the IUPAC name level despite both groups of patients presenting common symptomatology. Special attention should be placed to common prescriptions as they may more readily allow for identifying the effects of drugs on miRNA levels over disease-related changes.

Table 3. Classification of drugs commonly prescribed to FM patients.

Family	Subfamily	Active Principle	IUPAC Name	Reference
Antidepressants	Serotonin-Norepinephrine reuptake inhibitors (SNRIs)	Milnacipran	(±)-(1R,2S)-rel-2-(Aminomethyl)-N,N-diethyl-1-phenylcyclopropane-1-carboxamide	Cording M et al., 2015 [76]
		Duloxetine	(+)-(S)-N-Methyl-3-(naphthalen-1-yloxy)-3-(thiophen-2-yl)propan-1-amina	Lunn MP et al., 2014 [77]
	Selective serotonin reuptake inhibitors (SSRIs)	Citalopram	(RS)-1-[3-(dimethylamino) propyl]-1-(4-fluorophenyl)-1,3-dihydroisobenzofuran-5-carbonitrile	Walitt B et al., 2015 [78]
		Fluoxetine	**(RS)-N-Methyl-3-phenyl-3-(4-trifluoromethylphenoxy) propylamine**	
		Paroxetine	(3S, 4R)-3-[(1,3-Benzodioxol-5-yl oxy) methyl]-4-(4-fluorophenyl) piperidine	
		Tryptophan	2-amino-3-(1H-indol-3-yl) propanoic acid	
		Escitalopram	(S)-1-[3-(Dimethylamino)propyl]-1-(4-fluorophenyl)-1,3-dihydroisobenzofuran-5-carbonitrile	Riera R, 2015 [79]
		Sertraline	(1S,4S)-4-(3,4-dichlorophenyl)-N-methyl-1,2,3,4-tetrahydronaphthalen-1-amine	
	Tricyclic antidepressants	Amitriptyline	8-methyl-2,3,3a,4,5,6-hexahydro-1H-pyrazino[3,2,1-jk]carbazole	Moore RA et al., 2015 [80]
		Pirlindole	8-methyl-2,3,3a,4,5,6-hexahydro-1H-pyrazino[3,2,1-jk]carbazole	Tort S et al., 2012 [81]
	Monoamine oxidase inhibitors (MAOIs)	Moclobemide	4-chloro-N-(2-morpholin-4-ylethyl) benzamide	Welsch P et al., 2018 [82]
		Mirtazapine	(RS)-1,2,3,4,10,14b-Hexahydro-2-methylpyrazino[2,1-a]pyrido[2,3-c][2]benzazepine	Birse F et al., 2012 [83]
Antiepileptics	1st Generation	Phenytoin	5,5-diphenylimidazolidine-2,4-dione	Gill D et al., 2011 [84]
	2nd Generation	Valproic acid (Sodium valproate)	2-propylpentanoic acid	
		Clonazepam	5-(2-Chlorophenyl)-7-nitro-1,3-dihydro-1,4-benzodiazepin-2-one	Corrigan R et al., 2012 [85]
	3rd Generation	Pregabalin	(S)-3-(aminomethyl)-5-methylhexanoic acid	Derry S et al., 2016 [86]
		Gabapentin	2-[1-(aminomethyl)cyclohexyl]ethanoic acid	Wiffen PJ et al., 2017 [87]
		Lacosamide	N2-acetyl-N-benzyl-D-homoserinamide	Hearn L et al., 2016 [88]
		Topiramate	2,3: 4,5-Bis-O-(1-methylethylidene)-beta-D-fructopyranose sulfamate	Wiffen PJ et al., 2013 [89]
Antipsychotics	Atypical	Quetiapine	2-(2-(4-dibenzo [b,f] [1,4] thiazepine-11-yl-1-piperazinyl) ethoxy) ethanol	Walitt B et al., 2016 (Jun) [90]
Cannabinoids	Synthetic	Nabilone	(6aR,10aR)-rel-1-Hydroxy-6,6-dimethyl-3-(2-methyl-2-octanyl)-6,6a,7,8,10,10a-hexahydro-9H-benzo[c]chromen-9-one	Walitt B et al., 2016 (Jul) [91]
Nonsteroidal anti-inflammatory drugs (NSAIDs)	Selective inhibitor of Cyclooxygenase 2 (COX-2)	Etoricoxib	5-cloro-6'-metil-3-[4-(metilsulfonil)fenil]-2,3'-bipiridine	
	Inhibitor of prostaglandin synthesis	Ibuprofen	(RS)-2-(4-(2-Methylpropyl)phenyl)propanoic acid	Derry S et al., 2017 [92]
		Naproxen	(+)-(S)-2-(6-Methoxynaphthalen-2-yl)propanoic acid	
	Inhibitor of Cicloxygenase (COX-1 and COX-2)	Tenoxicam	(3E)-3-[hydroxy(pyridin-2-ylamino)methylene]-2-methyl-2,3-dihydro-4H-thieno[2,3-e] [1,2]thiazin-4-one 1,1-dioxide	
Opioids	Semi synthetic	Oxycodone	(5R,9R,13S,14S)-4,5-α-epoxy-14-hydroxy-3-methoxy-17-methyl-morphinan-6-one	Gaskell H et al., 2016 [93]

Drugs commonly prescribed to both FM and ME/CFS patients are bolded.

Table 4. Classification of drugs commonly prescribed to ME/CFS patients.

Family	Subfamily	Active Principle	IUPAC Name	Reference
Anticonvulsants	3rd Generation	Gabapentin	2-[1-(amynomethyl)cyclohexyl]ethanoic acid	Castro-Marrero J et al., 2017 [48]
		Pregabalin	(S)-3-(amynomethyl)-5-methylhexanoic acid	Collatz A et al., 2016 [46]
Antidepressants		Nafazodone	2-[3-[4-(3-chlorophenyl)piperazin-1-yl]propyl]-5-ethyl-4-(2-phenoxyethyl)-1,2,4-triazol-3-one	
		Buproprion	(RS)-2-(tert-Butylamino)-1-(3-chlorophenyl)propan-1-one	
	Selective serotonin reuptake inhibitors (SSRIs)	Citalopram	((RS)-1-[3-(Dimethylamino)propyl]-1-(4-fluorophenyl)-1,3-dihydroisobenzofuran-5-carbonitrile	Castro-Marrero J et al., 2017 [48]
		Escitalopram	(S)-1-[3-(Dimethylamino)propyl]-1-(4-fluorophenyl)-1,3-dihydroisobenzofuran-5-carbonitrile	
		Fluoxetine	**(RS)-N-Methyl-3-phenyl-3-(4-trifluoromethylphenoxy) propylamine**	
		Sertraline	(1S,4S)-4-(3,4-dichlorophenyl)-N-methyl-1,2,3,4-tetrahydronaphthalen-1-amine	
		Paroxetine	(3S, 4R)-3-[(1,3-Benzodioxol-5-yl oxy) methyl]-4-(4-fluorophenyl) piperidine	
		Methylphenidate	Methyl phenyl(piperidin-2-yl)acetate	Blockmans D and Persoons P, 2016 [97]; Castro-Marrero J et al., 2017 [48]
	Serotonin–norepinephrine reuptake inhibitors (SNRIs)	Duloxetine	(+)-(S)-N-Methyl-3-(naphthalen-1-yloxy)-3-(thiophen-2-yl)propan-1-amine	Castro-Marrero J et al., 2017 [48]
		Venlafaxine	(RS)-1-[2-dimethylamino-1-(4-methoxyphenyl)-ethyl]cyclohexanol	
		Amitriptyline	3-(10,11-dihydro-5H-dibenzo [a,d] cyclohepten-5-ylidene)-N, N-dimethyl-1-propanamine	
		Clomipramine	3-(2-chloro-5,6-dihydrobenzo[b][1]benzazepin-11-yl)-N,N-dimethylpropan-1-amine	
	Tricyclic antidepressants	Desipramine	3-(5,6-dihydrobenzo[b][1]benzazepin-11-yl)-N-methylpropan-1-amine	Castro-Marrero J et al., 2017 [48]
		Doxepin	(3E)-3-(6H-benzo[c][1]benzoxepin-11-ylidene)-N,N-dimethylpropan-1-amine	
		Imipramine	3-(5,6-dihydrobenzo[b][1]benzazepin-11-yl)-N,N-dimethylpropan-1-amine	
		Nortriptyline	3-(5,6-dihydrodibenzo[2,1-b:2′,1′-f][7]annulen-11-ylidene)-N-methylpropan-1-amine	
	Monoamine oxidase inhibitors (MAOIs)	Moclobemide	4-chloro-N-(2-morpholin-4-ylethyl)benzamide	Collatz A et al., 2016 [46]; Castro-Marrero J et al., 2017 [48]
		Phenelzine	2-phenylethylhydrazine	
		Selegiline	(R)-N-methyl-N-(1-pheny lpropan-2-yl)prop-2-yn-3-amine	Castro-Marrero J et al., 2017 [48]
	Noradrenergic and specific serotonin antagonist (NaSSAs)	Mirtazapine	(RS)-1,2,3,4,10,14b-Hexahydro-2-methylpyrazino[2,1-a]pyrido[2,3-c][2]benzazepine	Castro-Marrero J et al., 2017 [48]
	Monoaminergic stabilizer	(−)-OSU-6162	(RS)-3-[3-(methylsulfonyl)phenyl]-1-propylpiperidine	Nilsson MKL et al., 2017 [98]
	Stimulant to α2-Receptors	Clonidine hydrochloride	N-(2,6-dichlorophenyl)-4,5-dihydro-1H-imidazol-2-amine;hydrochloride	Collatz A et al., 2016 [46]
Antihypertensive	Angiotensin II receptor agonist	Olmesartan medoxomil	(5-metil-2-oxo-2H-1,3-dioxol-4-il)metil 4-(2-hidroxipropan-2-il)-2-propil-1-{[4-(2H-1,2,3,4-tetrazol-5-il)fenil][fenil]metil}-1H-imidazole-5-carboxilato	Proal AD et al., 2013 [99]
	Fatty acid oxidant	L-Carnitine	3-Hydroxy-4-(trimethylazaniumyl)butanoate	Plioplys AV and Plioplys S., 1997 [100]
Antioxidant	Ubiquinone	CoQ10	[(2E,6E,10E,14E,18E,22E,26E,30E,34E)-3,7,11,15,19,23,27,31,35,39-Decamethyltetraconta-2,6,10,14,18,22,26,30,34,38-decaenyl]-5,6-dimethoxy-3-methylcyclohexa-2,5-diene-1,4-dione	Castro-Marrero J et al., 2015 [101]
	Re-Dox Agent	NADH	Nicotine adenine dinucleotide	
		α-lipoic acid	(R)-5-(1,2-dithiolan-3-yl)pentanoic acid	
	Omega-3 fatty acid	Docosahexaenoic acid(DHA)	(4Z,7Z,10Z,13Z,16Z,19Z)-docosa-4,7,10,13,16,19-hexaenoic acid	Castro-Marrero J et al., 2017 [48]
	Vitamins	Vitamin C	(2R)-2-[(1S)-1,2-dihydroxyethyl]-3,4-dihydroxy-2H-furan-5-one	
		Folate (Vitamin B9) Hydroxycobalamin Vitamin B12)	(2S)-2-[[4-[(2-Amino-4-oxo-1H-pteridin-6-yl)methylamino]benzoyl]amino]pentanedioic acid Coα-[α-(5,6-dimethylbenzimidazolyl)]-Coβ-hydroxocobamide	

Table 4. Cont.

Family	Subfamily	Active Principle	IUPAC Name	Reference
Antiviral	Blocking adhesion and viral penetration	Amantadine	1-amino-adamantane	Plioplys AV and Plioplys S., 1997 [100]
	Acid nucleics analogs	Valganciclovir	[2-[(2-amino-6-oxo-3H-purin-9-yl)methoxy]-3-hydroxypropyl] (2S)-2-amino-3-methylbutanoate	Collatz A et al., 2016 [46]; Castro-Marrero J et al., 2017 [48]
		Acyclovir	2-amino-9-(2-hydroxyethoxymethyl)-3H-purin-6-one	Castro-Marrero J et al., 2017 [48]
		Valacyclovir	2-[[(2-amino-6-oxo-3H-purin-9-yl)methoxy]ethyl (2S)-2-amino-3-methylbutanoate	
Corticoids	Glucocorticoid	Hydrocortisone	(11β)-11,17,21-trihydroxypregn-4-ene-3,20-dione	Blockmans D et al., 2003 [102]; Collatz A et al., 2016 [46]
		Fludrocortisone	(8S,9R,10S,11S,13S,14S,17R)-9-fluoro-11,17-dihydroxy-17-(2-hydroxyacetyl)-10,13-dimethyl-1,2,6,7,8,11,12,14,15,16-decahydrocyclopenta[a]phenanthren-3-one	Blockmans D et al., 2003 [102]
Nonsteroidal Anti-Inflammatory Drugs (NSAIDs)	Inhibitor of prostaglandin synthesis	Ibuprofen	(RS)-2-(4-(2-Methylpropyl)phenyl)propanoic acid	Castro-Marrero J et al., 2017 [48]
		Naproxen	(+)-(S)-2-(6-Methoxynaphthalen-2-yl)propanoic acid	
	Immunomodulatory double stranded RNA	Rintatolimod	5′-Inosinic acid, homopolymer, complex with 5′-cytidylic acid polymer with 5′-uridylic acid (1:1)	Strayer DR et al., 2012 [103]
	Anti-neoplastic	Sodium dichloroacetate	Dichloroacetic acid	Comhaire F., 2018 [104]
	Ig gamma-1 chain C region	Rituximab	Lithium;4-[2-(diethylamino)ethylcarbamoyl]-2-iodobenzoate	
Others	Proliferation inductor from B cells	Intravenous immunoglobulin (Immunoglobulin G)	(2S)-2-[[(2S)-1-[[(2S)-6-amino-2-[[(2S,3R)-2-[[(2S)-2-amino-2-[[(2S)-4-amino-2-[[(2S)-2-amino-3-(1H-indol-3-yl)propanoyl]amino]-4-oxobutanoyl]amino]propanoyl]amino]hexanoyl]amino]-3-hydroxybutanoyl]amino]hexanoyl]pyrrolidine-2-carbonyl]amino]-5-(diaminomethylideneamino)pentanoic acid	Collatz A et al., 2016 [46]
	Hormone	Growth hormone (Somatotropin)	191 amino acid peptide (IUPAC name N/A)	
	Wakefulness-promoting	Modafinil	2-[(diphenylmethyl)sulfinyl]acetamide	
	Peripherally-selective antihistamine	Terfenadine	1-(4-tert-butylphenyl)-4-[4-[hydroxy(diphenyl)methyl]piperidin-1-yl]butan-1-ol	
	Precursor of Creatine	Guanidinoacetic acid (Glycocyamine)	2-(diaminomethylideneamino)acetic acid	Ostojic SM et al., 2016 [105]
Pain	Opiate	Codeine	(5α,6α)-7,8-didehydro-4,5-epoxy-3-methoxy-17-methylmorphinan-6-ol	
		Morphine	(4R,4aR,7S,7aR,12bS)-3-Methyl-2,3,4,4a,7,7a-hexahydro-1H-4,12-methanobenzofuro[3,2-e]isoquinoline-7,9-diol	Castro-Marrero J et al., 2017 [48]
	Opiod	Tramadol	(±)-cis-2-[(dimetilamino)metil]-1-(3-metoxifenil) ciclohexanol hidrocloruro	
Psycho-pharmaceutical	Benzodiazepine	Galantamine hidrobromide	(4aS,6R,8aS)-5,6,9,10,11,12-Hexahydro-3-methoxy-11-methyl-4aH-[1]benzofuro[3a,3,2-ef][2]benzazepin-6-ol	Collatz A et al., 2016 [46]
	Psychostimulant	Dextroamphetamine	(2S)-1-phenylpropan-2-amine	

Drugs commonly prescribed to both FM and ME/CFS patients are bolded.

3.3. miRNA–Drug Interactions in FM and ME/CFS

With the intention to discriminate whether the miRNomes proposed to associate with FM or with ME/CFS are derived from drug intake differences between the patient and control groups, we performed a screen of drugs that could alter any of the miRNAs in these miRNomes using the SM2miR web server [65] and each of the individual DE miRNAs or disease miRNome as the input, as previously detailed in the Methods section.

The SM2miR drug output file (Table S2) was contrasted with the FM and ME/CFS polypharmacy tables (Tables 3 and 4), and it was found that five of the commonly prescribed drugs for FM or ME/CFS (DHA, fluoxetine, glucocorticoids, morphine, and valproate) are estimated to alter the levels of one or more of the miRNAs found DE in FM or ME/CFS screenings (potential disease-associated miRNomes) and therefore these drugs could constitute confounding variables of the assay (Table 5) [106–111]. Overlapping tendencies may suggest that the detected differences between studied groups associate with treatment rather than constituting potential biomarkers of disease, while opposed tendencies might reflect additional factors leading to differential expression other than drug intake, disease status included. Importantly, as summarized in Table 5, the expression of miRNA-27b reported in miRNomes of both FM and ME/CFS in more than one report [67,74] is affected by the only overlapping compound commonly prescribed for treatment of both diseases (fluoxetine), indicating a potential drug–interference effect. Three additional miRNAs reported as miRNomes of ME/CFS by more than one study (miR-26a, miR-126, and miR-191) are also affected by drugs frequently prescribed to ME/CFS patients, so special attention should be paid when interpreting miRNome results including these miRNAs.

It must be pointed out that, in an effort to complete the search as much as possible, the list of DE miRNAs in FM and ME/CFS used in the SM2miR search not only included the miRNAs listed in Tables 1 and 2 but also those documented in the supplementary tables of the listed literature [67–74].

3.4. Drug–Disease Interactions Based on FM and ME/CFS miRNomes

To evaluate potential biased responses of FM and ME/CFS patients to pharmacotherapy in general, due to their DE miRNA profiles, we searched for diseases commonly treated with small-molecule drugs that depend on gene sets linked to FM or ME/CFS miRNomes (miRNA–gene–drug datasets). With this purpose, individual DE miRNAs in FM or ME/CFS were used as input in the Pharmaco-miR web search tool [50]. The output constituted a list of genes whose expression is dependent on FM and ME/CFS DE miRNAs (Table S3) and a third column facilitating small molecule drug associations for these gene lists. Among the 709 small molecules linked to FM miRNome, only 595 appeared registered in the Drugbank database. Out of the 668 small molecules associating with ME/CFS miRNomes, 557 appeared registered in Drugbank [64].

Finally, Drugbank numbers of these small molecules were used as the input to search repoDB, a database of small drugs developed by Brown and Patel to facilitate screenings for drug repositioning [66]. The results (Table S3, miRNome–drug–disease tabs) show 1480 and 1455 diseases treated with small molecules, respectively, associating with FM or ME/CFS miRNomes after filtering out duplications. Out of these diseases potentially impacting individualized medicine programs for FM and ME/CFS patients, more than 30% corresponded to cancer of some type. Within cancer, 13% corresponded to lymphoma, and 14% to lymphoma plus leukemia. This seems to indicate that quite possibly FM and ME/CFS patients may respond differently to treatments for these diseases with respect to non-FM and non-ME/CFS patients, so it is advised that attention be paid to individualized medicine programs for the treatment of these cancers in the case of FM and CFS/ME patients.

Table 5. Effect of FM and ME/CFS polypharmacy on miRNomes associated with disease.

Prescribed Drugs	miR Affected	Disease	miR Levels in Patients	Treatment Effect	Reference
Docosahexaenoic acid (DHA)	miR-30c	ME/CFS	↑ (PBMCs) [74]	Upregulated	Gil-Zamorano J et al., 2014 [106]
	miR-143-3p	ME/CFS	↑ (Plasma) [73]	Upregulated	
	miR-181a-5p	ME/CFS	↑ (PBMCs) [74]	Upregulated	
	miR-330	ME/CFS	↑ (PBMCs) [74]	Upregulated	
Fluoxetine	<u>miR-27b</u>	FM	↓ (CSF) [67]	Upregulated	Rodrigues AC et al., 2011 [107]
		ME/CFS	↑ (PBMCs) [74]		
Glucocorticoid	miR-16	ME/CFS	↓ (Plasma) [73]	Upregulated	Rainer J et al., 2009 [108]
	miR-19b	ME/CFS	↑ (PBMCs) [74]	Upregulated	
	miR-181a	ME/CFS	↑ (PBMCs) [74]	Upregulated	Rainer J et al., 2009 [108]; Lu S et al., 2012 [109]
	miR-223	ME/CFS	↓ (NK cells) [72]	Upregulated	
	miR-21	ME/CFS	↓ (NK cells) [72]	Upregulated	
	miR-10a	ME/CFS	↓ (NK cells) [72]	Upregulated	
	miR-27a	ME/CFS	↑ (PBMCs) [74]	Upregulated	
	miR-99b	ME/CFS	↑ (PBMCs) [74]	Upregulated	
	miR-126	ME/CFS	↓ (Plasma) [73] ↑ (PBMCs) [74]	Upregulated	Lu S et al., 2012 [109]
	miR-145	ME/CFS	↑ (PBMCs) [74]	Upregulated	
	miR-146a	ME/CFS	↓ (NK cells) [72]	Upregulated	
	miR-324-5p	ME/CFS	↑ (PBMCs) [74]	Upregulated	
	miR-339-3p	ME/CFS	↑ (PBMCs) [74]	Upregulated	
Morphine	miR-16	ME/CFS	↓ (Plasma) [73]	Upregulated	Dave R.S & Khalili K., 2010 [110]
	miR-24	ME/CFS	↑ (PBMCs) [74]	Upregulated	
	miR-30c	ME/CFS	↑ (PBMCs) [74]	Upregulated	
	miR-146a	ME/CFS	↓ (NK cells) [72]	Upregulated	
	miR-21	ME/CFS	↓ (NK cells) [72]	Downregulated	
	miR-26a	ME/CFS	↓ (NK cells) [72] ↑ (PBMCs) [74]	Downregulated	
	miR-99b	ME/CFS	↑ (PBMCs) [74]	Downregulated	
	miR-191	ME/CFS	↓ (NK cells) [72] ↑ (PBMCs) [74]	Downregulated	
	miR-320a	ME/CFS	↑ (PBMCs) [74]	Downregulated	
	miR-320c	ME/CFS	↑ (PBMCs) [74]	Downregulated	
	miR-423-5p	ME/CFS	↑ (PBMCs) [74]	Downregulated	
Valproate	miR-21	FM	↓ (PBMCs) [69]	Upregulated	Fayyad-Kazan H et al., 2010 [111]
	miR-125a	FM	↑ (WBC*) [71]	Downregulated	

* WBC: white blood cells. Bolded miRs correspond to miRs DE according to more than one ME/CFS study. Underlined miRs correspond to miRs DE in FM and ME/CFS studies.

4. Discussion

This paper is the first to evaluate the relationship between commonly prescribed drugs for FM and ME/CFS and miRNA expression and compares these profiles to FM- and ME/CFS-reported miRNomes in an effort to discern miRNAs presenting differential expression due to medication from differences more likely related to disease. The resources used in this study are limited and therefore it is expected that the evidence presented here will be refined as more data becomes available. The topic is not exclusive to FM and ME/CFS, as it can be extended to any other study evaluating miRNomes associated with disease. However, the fact that FM and ME/CFS patients are usually polymedicated to palliate the multiple symptoms that associate with these illnesses extends this concern to higher levels, particularly demanding careful registry of study participants' medication, when restrictive medication inclusion criteria is not an option. In this sense, the ME/CFS Common Data Elements initiative [49] has made publicly available medication guidelines and CRFs at the disposition of researchers, which may help standardize medication registry in ME/CFS studies.

Although some researchers have expressed their concern of the impact of drug use by FM and ME/CFS patients on the study of molecular markers and although recent work in the area is already reporting the medication used by participants [71,112], the information of registered drugs is not yet used to evaluate potential interference or bias of results. To elevate biomarker screenings of FM and ME/CFS based on miRNA profiles, complex stratified analysis to filter out potential drug and other confounding variables will be required. The complexity and limitations of this analysis is served by the fact that miRNA expression responds to many cues, such as exercise and diet, hormones, sex, and aging [38–43].

A commonly used approach to minimize confounding variables, although not free of certain difficulties for sampling, is to set restrictive inclusion criteria including sex selection, narrow age range, and BMI. This is important in miRNA screenings as these parameters are known to affect miRNA profiles [113]. Additional sampling details such as fasting blood draw and the selection of sedentary healthy controls may improve study outcomes. Some authors have even taken into account time of blood collection to reduce circadian variation [71], but it may not be possible to eliminate polypharmacy, particularly in studies including severely affected FM and ME/CFS patients.

Prescriptions for other common health problems such as diabetes or high cholesterol, diet supplements and some recreational drugs alter the expression of some miRNAs in FM and ME/CFS miRNomes (Table S4) [107,114–125]. Hormones and other natural compounds also impact FM and ME/CFS miRNomes (Table S5) [106,126–136], stressing the necessity for researchers to collect complete medical histories of participants to accurately evaluate miRNAs as biomarkers of these diseases.

Though FM and ME/CFS miRNomes relate to disease or derive from chronic polypharmacy use, DE miRs should represent a relevant factor to take into account when treatments for other diseases such as cancer are due. Here, we performed an analysis of the diseases whose treatment response could differ in the context of FM and ME/CFS miRNomes, and found a broad range of them. The major representation of cancer (above 35%) might merely reflect the fact that more studies are registered in the field, biasing databases. Importantly, a relevant number of hits associated with lymphoma, a type of cancer appearing at higher incidence among ME/CFS patients [137], is possibly due to associated immune dysfunctions of this disease.

Personalized medicine programs considering miRNome backgrounds may more adequately select effective treatments with reduced side effects. It is therefore envisioned that future improved therapeutic analysis, including pharmacogenomics and pharmacoepigenomics (precision medicine programs), will rely on complex software tools fed with large datasets. Further miRNA profiling studies including a larger number of samples are required to build on the scarce available FM and ME/CFS miRNome data. Since technical variability in miRNA qPCR replicates has been documented, with TaqMan overweighing qScript PCR [138], future studies should include repeated independent measures or either use alternative enzyme-free approaches such as NanoString [139].

In general, we have evaluated the effects of polypharmacy and miRNomes at individual levels, meaning that the information obtained here corresponds to the effects of a single drug on DE miRNAs or the impact of an individual miRNA on drug performance, but the effects of combined therapies on miRNA profiles or sets of DE miRNAs on drug response may not replicate or be additive of single events, highlighting the limitation of our study. In addition, most molecular data come from analysis of blood or other body fluid samples and more sparingly from non-cancerous solid tissues, limiting the validity of our results, as miRNA profiles are known to be tissue-restricted [140]. Drug assays are performed in either animal models or tumor cell lines leading to results that may not replicate in other systems, especially since many miRNAs are primate or human-specific [63,141].

In summary, as larger data sets become available to nurture databanks, biomarker discovery will be facilitated and personalized medicine programs will be refined, upgrading current diagnostic tools and clinical treatments. Drug–transcriptome interactions are key factors in either context, particularly in diseases subject to polypharmacy such as FM and ME/CFS.

5. Conclusions

The analysis presented here seem to support a potential impact of FM and ME/CFS polypharmacy in the discovery of miRNomes associating with these diseases. Based on this possibility, caution is advised when designing studies aimed at determining DE miRNAs linked to these diseases, including complete drug registry to permit stratified analysis.

FM and ME/CFS miRNomes may predispose patients to respond differently to a large variety of drug-based treatments, including those used for a large number of cancers, highlighting the importance of considering this epigenomic bias in refined personalized programs towards improving a patient's response to clinical treatments while minimizing toxicity. It is estimated that more sophisticated informatic tools will help with these predictions, but the paucity of molecular studies in FM and ME/CFS currently limits their development.

The results presented here are not definitive at this stage, but their observations should stimulate additional studies to further explore miRNA–drug interactions in the context of FM and ME/CFS.

Supplementary Materials: The following are available online at http://www.mdpi.com/1999-4923/11/3/126/s1. Table S1: PRISMA based search of FM and ME/CFS miRNA profiling studies; Table S2: FM and ME/CFS miRNomes SM2miR-based drug search; Table S3: FM and ME/CFS miRNomes Pharmaco-miR-based gene-drug associations and repoDB-drug-disease screening; Table S4: Effect of additional drugs, supplements and recreational drugs on FM and ME/CFS miRNomes and Table S5: Effect of hormones and other natural compounds on FM and ME/CFS miRNomes.

Author Contributions: Individual author contributions are as follows: conceptualization, E.O.; methodology, E.A.-P.; T.S.-F.; T.O.; L.N., and E.O.; software, formal analysis, and data curation, E.A.-P.; T.S.-F.; T.O.; L.N., and E.O.; writing—original draft preparation, E.O.; writing—review and editing, E.A.-P.; T.S.-F.; T.O.; L.N., and E.O.; funding acquisition, E.O.

Funding: This research was funded by Universidad Católica de Valencia San Vicente Mártir research grant 2018-270-01 to E.O.

Conflicts of Interest: The authors declare no conflict of interest. The funders had no role in the design of the study; in the collection, analyses, or interpretation of data; in the writing of the manuscript; or in the decision to publish the results.

Abbreviations

Fibromyalgia (FM); myalgic encephalomyelitis/chronic fatigue syndrome (ME/CFS); microRNAs (miRs); differentially expressed (DE); American College of Rheumatology (ACR); gene ontology (GO); Preferred Reporting Items for Systematic Reviews and Meta-Analyses criteria (PRISMA); International Classification of Diseases (ICD); non-steroidal anti-inflammatory drugs (NSAIDs); cognitive behaviour therapy (CBT); International Union of Pure and Applied Chemistry (IUPAC); concept unique identifiers (CUIs); national clinical trial (NCT); Common Data Elements (CDE); case report forms (CRFs); National Institute of Health (NIH); absorption, distribution, metabolism, and excretion (ADME); selective serotonin reuptake inhibitor (SSRI); serotonin-norepinephrine reuptake inhibitors (SNRIs); monoamine oxidase inhibitors (MAOIs).

References

1. Wolfe, F.; Smythe, H.A.; Yunus, M.B.; Bennett, R.M.; Bombardier, C.; Goldenberg, D.L.; Tugwell, P.; Campbell, S.M.; Abeles, M.; Clark, P.; et al. The American College of Rheumatology 1990 criteria for the classification of fibromyalgia. Report of the multicenter criteria committee. *Arthritis Rheum.* **1990**, *33*, 160–172. [CrossRef] [PubMed]
2. Wolfe, F.; Clauw, D.J.; Fitzcharles, M.A.; Goldenberg, D.L.; Katz, R.S.; Mease, P.; Russell, A.S.; Russell, I.J.; Winfield, J.B.; Yunus, M.B. The American College of Rheumatology preliminary diagnostic criteria for fibromyalgia and measurement of symptom severity. *Arthritis Care Res. (Hoboken)* **2010**, *62*, 600–610. [CrossRef]

3. Jahan, F.; Nanji, K.; Qidwai, W.; Qasim, R. Fibromyalgia syndrome: An overview of pathophysiology, diagnosis and management. *Oman Med. J.* **2012**, *27*, 192–195. [CrossRef] [PubMed]
4. Arnold, L.M.; Bennett, R.M.; Crofford, L.J.; Dean, L.E.; Clauw, D.J.; Goldenberg, D.L.; Fitzcharles, M.A.; Paiva, E.S.; Staud, R.; Sarzi-Puttini, P.; et al. AAPT Diagnostic Criteria for Fibromyalgia. *J. Pain.* **2018**. [CrossRef] [PubMed]
5. Abbi, B.; Natelson, B.-H. Is chronic fatigue syndrome the same illness as fibromyalgia: Evaluating the 'single syndrome' hypothesis. *QJM* **2013**, *106*, 3–9. [CrossRef]
6. Fukuda, K.; Straus, S.E.; Hickie, I.; Sharpe, M.C.; Dobbins, J.G.; Komaroff, A. The chronic fatigue syndrome: A comprehensive approach to its definition and study. International Chronic Fatigue Syndrome Study Group. *Ann. Intern. Med.* **1994**, *121*, 953–959. [CrossRef]
7. Carruthers, B.M.; Jain, A.K.; De Meirleir, K.L.; Peterson, D.L.; Klimas, N.G.; Lerner, A.; Bested, A.C.; Flor-Henry, P.; Joshi, P.; Powles, A.C.P.; et al. Myalgic encephalomyelitis/chronic fatigue syndrome: Clinical working case definition, diagnostic and treatment protocols. *J. Chronic Fatigue Syndr.* **2003**, *11*, 7–115. [CrossRef]
8. Carruthers, B.M.; van de Sande, M.I.; De Meirleir, K.L.; Klimas, N.G.; Broderick, G.; Mitchell, T.; Staines, D.; Powles, A.C.P.; Speight, N.; Vallings, R.; et al. Myalgic encephalomyelitis: International Consensus Criteria. *J. Intern. Med.* **2011**, *270*, 3273–3278. [CrossRef]
9. Committee on the Diagnostic Criteria for Myalgic Encephalomyelitis/Chronic Fatigue Syndrome, Board on the Health of Select Populations, Institute of Medicine. *Beyond Myalgic Encephalomyelitis/Chronic Fatigue Syndrome: Redefining an Illness*; National Academies Press (US): Washington, DC, USA, 2015. [PubMed]
10. Clayton, E.W. Beyond myalgic encephalomyelitis/chronic fatigue syndrome: A IOM report on redefining an illness. *JAMA* **2015**, *313*, 1101–1102. [CrossRef] [PubMed]
11. Jason, L.A.; McManimen, S.; Sunnquist, M.; Newton, J.L.; Strand, E.B. Clinical criteria versus a possible research case definition in chronic fatigue syndrome/myalgic encephalomyelitis. *Fatigue* **2017**, *5*, 89–102. [CrossRef]
12. Boerma, T.; Harrison, J.; Jakob, R.; Mathers, C.; Schmider, A.; Weber, S. Revising the ICD: Explaining the WHO approach. *Lancet* **2016**, *388*, 2476–2477. [CrossRef]
13. Jones, G.T.; Atzeni, F.; Beasley, M.; Flüß, E.; Sarzi-Puttini, P.; Macfarlane, G.J. The prevalence of fibromyalgia in the general population—A comparison of the American College of Rheumatology 1990, 2010 and modified 2010 classification criteria. *Arthritis Rheumatol.* **2014**. [CrossRef]
14. Cabo-Meseguer, A.; Cerdá-Olmedo, G.; Trillo-Mata, J.L. Fibromyalgia: Prevalence, epidemiologic profiles and economic costs. *Med. Clin. (Barc)* **2017**, *149*, 441–448. [CrossRef] [PubMed]
15. Reyes, M.; Nisenbaum, R.; Hoaglin, D.C.; Unger, E.R.; Emmons, C.; Randall, B.; Stewart, J.A.; Abbey, S.; Jones, J.F.; Gantz, N.; et al. Prevalence and incidence of chronic fatigue syndrome in Wichita, Kansas. *Arch. Intern. Med.* **2003**, *163*, 1530–1536. [CrossRef]
16. Jason, L.A.; Richman, J.A.; Rademaker, A.W.; Jordan, K.M.; Plioplys, A.V.; Taylor, R.R.; McCready, W.; Huang, C.-F.; Plioplys, S. A community-based study of chronic fatigue syndrome. *Arch. Intern. Med.* **1999**, *159*, 2129–2137. [CrossRef] [PubMed]
17. Estévez-López, F.; Castro-Marrero, J.; Wang, X.; Bakken, I.J.; Ivanovs, A.; Nacul, L.; Sepúlveda, N.; Strand, E.B.; Pheby, D.; Alegre, J.; et al. European Network on ME/CFS (EUROMENE). Prevalence and incidence of myalgic encephalomyelitis/chronic fatigue syndrome in Europe-the Euro-epiME study from the European network EUROMENE: A protocol for a systematic review. *BMJ Open.* **2018**, *8*, e020817. [CrossRef]
18. Crawley, E. Pediatric chronic fatigue syndrome: Current perspectives. *Pediatr. Health Med. Ther.* **2018**, *9*, 27–33. [CrossRef]
19. McManimen, S.L.; Jason, L.A. Post-Exertional Malaise in Patients with ME and CFS with Comorbid Fibromyalgia. *SRL Neurol. Neurosurg.* **2017**, *3*, 22–27.
20. Naschitz, J.E.; Rozenbaum, M.; Rosner, I.; Sabo, E.; Priselac, R.M.; Shaviv, N.; Ahdoot, A.; Ahdoot, M.; Gaitini, L.; Eldar, S.; et al. Cardiovascular response to upright tilt in fibromyalgia differs from that in chronic fatigue syndrome. *J. Rheumatol.* **2001**, *28*, 1356–1360.
21. Naschitz, J.E.; Slobodin, G.; Sharif, D.; Fields, M.; Isseroff, H.; Sabo, E.; Rosner, I. Electrocardiographic QT interval and cardiovascular reactivity in fibromyalgia differ from chronic fatigue syndrome. *Eur. J. Intern. Med.* **2008**, *19*, 187–191. [CrossRef]

22. Korszun, A.; Sackett-Lundeen, L.; Papadopoulos, E.; Brucksch, C.; Masterson, L.; Engelberg, N.C.; Haus, E.; Demitrack, M.A.; Crofford, L. Melatonin levels in women with fibromyalgia and chronic fatigue syndrome. *J. Rheumatol.* **1999**, *26*, 2675–2680. [PubMed]
23. Crofford, L.J.; Young, E.A.; Engleberg, N.C.; Korszun, A.; Brucksch, C.B.; McClure, L.A.; Brown, M.B.; Demitrack, M.A. Basal circadian and pulsatile ACTH and cortisol secretion in patients with fibromyalgia and/or chronic fatigue syndrome. *Brain Behav. Immun.* **2004**, *18*, 314–325. [CrossRef] [PubMed]
24. Light, A.R.; Bateman, L.; Jo, D.; Hughen, R.W.; Vanhaitsma, T.A.; White, A.T.; Light, K.C. Gene expression alterations at baseline and following moderate exercise in patients with Chronic Fatigue Syndrome and Fibromyalgia Syndrome. *J. Intern. Med.* **2012**, *271*, 64–81. [CrossRef] [PubMed]
25. Scheibenbogen, C.; Freitag, H.; Blanco, J.; Capelli, E.; Lacerda, E.; Authier, J.; Meeus, M.; Marrero, J.C.; Nora-Krukle, Z.; Oltra, E.; et al. The European ME/CFS Biomarker Landscape project: An initiative of the European network EUROMENE. *J. Transl. Med.* **2017**, *15*, 162. [CrossRef] [PubMed]
26. Xiao, C.; Rajewsky, K. MicroRNA control in the immune system: Basic principles. *Cell.* **2009**, *137*, 26–36, Erratum in: *Cell* **2009**, *137*, 380. [CrossRef] [PubMed]
27. Emde, A.; Hornstein, E. miRNAs at the interface of cellular stress and disease. *EMBO J.* **2014**, *33*, 1428–1437. [CrossRef] [PubMed]
28. Puik, J.R.; Meijer, L.L.; Le Large, T.Y.; Prado, M.M.; Frampton, A.E.; Kazemier, G.; Giovannetti, E. miRNA profiling for diagnosis, prognosis and stratification of cancer treatment in cholangiocarcinoma. *Pharmacogenomics* **2017**, *18*, 1343–1358. [CrossRef]
29. Filipowicz, W.; Bhattacharyya, S.N.; Sonenberg, N. Mechanisms of post-transcriptional regulation by microRNAs: Are the answers in sight? *Nat. Rev. Genet.* **2008**, *9*, 102–114. [CrossRef]
30. Vasudevan, S. Posttranscriptional upregulation by microRNAs. *Wiley Interdiscip. Rev. RNA* **2012**, *3*, 311–330. [CrossRef] [PubMed]
31. Xia, T.; Li, J.; Cheng, H.; Zhang, C.; Zhang, Y. Small-Molecule Regulators of MicroRNAs in Biomedicine. *Drug Dev. Res.* **2015**, *76*, 375–381. [CrossRef]
32. Cha, W.; Fan, R.; Miao, Y.; Zhou, Y.; Qin, C.; Shan, X.; Wan, X.; Cui, T. MicroRNAs as novel endogenous targets for regulation and therapeutic treatments. *MedChemComm* **2017**, *9*, 396–408. [CrossRef]
33. Melo, S.; Villanueva, A.; Moutinho, C.; Davalos, V.; Spizzo, R.; Ivan, C.; Rossi, S.; Setien, F.; Casanovas, O.; Simo-Riudalbas, L.; et al. Small molecule enoxacin is a cancer-specific growth inhibitor that acts by enhancing TAR RNA-binding protein 2-mediated microRNA processing. *Proc. Natl. Acad. Sci. USA* **2011**, *108*, 4394–4399, Erratum in: *Proc. Natl. Acad. Sci. USA* **2017**. [CrossRef]
34. Watashi, K.; Yeung, M.L.; Starost, M.F.; Hosmane, R.S.; Jeang, K.T. Identification of small molecules that suppress microRNA function and reverse tumorigenesis. *J. Biol. Chem.* **2010**, *285*, 24707–24716. [CrossRef]
35. Qiu, C.; Chen, G.; Cui, Q. Towards the understanding of microRNA and environmental factor interactions and their relationships to human diseases. *Sci. Rep.* **2012**, *2*, 318. [CrossRef]
36. Yang, Q.; Qiu, C.; Yang, J.; Wu, Q.; Cui, Q. miREnvironment database: Providing a bridge for microRNAs, environmental factors and phenotypes. *Bioinformatics* **2011**, *27*, 3329–3330. [CrossRef]
37. Luo, H.; Lan, W.; Chen, Q.; Wang, Z.; Liu, Z.; Yue, X.; Zhu, L. Inferring microRNA-environmental factor interactions based on multiple biological information fusion. *Molecules* **2018**, *23*, 2439. [CrossRef]
38. Peng, C.; Wang, Y.L. Editorial: MicroRNAs as new players in endocrinology. *Front Endocrinol. (Lausanne)* **2018**, *9*, 459. [CrossRef]
39. Smith-Vikos, T.; Slack, F.J. MicroRNAs and their roles in aging. *J. Cell Sci.* **2012**, *125 Pt 1*, 7–17. [CrossRef]
40. Rani, A.; O'Shea, A.; Ianov, L.; Cohen, R.A.; Woods, A.J.; Foster, T.C. miRNA in Circulating Microvesicles as Biomarkers for Age-Related Cognitive Decline. *Front Aging Neurosci.* **2017**, *9*, 323. [CrossRef]
41. Vienberg, S.; Geiger, J.; Madsen, S.; Dalgaard, L.T. MicroRNAs in metabolism. *Acta Physiol. (Oxf.)* **2017**, *219*, 346–361. [CrossRef]
42. Lopez, S.; Bermudez, B.; Montserrat-de la Paz, S.; Abia, R.; Muriana, F.J.G. A microRNA expression signature of the postprandial state in response to a high-saturated-fat challenge. *J. Nutr. Biochem.* **2018**, *57*, 45–55. [CrossRef] [PubMed]
43. Sapp, R.M.; Shill, D.D.; Roth, S.M.; Hagberg, J.M. Circulating microRNAs in acute and chronic exercise: More than mere biomarkers. *J. Appl. Physiol.* **2017**, *122*, 702–717. [CrossRef] [PubMed]
44. Häuser, W.; Welsch, P.; Klose, P.; Derry, S.; Straube, S.; Wiffen, P.J.; Moore, R. Pharmacological therapies for fibromyalgia in adults—An overview of Cochrane Reviews. *Cochrane Database Syst. Rev.* **2018**. [CrossRef]

45. Thorpe, J.; Shum, B.; Moore, R.A.; Wiffen, P.J.; Gilron, I. Combination pharmacotherapy for the treatment of fibromyalgia in adults. *Cochrane Database Syst. Rev.* **2018**. [CrossRef]
46. Collatz, A.; Johnston, S.C.; Staines, D.R.; Marshall-Gradisnik, S.M. A Systematic Review of Drug Therapies for Chronic Fatigue Syndrome/Myalgic Encephalomyelitis. *Clin. Ther.* **2016**, *38*, 1263–1271. [CrossRef]
47. Smith, M.E.; Haney, E.; McDonagh, M.; Pappas, M.; Daeges, M.; Wasson, N.; Fu, R.; Nelson, H.D. Treatment of Myalgic Encephalomyelitis/Chronic Fatigue Syndrome: A Systematic Review for a National Institutes of Health Pathways to Prevention Workshop. *Ann. Intern. Med.* **2015**, *162*, 841–850. [CrossRef] [PubMed]
48. Castro-Marrero, J.; Sáez-Francàs, N.; Santillo, D.; Alegre, J. Treatment and management of chronic fatigue syndrome/myalgic encephalomyelitis: All roads lead to Rome. *Br. J. Pharmacol.* **2017**, *174*, 345–369. [CrossRef]
49. NINDS. Common Data Elements. Available online: https://www.commondataelements.ninds.nih.gov/MECFS.aspx#tab=Data_Standards (accessed on 15 November 2018).
50. Rukov, J.L.; Wilentzik, R.; Jaffe, I.; Vinther, J.; Shomron, N. Pharmaco-miR: Linking microRNAs and drug effects. *Brief Bioinform.* **2014**, *15*, 648–659. [CrossRef]
51. Russo, F.; Di Bella, S.; Bonnici, V.; Laganà, A.; Rainaldi, G.; Pellegrini, M.; Pulvirenti, A.; Giugno, R.; Ferro, A.; et al. A knowledge base for the discovery of function, diagnostic potential and drug effects on cellular and extracellular miRNAs. *BMC Genom.* **2014**, *15* (Suppl. 3), S4. [CrossRef] [PubMed]
52. Zhang, G.; Nebert, D.W. Personalized medicine: Genetic risk prediction of drug response. *Pharmacol Ther.* **2017**, *175*, 75–90. [CrossRef]
53. Lloyd, R.A.; Hotham, E.; Hall, C.; Williams, M.; Suppiah, V. Pharmacogenomics and patient treatment parameters to opioid treatment in chronic pain: A focus on Morphine, Oxycodone, Tramadol, and Fentanyl. *Pain Med.* **2017**, *18*, 2369–2387. [CrossRef] [PubMed]
54. Rukov, J.L.; Shomron, N. MicroRNA pharmacogenomics: Post-transcriptional regulation of drug response. *Trends Mol. Med.* **2011**, *17*, 412–423. [CrossRef] [PubMed]
55. Bracco, L.; Kearsey, J. The relevance of alternative RNA splicing to pharmacogenomics. *Trends Biotechnol.* **2003**, *21*, 346–353. [CrossRef]
56. Ivanov, M.; Kacevska, M.; Ingelman-Sundberg, M. Epigenomics and interindividual differences in drug response. *Clin. Pharmacol. Ther.* **2012**, *92*, 727–736. [CrossRef] [PubMed]
57. Hu, H.; Baines, C. Recent insights into 3 underrecognized conditions: Myalgic encephalomyelitis-chronic fatigue syndrome, fibromyalgia, and environmental sensitivities-multiple chemical sensitivity. *Can. Fam. Physician* **2018**, *64*, 413–415.
58. Liberati, A.; Altman, D.G.; Tetzlaff, J.; Mulrow, C.; Gøtzsche, P.C.; Ioannidis, J.P.; Clarke, M.; Devereaux, P.J.; Kleijnen, J.; Moher, D. The PRISMA statement for reporting systematic reviews and meta-analyses of studies that evaluate health care interventions: Explanation and elaboration. *PLoS Med.* **2009**, *6*, e1000100. [CrossRef]
59. PubMed US National Library of Medicine National Institutes of Health. Available online: https://www.ncbi.nlm.nih.gov/pubmed (accessed on 10 October 2018).
60. FECYT. Fundación Española para la Ciencia y la Tecnología. Web of Science (WOS). Available online: https://www.fecyt.es/es/recurso/web-science (accessed on 10 October 2018).
61. Pubmed Labs. Bethesda (MD): National Library of Medicine (US), National Center for Biotechnology Information. 2018. Available online: https://www.ncbi.nlm.nih.gov/labs/pubmed/ (accessed on 10 October 2018).
62. Cochrane Library. Available online: https://www.cochranelibrary.com (accessed on 11 October 2018).
63. Kozomara, A.; Griffiths-Jones, S. miRBase: Integrating microRNA annotation and deep-sequencing data. *Nucleic Acids Res.* **2011**, *39*, D152–D157. [CrossRef]
64. Wishart, D.S.; Feunang, Y.D.; Guo, A.C.; Lo, E.J.; Marcu, A.; Grant, J.R.; Sajed, T.; Johnson, D.; Li, C.; Sayeeda, Z.; et al. DrugBank 5.0: A major update to the DrugBank database for 2018. *Nucleic Acids Res.* **2018**, *46*, D1074–D1082. [CrossRef]
65. Liu, X.; Wang, S.; Meng, F.; Wang, J.; Zhang, Y.; Dai, E.; Yu, X.; Li, X.; Jiang, W. SM2miR: A database of the experimentally validated small molecules' effects on microRNA expression. *Bioinformatics* **2013**, *29*, 409–411. [CrossRef]
66. Brown, A.S.; Patel, C.J. A standard database for drug repositioning. *Sci Data* **2017**, *4*, 170029. [CrossRef]
67. Bjersing, J.L.; Lundborg, C.; Bokarewa, M.I.; Mannerkorpi, K. Profile of cerebrospinal microRNAs in fibromyalgia. *PLoS ONE* **2013**, *8*, e78762. [CrossRef]

68. Bjersing, J.L.; Bokarewa, M.I.; Mannerkorpi, K. Profile of circulating microRNAs in fibromyalgia and their relation to symptom severity: An exploratory study. *Rheumatol. Int.* **2015**, *35*, 635–642. [CrossRef]
69. Cerdá-Olmedo, G.; Mena-Durán, A.V.; Monsalve, V.; Oltra, E. Identification of a microRNA signature for the diagnosis of fibromyalgia. *PLoS ONE* **2015**, *10*, e0121903. [CrossRef]
70. Masotti, A.; Baldassarre, A.; Guzzo, M.P.; Iannuccelli, C.; Barbato, C.; Di Franco, M. Circulating microRNA Profiles as Liquid Biopsies for the Characterization and Diagnosis of Fibromyalgia Syndrome. *Mol. Neurobiol.* **2017**, *54*, 7129–7136. [CrossRef]
71. Leinders, M.; Doppler, K.; Klein, T.; Deckart, M.; Rittner, H.; Sommer, C.; Üçeyler, N. Increased cutaneous miR-let-7d expression correlates with small nerve fiber pathology in patients with fibromyalgia syndrome. *Pain* **2016**, *157*, 2493–2503. [CrossRef]
72. Brenu, E.W.; Ashton, K.J.; van Driel, M.; Staines, D.R.; Peterson, D.; Atkinson, G.M.; Marshall-Gradisnik, S.M. Cytotoxic lymphocyte microRNAs as prospective biomarkers for Chronic Fatigue Syndrome/Myalgic Encephalomyelitis. *J. Affect Disord.* **2012**, *141*, 261–269. [CrossRef]
73. Brenu, E.W.; Ashton, K.J.; Batovska, J.; Staines, D.R.; Marshall-Gradisnik, S.M. High-throughput sequencing of plasma microRNA in chronic fatigue syndrome/myalgic encephalomyelitis. *PLoS ONE* **2014**, *9*, e102783. [CrossRef]
74. Petty, R.D.; McCarthy, N.E.; Le Dieu, R.; Kerr, J.R. MicroRNAs hsa-miR-99b, hsa-miR-330, hsa-miR-126 and hsa-miR-30c: Potential diagnostic biomarkers in Natural Killer (NK) cells of patients with Chronic Fatigue Syndrome (CFS)/Myalgic Encephalomyelitis (ME). *PLoS ONE* **2016**, *11*, e0150904. [CrossRef]
75. Baraniuk, J.N.; Shivapurkar, N. Exercise-induced changes in cerebrospinal fluid miRNAs in Gulf War Illness, Chronic Fatigue Syndrome and sedentary control subjects. *Sci. Rep.* **2017**, *7*, 15338, Erratum in: *Sci. Rep.* **2018**, *8*, 6455. [CrossRef]
76. Cording, M.; Derry, S.; Phillips, T.; Moore, R.A.; Wiffen, P.J. Milnacipran for pain in fibromyalgia in adults. *Cochrane Database Syst. Rev.* **2015**, CD008244. [CrossRef]
77. Lunn, M.P.; Hughes, R.A.; Wiffen, P.J. Duloxetine for treating painful neuropathy, chronic pain or fibromyalgia. *Cochrane Database Syst. Rev.* **2014**, CD007115. [CrossRef] [PubMed]
78. Walitt, B.; Urrútia, G.; Nishishinya, M.B.; Cantrell, S.E.; Häuser, W. Selective serotonin reuptake inhibitors for fibromyalgia syndrome. *Cochrane Database Syst. Rev.* **2015**, CD011735. [CrossRef]
79. Riera, R. Selective serotonin reuptake inhibitors for fibromyalgia syndrome. *Sao Paulo Med. J.* **2015**, *133*, 454. [CrossRef] [PubMed]
80. Moore, R.A.; Derry, S.; Aldington, D.; Cole, P.; Wiffen, P.J. Amitriptyline for neuropathic pain in adults. *Cochrane Database Syst. Rev.* **2015**, CD008242. [CrossRef] [PubMed]
81. Tort, S.; Urrútia, G.; Nishishinya, M.B.; Walitt, B. Monoamine oxidase inhibidors (MAOIs) for fibromyalgia syndrome. *Cochrane Database Syst. Rev.* **2012**, CD009807. [CrossRef]
82. Welsch, P.; Bernardy, K.; Derry, S.; Moore, R.A.; Häuser, W. Mirtazapine for fibromyalgia in adults. *Cochrane Database Syst. Rev.* **2018**, CD012708. [CrossRef]
83. Birse, F.; Derry, S.; Moore, R.A. Phenytoin for neuropathic pain and fibromyalgia in adults. *Cochrane Database Syst. Rev.* **2012**, CD009485. [CrossRef]
84. Gill, D.; Derry, S.; Wiffen, P.J.; Moore, R.A. Valproic acid and sodium valproate for neuropathic pain and fibromyalgia in adults. *Cochrane Database Syst. Rev.* **2011**, CD009183. [CrossRef]
85. Corrigan, R.; Derry, S.; Wiffen, P.J.; Moore, R.A. Clonazepam for neuropathic pain and fibromyalgia in adults. *Cochrane Database Syst. Rev.* **2012**, CD009486. [CrossRef] [PubMed]
86. Derry, S.; Cording, M.; Wiffen, P.J.; Law, S.; Phillips, T.; Moore, R.A. Pregabalin for pain in fibromyalgia in adults. *Cochrane Database Syst. Rev.* **2016**, CD011790. [CrossRef]
87. Wiffen, P.J.; Derry, S.; Bell, R.F.; Rice, A.S.; Tölle, T.R.; Phillips, T.; Moore, R.A. Gabapentin for chronic neuropathic pain in adults. *Cochrane Database Syst. Rev.* **2017**, CD007938. [CrossRef]
88. Hearn, L.; Derry, S.; Moore, R.A. Lacosamide for neuropathic pain and fibromyalgia in adults. *Cochrane Database Syst. Rev.* **2012**, CD009318. [CrossRef] [PubMed]
89. Wiffen, P.J.; Derry, S.; Lunn, M.P.; Moore, R.A. Topiramate for neuropathic pain and fibromyalgia in adults. *Cochrane Database Syst. Rev.* **2013**, CD008314. [CrossRef]
90. Walitt, B.; Klose, P.; Üçeyler, N.; Phillips, T.; Häuser, W. Antipsychotics for fibromyalgia in adults. *Cochrane Database Syst. Rev.* **2016**, CD011804. [CrossRef] [PubMed]

91. Walitt, B.; Klose, P.; Fitzcharles, M.A.; Phillips, T.; Häuser, W. Cannabinoids for fibromyalgia. *Cochrane Database Syst. Rev.* **2016**, CD011694. [CrossRef]
92. Derry, S.; Wiffen, P.J.; Häuser, W.; Mücke, M.; Tölle, T.R.; Bell, R.F.; Moore, R.A. Oral nonsteroidal anti-inflammatory drugs for fibromyalgia in adults. *Cochrane Database Syst. Rev.* **2017**, CD012332. [CrossRef] [PubMed]
93. Gaskell, H.; Moore, R.A.; Derry, S.; Stannard, C. Oxycodone for pain in fibromyalgia in adults. *Cochrane Database Syst. Rev.* **2016**, CD012329. [CrossRef] [PubMed]
94. Larun, L.; Brurberg, K.G.; Odgaard-Jensen, J.; Price, J.R. Exercise therapy for chronic fatigue syndrome. *Cochrane Database Syst. Rev.* **2017**, CD003200. [CrossRef]
95. Price, J.R.; Mitchell, E.; Tidy, E.; Hunot, V. Cognitive behaviour therapy for chronic fatigue syndrome in adults. *Cochrane Database Syst. Rev.* **2008**, CD001027. [CrossRef]
96. Adams, D.; Wu, T.; Yang, X.; Tai, S.; Vohra, S. Traditional Chinese medicinal herbs for the treatment of idiopathic chronic fatigue and chronic fatigue syndrome. *Cochrane Database Syst. Rev.* **2009**, CD006348. [CrossRef]
97. Blockmans, D.; Persoons, P. Long-term methylphenidate intake in chronic fatigue syndrome. *Acta Clin. Belg.* **2016**, *71*, 407–414. [CrossRef]
98. Nilsson, M.K.L.; Zachrisson, O.; Gottfries, C.G.; Matousek, M.; Peilot, B.; Forsmark, S.; Schuit, R.C.; Carlsson, M.L.; Kloberg, A.; Carlsson, A. A randomised controlled trial of the monoaminergic stabiliser (-)-OSU6162 in treatment of myalgic encephalomyelitis/chronic fatigue syndrome. *Acta Neuropsychiatr.* **2018**, *30*, 148–157. [CrossRef]
99. Proal, A.D.; Albert, P.J.; Marshall, T.G.; Blaney, G.P.; Lindseth, I.A. Immunostimulation in the treatment for chronic fatigue syndrome/myalgic encephalomyelitis. *Immunol. Res.* **2013**, *56*, 398–412. [CrossRef]
100. Plioplys, A.V.; Plioplys, S. Amantadine and L-carnitine treatment of Chronic Fatigue Syndrome. *Neuropsychobiology* **1997**, *35*, 16–23. [CrossRef]
101. Castro-Marrero, J.; Cordero, M.D.; Segundo, M.J.; Sáez-Francàs, N.; Calvo, N.; Román-Malo, L.; Aliste, L.; Fernández de Sevilla, T.; Alegre, J. Does oral coenzyme Q10 plus NADH supplementation improve fatigue and biochemical parameters in chronic fatigue syndrome? *Antioxid. Redox Signal.* **2015**, *22*, 679–685. [CrossRef]
102. Blockmans, D.; Persoons, P.; Van Houdenhove, B.; Lejeune, M.; Bobbaers, H. Combination therapy with hydrocortisone and fludrocortisone does not improve symptoms in chronic fatigue syndrome: A randomized, placebo-controlled, double-blind, crossover study. *Am. J. Med.* **2003**, *114*, 736–741. [CrossRef]
103. Strayer, D.R.; Carter, W.A.; Stouch, B.C.; Stevens, S.R.; Bateman, L.; Cimoch, P.J.; Lapp, C.W.; Peterson, D.L. Chronic Fatigue Syndrome AMP-516 Study Group; Mitchell WM. A double-blind, placebo-controlled, randomized, clinical trial of the TLR-3 agonist rintatolimod in severe cases of chronic fatigue syndrome. *PLoS ONE* **2012**, *7*, e31334. [CrossRef]
104. Comhaire, F. Treating patients suffering from myalgic encephalopathy/chronic fatigue syndrome (ME/CFS) with sodium dichloroacetate: An open-label, proof-of-principle pilot trial. *Med. Hypotheses.* **2018**, *114*, 454–458. [CrossRef]
105. Ostojic, S.M.; Stojanovic, M.; Drid, P.; Hoffman, J.R.; Sekulic, D.; Zenic, N. Supplementation with Guanidinoacetic Acid in Women with Chronic Fatigue Syndrome. *Nutrients* **2016**, *8*, 72. [CrossRef]
106. Gil-Zamorano, J.; Martin, R.; Daimiel, L.; Richardson, K.; Giordano, E.; Nicod, N.; García-Carrasco, B.; Soares, S.M.; Iglesias-Gutiérrez, E.; Lasunción, M.A.; et al. Docosahexaenoic acid modulates the enterocyte Caco-2 cell expression of microRNAs involved in lipid metabolism. *J. Nutr.* **2014**, *144*, 575–585. [CrossRef] [PubMed]
107. Rodrigues, A.C.; Li, X.; Radecki, L.; Pan, Y.Z.; Winter, J.C.; Huang, M.; Yu, A.M. MicroRNA expression is differentially altered by xenobiotic drugs in different human cell lines. *Biopharm. Drug. Dispos.* **2011**, *32*, 355–367. [CrossRef]
108. Rainer, J.; Ploner, C.; Jesacher, S.; Ploner, A.; Eduardoff, M.; Mansha, M.; Wasim MPanzer-Grümayer, R.; Trajanoski, Z.; Niederegger, H.; et al. Glucocorticoid-regulated microRNAs and mirtrons in acute lymphoblastic leukemia. *Leukemia* **2009**, *23*, 746–752. [CrossRef] [PubMed]
109. Lu, S.; Mukkada, V.A.; Mangray, S.; Cleveland, K.; Shillingford, N.; Schorl, C.; Brodsky, A.S.; Resnick, M.B. MicroRNA profiling in mucosal biopsies of eosinophilic esophagitis patients pre and post treatment with steroids and relationship with mRNA targets. *PLoS ONE* **2012**, *7*, e40676. [CrossRef] [PubMed]

110. Dave, R.S.; Khalili, K. Morphine treatment of human monocyte-derived macrophages induces differential miRNA and protein expression: Impact on inflammation and oxidative stress in the central nervous system. *J. Cell Biochem.* **2010**, *110*, 834–845. [CrossRef]
111. Fayyad-Kazan, H.; Rouas, R.; Merimi, M.; El Zein, N.; Lewalle, P.; Jebbawi, F.; Mourtada, M.; Badran, H.; Ezzeddine, M.; Salaun, B.; et al. Valproate treatment of human cord blood CD4-positive effector T cells confers on them the molecular profile (microRNA signature and FOXP3 expression) of natural regulatory CD4-positive cells through inhibition of histone deacetylase. *J. Biol. Chem.* **2010**, *285*, 2048–2191. [CrossRef]
112. Lukkahatai, N.; Walitt, B.; Deandrés-Galiana, E.J.; Fernández-Martínez, J.L.; Saligan, L.N. A predictive algorithm to identify genes that discriminate individuals with fibromyalgia syndrome diagnosis from healthy controls. *J. Pain Res.* **2018**, *11*, 2981–2990. [CrossRef]
113. Ameling, S.; Kacprowski, T.; Chilukoti, R.K.; Malsch, C.; Liebscher, V.; Suhre, K.; Pietzner, M.; Friedrich, N.; Homuth, G.; Hammer, E.; et al. Associations of circulating plasma microRNAs with age, body mass index and sex in a population-based study. *BMC Med. Genom.* **2015**, *8*, 61. [CrossRef]
114. Peng, X.; Li, W.; Yuan, L.; Mehta, R.G.; Kopelovich, L.; McCormick, D.L. Inhibition of proliferation and induction of autophagy by atorvastatin in PC3 prostate cancer cells correlate with downregulation of Bcl2 and upregulation of miR-182 and p21. *PLoS ONE* **2013**, *8*, e70442. [CrossRef]
115. Minami, Y.; Satoh, M.; Maesawa, C.; Takahashi, Y.; Tabuchi, T.; Itoh, T.; Nakamura, M. Effect of atorvastatin on microRNA 221/222 expression in endothelial progenitor cells obtained from patients with coronary artery disease. *Eur. J. Clin. Investig.* **2009**, *39*, 359–367. [CrossRef]
116. Saito, Y.; Suzuki, H.; Imaeda, H.; Matsuzaki, J.; Hirata, K.; Tsugawa, H.; Hibino, S.; Kanai, Y.; Saito, H.; Hibi, T. The tumor suppressor microRNA-29c is downregulated and restored by celecoxib in human gastric cancer cells. *Int. J. Cancer* **2013**, *132*, 1751–1760. [CrossRef]
117. Li, Y.; Kong, D.; Ahmad, A.; Bao, B.; Dyson, G.; Sarkar, F.H. Epigenetic deregulation of miR-29a and miR-1256 by isoflavone contributes to the inhibition of prostate cancer cell growth and invasion. *Epigenetics* **2012**, *7*, 940–949. [CrossRef] [PubMed]
118. Li, Y.; Kong, D.; Ahmad, A.; Bao, B.; Sarkar, F.H. Targeting bone remodeling by isoflavone and 3,3′-diindolylmethane in the context of prostate cancer bone metastasis. *PLoS ONE* **2012**, *7*, e33011. [CrossRef] [PubMed]
119. Bao, B.; Wang, Z.; Ali, S.; Ahmad, A.; Azmi, A.S.; Sarkar, S.H.; Banerjee, S.; Kong, D.; Li, Y.; Thaku, S.; et al. Metformin inhibits cell proliferation, migration and invasion by attenuating CSC function mediated by deregulating miRNAs in pancreatic cancer cells. *Cancer Prev. Res. (Phila)* **2012**, *5*, 355–364. [CrossRef]
120. Chandrasekar, V.; Dreyer, J.L. microRNAs miR-124, let-7d and miR-181a regulate cocaine-induced plasticity. *Mol. Cell Neurosci.* **2009**, *42*, 350–362. [CrossRef]
121. Mantri, C.K.; Mantri, J.V.; Pandhare, J.; Dash, C. Methamphetamine inhibits HIV-1 replication in CD4+ T cells by modulating anti-HIV-1 miRNA expression. *Am. J. Pathol.* **2014**, *184*, 92–100. [CrossRef]
122. Guo, Y.; Chen, Y.; Carreon, S.; Qiang, M. Chronic intermittent ethanol exposure and its removal induce a different miRNA expression pattern in primary cortical neuronal cultures. *Alcohol Clin. Exp. Res.* **2012**, *36*, 1058–1066. [CrossRef]
123. Shin, V.Y.; Jin, H.; Ng, E.K.; Cheng, A.S.; Chong, W.W.; Wong, C.Y.; Leung, W.K.; Sung, J.J.Y.; Chu, K.-M. NF-κB targets miR-16 and miR-21 in gastric cancer: Involvement of prostaglandin E receptors. *Carcinogenesis* **2011**, *32*, 240–245. [CrossRef] [PubMed]
124. Zhang, Y.; Pan, T.; Zhong, X.; Cheng, C. Nicotine upregulates microRNA-21 and promotes TGF-β-dependent epithelial-mesenchymal transition of esophageal cancer cells. *Tumour Biol.* **2014**, *35*, 7063–7072. [CrossRef]
125. Maccani, M.A.; Avissar-Whiting, M.; Banister, C.E.; McGonnigal, B.; Padbury, J.F.; Marsit, C.J. Maternal cigarette smoking during pregnancy is associated with downregulation of miR-16, miR-21, and miR-146a in the placenta. *Epigenetics* **2010**, *5*, 583–589. [CrossRef]
126. Bhat-Nakshatri, P.; Wang, G.; Collins, N.R.; Thomson, M.J.; Geistlinger, T.R.; Carroll, J.S.; Brown, M.; Hammond, S.; Srour, E.F.; Liu, Y.; et al. Estradiol-regulated microRNAs control estradiol response in breast cancer cells. *Nucleic Acids Res.* **2009**, *37*, 4850–4861. [CrossRef]
127. Tilghman, S.L.; Bratton, M.R.; Segar, H.C.; Martin, E.C.; Rhodes, L.V.; Li, M.; McLachlan, J.A.; Wiese, T.E.; Nephew, K.P.; Burow, M.E. Endocrine disruptor regulation of microRNA expression in breast carcinoma cells. *PLoS ONE* **2012**, *7*, e32754. [CrossRef]

128. Wickramasinghe, N.S.; Manavalan, T.T.; Dougherty, S.M.; Riggs, K.A.; Li, Y.; Klinge, C.M. Estradiol downregulates miR-21 expression and increases miR-21 target gene expression in MCF-7 breast cancer cells. *Nucleic Acids Res.* **2009**, *37*, 2584–2595. [CrossRef]
129. Waltering, K.K.; Porkka, K.P.; Jalava, S.E.; Urbanucci, A.; Kohonen, P.J.; Latonen, L.M.; Kallioniemi, O.P.; Jenster, G.; Visakorpi, T. Androgen regulation of micro-RNAs in prostate cancer. *Prostate* **2011**, *71*, 604–614. [CrossRef] [PubMed]
130. Yu, X.; Zhang, X.; Dhakal, I.B.; Beggs, M.; Kadlubar, S.; Luo, D. Induction of cell proliferation and survival genes by estradiol-repressed microRNAs in breast cancer cells. *BMC Cancer* **2012**, *12*, 29. [CrossRef] [PubMed]
131. Feng, B.; Cao, Y.; Chen, S.; Ruiz, M.; Chakrabarti, S. miRNA-1 regulates endothelin-1 in diabetes. *Life Sci.* **2014**, *98*, 18–23. [CrossRef] [PubMed]
132. Du, B.; Ma, L.M.; Huang, M.B.; Zhou, H.; Huang, H.L.; Shao, P.; Chen, Y.Q.; Qu, L.H. High glucose down-regulates miR-29a to increase collagen IV production in HK-2 cells. *FEBS Lett.* **2010**, *584*, 811–816. [CrossRef] [PubMed]
133. Bae, J.; Won, M.; Kim, D.Y.; Kim, J.H.; Kim, Y.M.; Kim, Y.T.; Nam, J.H.; Suh, D.S. Identification of differentially expressed microRNAs in endometrial cancer cells after progesterone treatment. *Int. J. Gynecol. Cancer* **2012**, *22*, 561–565. [CrossRef] [PubMed]
134. Cochrane, D.R.; Jacobsen, B.M.; Connaghan, K.D.; Howe, E.N.; Bain, D.L.; Richer, J.K. Progestin regulated miRNAs that mediate progesterone receptor action in breast cancer. *Mol. Cell Endocrinol.* **2012**, *355*, 15–24. [CrossRef]
135. Wang, W.L.; Chatterjee, N.; Chittur, S.V.; Welsh, J.; Tenniswood, M.P. Effects of 1α,25 dihydroxyvitamin D3 and testosterone on miRNA and mRNA expression in LNCaP cells. *Mol. Cancer* **2011**, *10*, 58. [CrossRef] [PubMed]
136. Jorde, R.; Svartberg, J.; Joakimsen, R.M.; Coucheron, D.H. Plasma profile of microRNA after supplementation with high doses of vitamin D3 for 12 months. *BMC Res. Notes* **2012**, *5*, 245. [CrossRef] [PubMed]
137. Chang, C.M.; Warren, J.L.; Engels, E.A. Chronic fatigue syndrome and subsequent risk of cancer among elderly US adults. *Cancer* **2012**, *118*, 5929–5936. [CrossRef] [PubMed]
138. Daniels, S.I.; Sillé, F.C.; Goldbaum, A.; Yee, B.; Key, E.F.; Zhang, L.; Smith, M.T.; Thomas, R. Improving power to detect changes in blood miRNA expression by accounting for sources of variability in experimental designs. *Cancer Epidemiol. Biomarkers Prev.* **2014**, *23*, 2658–2666. [CrossRef] [PubMed]
139. Foye, C.; Yan, I.K.; David, W.; Shukla, N.; Habboush, Y.; Chase, L.; Smith, M.T.; Thomas, R. Comparison of miRNA quantitation by Nanostring in serum and plasma samples. *PLoS ONE* **2017**, *12*, e0189165. [CrossRef] [PubMed]
140. Ludwig, N.; Leidinger, P.; Becker, K.; Backes, C.; Fehlmann, T.; Pallasch, C.; Rheinheimer, S.; Meder, B.; Stähler, C.; Meese, E.; et al. Distribution of miRNA expression across human tissues. *Nucleic Acids Res.* **2016**, *44*, 3865–3877. [CrossRef] [PubMed]
141. Awan, H.M.; Shah, A.; Rashid, F.; Shan, G. Primate-specific Long Non-coding RNAs and MicroRNAs. *Genom. Proteom. Bioinform.* **2017**, *15*, 1871–1895. [CrossRef]

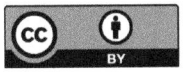

© 2019 by the authors. Licensee MDPI, Basel, Switzerland. This article is an open access article distributed under the terms and conditions of the Creative Commons Attribution (CC BY) license (http://creativecommons.org/licenses/by/4.0/).

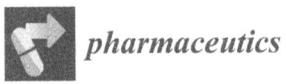

Review

DPYD and Fluorouracil-Based Chemotherapy: Mini Review and Case Report

Theodore J. Wigle [1,2], Elena V. Tsvetkova [3], Stephen A. Welch [3] and Richard B. Kim [1,2,*]

1. Department of Physiology and Pharmacology, Schulich School of Medicine & Dentistry, Western University, London, ON N6A 3K7, Canada; twigle@uwo.ca
2. Division of Clinical Pharmacology, Department of Medicine, Schulich School of Medicine & Dentistry, Western University, London, ON N6A 3K7, Canada
3. Division of Medical Oncology, Department of Oncology, Schulich School of Medicine & Dentistry, Western University, London, ON N6A 3K7, Canada; elena.tsvetkova@lhsc.on.ca (E.V.T.); stephen.welch@lhsc.on.ca (S.A.W.)
* Correspondence: Richard.Kim@lhsc.on.ca; Tel.: +519-685-8500 (ext. 33553); Fax: +519-663-3090

Received: 2 April 2019; Accepted: 23 April 2019; Published: 1 May 2019

Abstract: 5-Fluorouracil remains a foundational component of chemotherapy for solid tumour malignancies. While considered a generally safe and effective chemotherapeutic, 5-fluorouracil has demonstrated severe adverse event rates of up to 30%. Understanding the pharmacokinetics of 5-fluorouracil can improve the precision medicine approaches to this therapy. A single enzyme, dihydropyrimidine dehydrogenase (DPD), mediates 80% of 5-fluorouracil elimination, through hepatic metabolism. Importantly, it has been known for over 30-years that adverse events during 5-fluorouracil therapy are linked to high systemic exposure, and to those patients who exhibit DPD deficiency. To date, pre-treatment screening for DPD deficiency in patients with planned 5-fluorouracil-based therapy is not a standard of care. Here we provide a focused review of 5-fluorouracil metabolism, and the efforts to improve predictive dosing through screening for DPD deficiency. We also outline the history of key discoveries relating to DPD deficiency and include relevant information on the potential benefit of therapeutic drug monitoring of 5-fluorouracil. Finally, we present a brief case report that highlights a limitation of pharmacogenetics, where we carried out therapeutic drug monitoring of 5-fluorouracil in an orthotopic liver transplant recipient. This case supports the development of robust multimodality precision medicine services, capable of accommodating complex clinical dilemmas.

Keywords: dihydropyrimidine dehydrogenase; *DPYD*; 5-fluorouracil; fluoropyrimidine; therapeutic drug monitoring; orthotopic liver transplant

---

1. Introduction to Fluoropyrimidines

5-fluorouracil (5-FU) has remained an important antineoplastic agent since the first description of the fluoropyrimidine class in 1957, and approval for testing in humans in 1962 [1,2]. Fluoropyrimidines, including 5-fluorouracil and its oral pre-prodrug capecitabine, serve as core components in the treatment of colorectal, pancreatic, gastric, breast, head and neck cancers [2–4]. However, the use of fluoropyrimidines carries an unfortunate risk of severe adverse events (AEs) of up to 30% [5,6]. Common AEs observed with fluoropyrimidine chemotherapies include non-bloody diarrhea, mucosal ulceration, immune suppression, and a painful skin condition known as hand-foot syndrome. Through optimizing the delivery methods, dosing schedules, and concomitant antineoplastic agents, a number of modern combination regimens with a fluoropyrimidine backbone have emerged including FOLFOX, FOLFIRINOX, CAPOX, and FLOT. Nevertheless, clinical trials using fluoropyrimidine-based chemotherapies continue to show severe AE rates up to 23% [7–10]. Accordingly, delineating the genetic and non-genetic determinants of fluoropyrimidine metabolism and efficacy, is essential to the implementation of precision medicine approaches for fluoropyrimidine-based chemotherapy.

Fluoropyrimidines are an antimetabolite class of chemotherapeutic. As antimetabolites, they target replicating cells. Fluoropyrimidines act primarily through conversion of 5-FU to fluoro-deoxyuridine monophosphate (FdUMP). FdUMP acts as an irreversible inhibitor of the thymidylate synthase enzyme this is stabilized by forming a ternary complex with the reduced folate species methylene-tetrahydrofolate. Thymidylate synthase plays an important role in regulating the nucleotide pool by converting deoxyuridine monophosphate (dUMP) to deoxythymidine monoposhpate (dTMP), providing this pyrimidine building block for DNA synthesis. When thymidylate synthase is inhibited, the buildup of dUMP nucleotides leads to their incorporation into DNA, which overwhelms DNA repair mechanisms and eventually leads to cell-death. Thymidylate synthase inhibition is the major canonical mechanism of action of fluoropyrimidines, in addition they can exert antineoplastic effects through at least two additional pathways. First, active fluoropyrimidine (FdUMP) can also be incorrectly incorporated into DNA in place of dTMP leading to both single strand and double strand breaks. The resultant DNA damage induces cell cycle arrest and death. Second, 5-FU is converted to fluorouridine triphosphate (FUTP) and incorrectly incorporated in RNA. The combination of RNA damage, DNA damage, and inhibition of cell cycle provide the mechanistic basis for the antineoplastic effects of fluoropyrimidines (Figure 1, for review see [11]). The antimetabolite properties of 5-FU support the antineoplastic effects, but a lack of specificity underpins the AEs seen with this therapy. The classic fluoropyrimidine toxicities occur in rapidly regenerating tissues such as the mucosal membranes, skin, and bone marrow. Therefore, the effective but nonspecific nature of fluoropyrimidines is the likely culprit for numerous AEs. Appropriately balancing the therapeutic benefit vs. toxicity of this class of antineoplastic drugs has proved to be a major challenge, requiring a detailed understanding of the pharmacology.

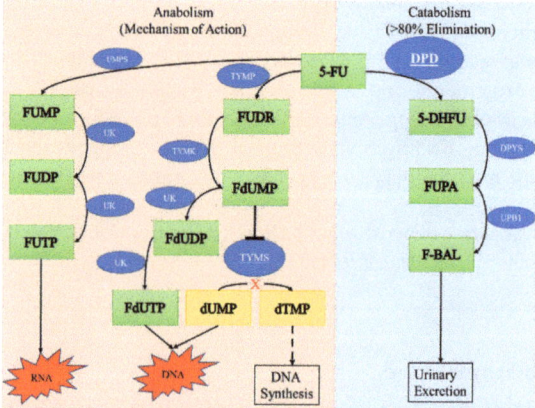

Figure 1. A simplified metabolism of 5-fluorouracil (5-FU). Thymidylate phosphorylase (TYMP) generates fluorouridine (FUDR), which is converted to Fluoro-deoxyuridine monophosphate (FdUMP) by thymidylate kinase (TYMK). FdUMP inhibits thymidylate synthase (TYMS) causing an imbalance of deoxyuridine monophosphate (dUMP) and deoxythymidine monophosphate (dTMP). Incorporation of dUMP into DNA causes damage and leads to cell death. 5-FU is converted to fluorouridine monophosphate (FUMP) by uridine monophosphate synthetase (UMPS) with further phosphorylation by uridine kinase (UK). Incorporation of fluorinated nucleotides (FUTP or FdUMP) into both RNA and DNA respectively leads to cell death. Inactivation of 5-FU occurs through dihydropyrimidine dehydrogenase (DPD) conversion to 5-dihydrofluorouracil (5-DHFU). Dihydropyrmidinase (DPYS) catalyzes the creation of fluoro-beta-ureidopropionate (FUPA) and beta-ureidopropionase (UPB1) activity culminates in urinary elimination of fluoro-beta-alanine (FBAL).

2. Metabolism and Clearance of 5-FU

Understanding the metabolism of 5-FU took nearly 35 years to flesh out. Heidelberger and colleagues knew from early stages that 5-FU was rapidly metabolized [1,12], and from human pharmacologic studies we now know that 5-FU has a half-life ranging from 8 to 20 min, varying with route of administration [13]. Heidelberger and colleagues were unable to completely parse out the different effects of the catabolic and anabolic pathways on 5-FU metabolism. The anabolic pathway is directly related to the fluoropyrimidine mechanism of action through generation of FdUMP, and initially it was believed this pathway was also responsible for the elimination of 5-FU. However, the earliest studies were limited by the sensitivity of available analytical assays and the rapid degradation of 5-FU metabolites, thereby producing conflicting results [14]. With the development of a new high-pressure liquid chromatography technique, researchers were then able to accurately measure 5-FU metabolites [15]. These studies confirmed dihydropyrimidine dehydrogenase (DPD; EC 1.3.1.2, encoded by *DPYD*) to be the first and rate-limiting enzyme in the catabolic cascade of 5-FU, but did not establish the clinical significance of these findings [15,16]. The pivotal role of DPD activity in fluoropyrimidine catabolism and the implications of DPD deficiency for fluoropyrimidine-related AEs were identified in the clinical literature shortly thereafter. The first case report presented a patient treated with 5-FU who had oral ulceration, neurotoxicity, and severe myelosuppression leading to hospitalization. This patient, and a first degree relative, were found to have familial pyrimidinemia and pyrimidinuria—characterized by elevated uracil and thymine in both blood and urine [17]. This first case report provided the initial link between an inborn error of metabolism and fluoropyrimidine-related AEs. While Tuchman et al. were not able to directly assess DPD activity in this patient, a key corollary of their findings is the knowledge that the endogenous function of DPD is the metabolism of both uracil and thymine [18]. Within two years, a pharmacokinetic analysis of 5-FU metabolism in cancer patients demonstrated that the primary process of 5-FU elimination occurred through DPD-dependent catabolism. This study found that the catabolic pathway is responsible for the elimination of over 80% of systemic 5-FU, with 95% of the final metabolite being eliminated in the urine (Figure 1) [19]. Following this confirmation of DPD as the key metabolic enzyme responsible for 5-FU elimination, Diasio et al., published a case report of severe fluoropyrimidine induced neurotoxicity in a female patient with familial DPD deficiency. This patient also developed profound neutropenia requiring hospitalization [20]. There were a number of case reports that followed this publication and supported the link between DPD deficiency and fluoropyrimidine toxicities [21–23]. Cloning of *DPYD* set the stage for identifying the molecular basis of this hereditary defect [24]. It was identified that the most common familial DPD deficiency was linked to a defect in processing of the DPD precursor mRNA, namely an exon skipping variant resulting in the loss of 165 nucleotides from the fully spliced mRNA [25]. However, the first paper to identify the mechanistic cause of the deficiency failed to identify the point mutation responsible for this effect. The first DNA sequence level identification of this *DPYD* variant was published one year later by two different groups one-month apart, they presented the same findings in two unrelated families. They identified a single nucleotide polymorphism (SNP) within *DPYD* that introduced a new splice site, which resulted in exon 14 skipping. The resultant DPD protein has complete loss of function [26,27]. This variant is now commonly referred to as *DPYD**2A (also known as: c.1905+1G>A or rs3918290) and plays a major role in driving research of the pharmacogenetic influences of fluoropyrimidine-related AEs. The *DPYD**2A allele is present in approximately 2% of Caucasians of European descent. Heterozygous carriers of this allele exhibit a 50% reduction of DPD activity. While very rare (~1:1000), homozygous *DPYD**2A patients demonstrate complete DPD deficiency [28]. Complete DPD deficiency can remain undetected in otherwise healthy individuals. Unfortunately, the consequences of unrecognized DPD deficiency during fluoropyrimidine chemotherapy can be lethal. To this day there continue to be case reports of the lethal consequences of fluoropyrimidine chemotherapy in completely DPD deficient patients [29,30]. This disquieting reality of fluoropyrimidine chemotherapy has led to many efforts to understand and implement pre-treatment screening for DPD deficiency.

3. Understanding DPD Activity

Given the association between DPD deficiency and severe fluoropyrimidine-related AEs, there is a requirement to understand the baseline variation in DPD activity. It was first identified that DPD activity follows a circadian rhythm: DPD activity peaks near midnight, with trough DPD activity in the early afternoon [31]. This curious discovery was linked to variation in the systemic 5-FU exposure during prolonged continuous infusions, with a change in systemic 5-FU levels from peak to trough of 2.3-fold during a prolonged 5-day course [32]. However, there is little agreement on the value of predicting this chronological rhythm, or the rhythm's physiologic significance [33–35]. In general, it is now understood that hepatic DPD activity is responsible for the majority of 5-FU clearance [13], and on a population level follows a normal distribution [36]. Lu et al., quantified DPD activity from frozen liver sections using a radiolabeled biochemical assay. The authors showed a strong correlation between DPD protein level expression and enzyme activity [36]. Alternative attempts to quantify DPD activity sought to correlate mRNA expression with DPD activity. Initial studies showed a strong correlation between DPD mRNA and DPD activity in *DPYD* wild-type individuals [37,38]. However, eventually, this line of study was abandoned as it was realized that increased expression of mRNA would not compensate for a functionally inactive enzyme. Therefore, DPD mRNA levels would not be reflective of global DPD activity or provide sufficient understanding of 5-FU elimination. Given DPD is widely expressed, researchers have sought to understand population variation in DPD activity through the study of peripheral blood mononuclear cells (PBMCs). There was a significant but limited correlation between PBMC DPD activity and hepatocyte DPD activity $R^2 < 0.6$ [39,40], which makes interpreting the relevance of PBMC DPD activity studies more challenging. In addition, the correlation between PBMC DPD activity and systemic 5-FU clearance demonstrated even weaker associations than between PBMC DPD activity and hepatic DPD activity [39,41]. Finally, PBMC DPD activity demonstrated greater variation than was found in studies of hepatic DPD activity, where PBMC DPD activity demonstrated variation of activity between 8- to 21-fold depending on the study [41–44]. Therefore, the utility of PBMC DPD activity in characterizing the population variation of endogenous DPD activity remains difficult to interpret. In addition, DPD activity is known to differ between healthy and malignant tissues of the same organ [45]. The discrepancies between DPD activity in malignant neoplasms, inflamed mucosa and healthy tissue has led to some debate regarding which tissue type is of greatest importance for DPD activity during fluoropyrimidine chemotherapy. One branch of research chooses to focus on DPD activity in the malignant cells as a predictor of fluoropyrimidine efficacy [37,38,46]. The complimentary studies aim to interrogate global DPD activity, as a more relevant variable in the systemic clearance of 5-FU and therefore fluoropyrimidine-related AEs [47].

4. Evolution of DPD Activity Testing

The primary goal for pre-treatment DPD activity assessment is to accurately predict patients with deficient clearance of fluoropyrimidines who are at an increased risk for severe AEs. Given the predominantly hepatic catabolism of systemic fluoropyrimidines, pre-treatment testing needs to approximate the baseline status of hepatic metabolism. While liver biopsy for DPD activity determination has been performed experimentally [36] it is not a reasonable approach for scaling as a pre-treatment screening tool. Therefore, peripheral measurement of DPD activity has been pursued as a surrogate for hepatic metabolism. Most early studies focused on biochemical assays of DPD activity in PBMCs. The technique provided a minimally invasive method of directly assessing basal DPD activity, with high sensitivity [48]. However, this method has not garnered wide spread support due to several limitations. First as previously noted, there was a poor correlation between PBMC DPD activity, hepatic DPD activity and systemic 5-FU clearance casting doubt on the clinical relevance of this method [49]. As well incorporating this technique within clinical care is cumbersome for testing laboratories and requires significant infrastructure costs [48]. Therefore, alternative methods for assessing DPD activity have been developed. Endogenous metabolites of DPD activity could provide a physiologically relevant biomarker of DPD activity. With this premise in mind a number of studies have attempted to characterize systemic uracil and dihydrouracil concentrations as endogenous markers of DPD activity [33,35,50–61]. DPD converts uracil to dihydrouracil, thus the ratio of product: metabolite could serve as a marker of basal enzyme activity [18,62]. The techniques employed in testing this approach have evolved from labor intensive techniques such as metabolite challenges [55,61], to the pragmatic direct measurement of baseline plasma uracil concentration [59]. The assessment of pre-treatment uracil and dihydrouracil in plasma samples has produced promising results. These tests do not require as extensive an infrastructure and demonstrate predictive value for fluoropyrimidine-related AEs [53,60,63,64]. However, pre-treatment uracil concentration or the dihydrouracil: uracil ratio, has not yet been prospectively validated for predictive use. A recent prospective cohort study employing the dihydrouracil: uracil ratio as a component of a multiparametric pre-treatment testing approach, was unfortunately cancelled early due to safety concerns [65]. Another prospective validation will be completed as a secondary analysis of a recently completed trial of pretreatment *DPYD* genotyping in the Netherlands (clinicaltrials.gov, NCT02324452) [10]. We await the results of this trial and confirmatory results before suggesting the clinical validity of this test in the pre-treatment setting. All of the above assessments of DPD activity are still complicated by the known circadian rhythm of DPD activity. First, researchers need to establish the time of day that is an appropriate reference of global DPD activity. While many attempts have been made to assess the value of using chronicity in fluoropyrimidines, the field remains in a state of flux [49]. In summary, the predictors of fluoropyrimidine-related AEs described thus far have relied upon the direct phenotypic determination of DPD activity; however, a more comprehensive genetic approach may be of a significant clinical benefit.

There has been a parallel and often intertwined field of study testing the genetic variation within *DPYD* for clinical relevance. After the initial discovery of *DPYD**2A there have been numerous studies identifying additional *DPYD* variants and testing for their association with severe AEs in fluoropyrimidine therapy. Since this field was in its infancy during the 1990s, it has been understood that a single genetic variant could not account for the observed frequency of DPD deficiency in the population [21]. Currently there are over 200 *DPYD* variants that have been identified [66]. Leaders in this field have attempted to characterize the effects of many of these variants on DPD activity in vitro, to identify those that are clinically relevant [28,67,68]. This research has supported large scale association studies providing the basis for our current understanding of the field [69–76]. Through a series of systematic meta-analyses researchers have begun to validate the currently actionable *DPYD* variants [77–79]. As of 2011, the Royal Dutch Association for the Advancement of Pharmacy's 'Pharmacogenetics Working Group' published guidelines cautiously recommending fluoropyrimidine dose reductions for 14 *DPYD* variants [80]. This guideline has been improved upon and there is now an expert consensus guideline by the Clinical Pharmacogenomics Implementation Consortium (CPIC) that has limited the number of variants to only those with strong supporting evidence [81]. Therefore, the CPIC guideline for *DPYD* and fluoropyrimidines only states four *DPYD* variants as clinically actionable [28].

The four variants currently considered clinically actionable include *DPYD**2A, *DPYD**13, *DPYD*c.2846A>T, and *DPYD* haplotype-B3. We have previously discussed the discovery and characterization of first variant *DPYD**2A in DPD deficient patients [26,27]. Through in vitro assessment of DPD enzymatic activity, it has been shown that *DPYD**2A leads to complete loss of DPD enzymatic activity [67]. In addition, numerous clinical studies have supported the association between the *DPYD**2A variant and fluoropyrimidine-related AEs [72,74,75,82–84]. Given the observed complete loss of function and the known association with toxicity the recommendation of a 50% dose reduction was developed [28,81]. Prospective *DPYD**2A genotyping with dose reduction was also shown to reduce fluoropyrimidine-related AEs, while attaining cost-effectiveness [9]. The second clinically actionable variant is *DPYD**13 (also known as *DPYD*c.1679T>G, or rs55886062, or DPD p.I560S). *DPYD**13 was initially discovered through exploratory sequencing of a subset of *DPYD* exons in a single patient with known DPD deficiency [85]. The *DPYD**13 variant causes a serine for isoleucine substitution in a highly conserved region of the DPD protein. The interpretation of this change suggests the substitution of a hydrophilic base into an otherwise well-conserved hydrophobic region could lead to destabilizing the protein [82]. In vitro assessment of the *DPYD**13 variant demonstrated near complete ablation of DPD enzymatic activity [67]. In Caucasian populations this variant is very rare [28]. This has made the clinical associations for this variant more challenging, however in samples with sufficient power and a meta-analysis it is possible to confirm the *DPYD**13 variant is associated with an increased risk for toxicity [71,78,79]. The third actionable *DPYD* variant is *DPYD*c.2846A>T (also known as rs67376798, or DPD p.D949V) was also first identified through exploratory sequencing of *DPYD* exons, in patients that had experienced severe fluoropyrimidine-related AEs [82]. The substitution of valine for aspartic acid at position 560 is proposed to impact the interaction between DPD and its co-factors [82]. The in vitro functional assessment of *DPYD*c.2846A>T shows a 40–60% reduction in enzyme activity [67,68,86]. The partial loss of function is an important distinction between this variant and both *DPYD**2A and *DPYD**13. The partial reduction in function could alter the potential pharmacogenetic influence of *DPYD*c.2846A>T on fluoropyrimidine-related toxicities. However, there is substantial evidence linking *DPYD*c.2846A>T with increased fluoropyrimidine-related toxicities and the presence of *DPYD*c.2846A>T [69,72,74,75,78,79]. In the original guidelines carriers this variant was recommended to receive a 50% dose reduction of fluoropyrimidines [81]. However, when the guidelines were updated the dose recommendation was changed to state between 25–50%, to account for the functional data highlighting there is not a complete loss of function with this variant [29]. This may change again following recent data suggesting that 25% dose reduction does not sufficient reduce the risk for fluoropyrimidine-related AEs [10]. The fourth *DPYD* variant that is included in the updated pharmacogenetic guidelines is *DPYD* haplotype-B3 (also known as *DPYD*c.1129-5923C>G, or *DPYD*c.1236G>A, or rs75017182 or rs56276561). This haplotype was initially identified by Amstutz et al., in patients with fluoropyrimidine-related toxicities [87]. The characterization of this variant revealed that the variant reduces the mRNA splicing efficiency by 30%. This reduction in functional mRNA production was linked to a 35% reduction in DPD enzymatic activity [88,89]. As with *DPYD*c.2846A>T, *DPYD* haplotype-B3 is an incomplete loss of function with the same inherent implications for the pharmacogenetic relevance of this variant. However, combining the in vitro data with multiple clinical association studies the consensus opinion is that there is sufficient evidence to support *DPYD* Haplotype-B3 as an actionable variant [29,79]. Together these four variants form the base of the current pharmacogenetic guidelines for Caucasian populations. Building upon the consensus CPIC guidelines are strong prospective trials of *DPYD* genotype-guided dosing in fluoropyrimidine therapy, both demonstrating a reduction of severe fluoropyrimidine-related AEs while maintaining cost effectiveness [9,10,90]. This represents a major advancement in the field of pharmacogenetics and supports the wide spread implementation of *DPYD* genotyping pre-treatment.

Despite the recent advances in the pharmacogenetics of fluoropyrimidine-related AEs, the use of *DPYD* genotyping also has its limitations. When including the four actionable SNPs the sensitivity for severe AEs remains low and accounted for at most 30% of AEs [81], meaning that the causes of many AEs are unaccounted for by genotype testing alone. Furthermore, pharmacogenetic testing has not been widely accepted or recommended as a routine test in the pre-treatment period. While governing agencies concede the danger of fluoropyrimidines in DPD deficient patients they fail to recommend or require pre-treatment DPD testing as a routine test [2,3,91]. In part, the lack of uptake can be traced to concerns over which populations can benefit from the available knowledge, which fluoropyrimidine-containing regimens should be screened, a need for confirmatory cost-analysis, and the current lack of prospective survival outcomes data [92]. Retrospective studies have attempted to address these limitations, showing positive support for both the broad implementation of *DPYD* genotyping in various fluoropyrimidine regimens and non-inferiority in survival outcomes [93,94]. However, further prospective confirmatory studies are required to change the opinion of regulatory authorities. As well there have been important lessons learned from centers that have implemented pre-treatment testing. At our medical center, implementation of *DPYD* genotype testing started with a handful of patients referred to our Personalized Medicine Clinic after severe fluoropyrimidine-related AEs. It was clear from this early implementation that patients who exhibited severe toxicity were far more likely to be carriers of loss of function genetic variants in *DPYD* ~17% compared to the local population frequency ~4%. In the past 5 years, guidelines on the clinical implementation of *DPYD* genotype testing, along with recommended dose reduction have allowed for *DPYD* genotype-guided dosing to be more broadly and confidently provided to requesting physicians. At our center, pre-treatment *DPYD* genotype testing is incorporated into routine care through a prospective cohort study of pharmacogenetic technologies. A multidisciplinary team, including physicians, pharmacists, and nurses work together to provide *DPYD* genotype testing results within 24–48 h after the patient's initial assessment. Indeed, the ability to provide timely patient centered precision medicine, without delay in treatment timelines has been viewed as highly desirable and beneficial for patient care. Moreover, we now see a clear benefit of pre-treatment *DPYD* testing for preventing severe toxicity as well as cost-effectiveness. In a recent commentary, authors with 8-years experience of providing pre-treatment testing advocate for a multimodality approach to improve the sensitivity and eliminate some of the ambiguity of the *DPYD* genotype testing alone [95]. The concept of a multimodality genotype-phenotype approach has also been incorporated in recent guidelines by the Group of Clinical Pharmacology in Oncology (GPCO)-UNICANCER and the French Network of Pharmacogenetics [96]. Overall, there is strong evidence for the use of *DPYD* genotyping in the pre-treatment setting to reduce the risk of fluoropyrimidine-related AEs. However, this testing alone will not identify all patients with DPD deficiency and additional modalities should still be considered to further improve patient safety outcomes.

5. Therapeutic Drug Monitoring for 5-Fluorouracil

We have discussed a few of the known benefits and challenges, implicit in the use of DPD deficiency prediction for fluoropyrimidine-based therapy. Given the limited sensitivity of the available pre-treatment techniques, the use of therapeutic drug monitoring (TDM) may play an important role in promoting the safe and efficacious use of fluoropyrimidines. This work is founded on the early clinical pharmacokinetic literature that demonstrated high systemic 5-FU level was correlated with both disease response and toxicity [97,98]. Therefore, if the systemic drug level could be assessed during active treatment and actively feedback to the treating physicians, dose titration may alter the clinical outcomes for these patients. This work spurred efforts at the first 5-FU TDM trial by Santini et al. who used a retrospective control group and were able to show improvements in both disease response and fluoropyrimidine-related AEs [99]. The work by Santini et al. on head and neck cancers was complimented by comparable trials in colorectal cancers [100,101]. Further advancement led to randomized controlled trials in each disease site. Both trials confirmed the value of 5-FU TDM for both efficacy and AE reduction [102,103]. These trials established the first dose titration algorithms to maximize the therapeutic index of 5-FU. There have been many additional smaller studies of TDM in 5-FU summarized by Lee et al. [104]. The positive results from these studies drove the development of commercial products for 5-FU pharmacokinetic guided dose titrations available in the USA and France (My5-FU®, Saladax Biomedical Inc.; ODPM Protocol™, Onco Drug Personalized Medicine). Having analyzed post-marketing data of a commercial assay, Kaldate et al. provided an updated dosing algorithm with a more accessible target range [105]. A systematic review and meta-analysis combining four prospective trials in this field, demonstrated that TDM for 5-FU reduces the risk of severe AEs, while improving the clinical response [106]. The benefit of TDM over screening is directly connecting drug level to clinical outcomes, with continued follow-up allowing for feedback and dose correction. However, TDM carries the risk of first cycle toxicity and therefore does not fully eliminate the need for pre-treatment screening for DPD deficiency. Other drawbacks of TDM are difficulties in standardizing the approach and the inherent costs of employing such an intensive program. Some constructive suggestions to address these concerns include centralized testing [107], and prospective cost-analysis to add to the very limited retrospective model-based literature [108]. Upon review of the available literature in this field, the International Association of Therapeutic Drug Monitoring and Clinical Toxicology released a guideline in favor the use of TDM for 5-FU [109]. However, TDM is not a clinical standard, and still requires prospective validation to confirm its efficacy and cost-effectiveness in modern fluoropyrimidine-based regimens.

6. Clinical Dilemma

Given the complexity of this topic, it is not surprising that there are additional therapeutic dilemmas that are not accounted for in the literature. For example, within our center we operate a collaborative research program between the divisions of Clinical Pharmacology and Medical Oncology, in order to provide pre-treatment *DPYD* genotyping following the CPIC guidelines [28]. Recently we were requested to see a patient with planned fluoropyrimidine based therapy on the background of orthotopic liver transplant. This patient effectively possesses two genetic backgrounds. Given the liver serves as the primary site of 5-FU metabolism and we possessed no tissue to genotype, we were forced to go beyond our normal routine practice. We implemented TDM for this patient in real time with dose titration in accordance with published algorithms. The case report below details our process for implementing this without altering the treatment plan of the medical oncologists or delaying the patient's treatment.

7. Case Presentation

A 40-year-old Caucasian male presented with painless jaundice and two-month history of bowel irregularity. The patient described loose stools, increasing in frequency over a two-month period, which floated and were difficult to flush. Past medical history is remarkable for a 14-year history of ulcerative colitis (UC), in remission, and Primary Sclerosing Cholangitis (PSC). At the time of presentation, the patient was two years post orthotopic liver transplant with curative intent for end stage liver disease secondary to rapid progression of his PSC. The patient tolerated the transplant well without acute rejection or infective complications. His medications included tacrolimus and prednisone. A routine abdominal ultrasound identified an irregular mass in the pancreas that led to additional imaging studies, including an abdominal computed tomography (CT). The abdominal CT with contrast identified a large, bulky, poorly delineated mass in the head of the pancreas. The mass was found to be invading segment 1 and 2 of the duodenum and obliterating the common bile duct. CT thorax and pelvis did not report metastatic disease. Magnetic resonance study confirmed locally advanced disease, deemed to be borderline resectable at initial presentation. An endoscopic ultrasound guided biopsy confirmed poorly differentiated adenocarcinoma of the pancreas. At this time, the case was reviewed by the multidisciplinary team and treatment options were presented to the patient. The patient, understanding the gravity of the diagnosis, wished to pursue maximal therapy and undergo neoadjuvant FOLFIRINOX followed by reassessment for potential curative resection. This triggered referral to our Personalized Medicine Clinic for *DPYD* genotype testing, the patient was genotyped using DNA from PBMCs and found to be wild-type for the following *DPYD* SNPs c.1905+1G>A, c.2846A>T, c.1679G>T, and c.1236G>A, tested in accordance with the CPIC guideline [28]. However, it was identified that given the patient's history of orthotopic liver transplant of unknown *DPYD* status, there would be limited value in the genetic background of his PBMCs. Therefore, the treating medical oncologists proceeded with an initial dose reduction of 30% as a way of balancing the patient's desire for maximal therapy and the care team's desire to prevent early severe toxicity in this unknown setting.

We planned to employ TDM utilizing liquid-liquid extraction and a high-pressure liquid chromatography tandem mass spectrometry assay developed in our laboratory for research purposes, to verify the patient's systemic exposure was below the toxic threshold. Accordingly, for the first treatment of FOLFIRINOX, the patient received a 30% dose reduction of the 5-FU components. During the continuous infusion of 5-FU, a peripheral whole blood sample was collected from a venous puncture contralateral to the 5-FU infusion site. The sample was collected 2 h post initiation of the 5-FU continuous infusion pump. The sample was immediately placed on ice and the plasma was separated by centrifugation within 20 min at which time it was frozen to −80°C. We determined the patient's plasma concentration of 5-FU to be 204.97 ng/mL, given a 46-h infusion this equates to an area under the curve of 9.43 mg·h/L, considered to be a subtherapeutic concentration. Combined with clinical observation of the patient, this result provided reassurance that the patient was not demonstrating signs of frank DPD deficiency. The treating oncologist utilized these results and titrated the dose accordingly while using published titration algorithms for reference [97,99]. The patient was keen to proceed to full dose intensity and the treating oncologists elected to administer the full dose of 5-FU with the reassurance of the TDM. To ensure this was an appropriate course of action and the transplant liver responded appropriately to the larger dose, we continued to monitor the patient. During the second cycle the patient was seen 24 h into the infusion instead of 2 h into continuous infusion as in the first cycle. Despite the known intra-patient variation changing the time of sampling was required to accommodate the logistics of this patient. The decision was deemed appropriate as the measurement would be at the predicted peak systemic 5-FU level and still serve to prevent supratherapeutic dosing. During the second infusion we found the patient's plasma concentration of 5-FU to be 539.04 ng/mL, equating a predicted AUC of 24.8 mg·h/L. This falls directly within the known therapeutic range of 5-FU and provided confidence to the treating physician that the patient was now receiving optimal management with regards to the 5-FU component. The patient continued with FOLFIRINOX therapy, without developing any severe fluoropyrimidine-related AEs. Following this neoadjuvant course there was significant disease response and the patient proceeded to surgery with curative intent.

8. Discussion

In this case, we have presented a therapeutic dilemma whereby a patient with a complex medical history and mixed genetic background, identified a limitation of pharmacogenetics. Upon review of the literature we believe there is a clinically important niche of orthotopic liver transplant patients where fluoropyrimidine therapy would benefit patient care. Immunosuppression post organ transplant induces an increased risk for development of neoplasms including skin, lymphoid and solid organ malignancies [110,111]. The increased rate of de novo colorectal, head and neck cancers is especially noteworthy as these disease sites are primary targets of fluoropyrimidine-based chemotherapy [112]. This patient's medical history of ulcerative colitis and PSC pose additional risk factors for developing a de novo neoplasm. PSC is an aggressive disease often refractory to multiple therapies, ultimately the only curative treatment is orthotopic liver transplant [113]. PSC and ulcerative colitis are components of a constellation of diseases with an increased risk for the development of gastrointestinal malignancies [114]. PSC itself is directly related with an increased risk for solid tumour malignancies including cholangiocarcinoma, gall bladder carcinoma, colorectal cancer, and pancreatic adenocarcinoma [115]. With both an extensive history of ulcerative colitis and PSC this patient was a high-risk candidate to develop a post orthotopic liver transplant de novo neoplasm. Our patient developed pancreatic adenocarcinoma—known to have the highest mortality rate per case for malignant neoplasms—with median survival at diagnosis of 9 months [116]. Utilizing the most aggressive evidence-based approach in managing borderline resectable pancreatic adenocarcinoma, the treating oncologist used fluoropyrimidne-based chemotherapy in this complicated patient [117,118].

Unfortunately, due to the overall rarity of this condition, there is very little evidence for the effective use of fluoropyrimidines post orthotopic liver transplant. There is a limited body evidence for the use of fluoropyrimidines for adjuvant treatment in hepatocellular carcinoma treated with orthotopic liver transplant [119–121]. However, this data remains limited due to small sample size and the clinical preference for alternative treatment modalities in the treatment of hepatocellular carcinoma [122,123]. Therefore, there are no evidence-based recommendations for managing patients with this complex presentation. It is believed that practitioners should follow the same guidelines as with classical presentations [112]. This remains an intimidating dilemma owing to the known hepatotoxicity of fluoropyrimidines. There are case reports of both liver injury and graft rejection in liver transplant recipients receiving fluoropyrimidine-based chemotherapy [124,125]. These findings explain the caution with which the treating oncologists approached the care for this patient. We demonstrated that

TDM in a post orthotopic liver transplant patient receiving 5-FU infusion was possible, and attainable within the normal timeline of therapy. The resultant information provided reassurance to the patient and practitioner without delaying therapy. TDM for 5-FU should be considered for fluoropyrimidine chemotherapy in orthotopic liver transplant recipients. The implementation of TDM for a unique case such as this underlies the benefit of combining pharmacogenetics and classic pharmacokinetic approaches to improve patient care through precision medicine.

Funding: R.B.K. is supported by Wolfe Medical Research Chair in Pharmacogenomics and Ontario Research Fund-Research Excellence (Round 8)

Acknowledgments: The authors thank Cam Ross and Yinyin Liao for technical assistance. The authors would also like to thank the support staff of London Health Sciences Centre, London Regional Cancer Centre, and Lawson Health Research Institute for their continued support of ongoing projects.

Conflicts of Interest: The authors declare no conflict of interest.

References

1. Heidelberger, C.; Chaudhuri, N.; Danneberg, P.; Mooren, D.; Griesch, L.; Duschinsky, R.; Schnitzer, R.; Pleven, E.; Scheiner, J. Fluorinated Pyrimidines, A New Class of Tumour-Inhibitory Compounds. *Nature* **1957**, *179*, 663–666. [CrossRef] [PubMed]
2. Fluorouracil, USFDA Product Label. Available online: www.accessdata.fda.gov/drugsatfda_docs/label/2016/012209s040lbl.pdf (accessed on 22 March 2019).
3. Fluorouracil, Sandoz Canada Inc. Health Canada Approved Product Monograph. Available online: www.sandoz.ca/sites/www.sandoz.ca/files/Fluorouracil%20Product%20Monograph.pdf (accessed on 22 March 2019).
4. Peyrade, F.; Cupissol, D.; Geoffrois, L.; Rolland, F.; Borel, C.; Ciais, C.; Faivre, S.; Guigay, J. Systemic Treatment and Medical Management of Metastatic Squamous Cell Carcinoma of the Head and Neck: Review of the Literature and Proposal for Management Changes. *Oral Oncol.* **2013**, *49*, 482–491. [CrossRef]
5. Mikhail, S.E.; Sun, J.F.; Marshall, J.L. Safety of Capecitabine: A Review. *Expert Opin. Drug Saf.* **2010**, *9*, 831–841. [CrossRef] [PubMed]
6. Meta-analysis Group in Cancer; Lévy, E.; Piedbois, P.; Buyse, M.; Pignon, J.; Rougier, P.; Ryan, L.; Hansen, R.; Zee, B.; Weinerman, B.; et al. Toxicity of Fluorouracil in Patients with Advanced Colorectal Cancer: Effect of Administration Schedule and Prognostic Factors. *J. Clin.* **1998**, *16*, 3537–3541. [CrossRef]
7. Chionh, F.; Lau, D.; Yeung, Y.; Price, T.; Tebbutt, N. Oral versus Intravenous Fluoropyrimidines for Colorectal Cancer. *Cochrane Rev.* **2017**, *7*. [CrossRef]
8. Kim, S.; Baek, J.; Oh, J.; Park, S.; Sohn, D.; Kim, M.; Chang, H.; Kong, S.-Y.; Kim, D. A Phase II Study of Preoperative Chemoradiation with Tegafur-Uracil plus Leucovorin for Locally Advanced Rectal Cancer with Pharmacogenetic Analysis. *Radiat. Oncol.* **2017**, *12*, 62. [CrossRef]
9. Deenen, M.J.; Meulendijks, D.; Cats, A.; Sechterberger, M.K.; Severens, J.L.; Boot, H.; Smits, P.H.; Rosing, H.; Mandigers, C.; Soesan, M.; et al. Upfront Genotyping of *DPYD**2A to Individualize Fluoropyrimidine Therapy: A Safety and Cost Analysis. *J. Clin. Oncol.* **2015**, *34*, 227–234. [CrossRef]
10. Henricks, L.M.; Lunenburg, C.A.; de Man, F.M.; Meulendijks, D.; Frederix, G.W.; Kienhuis, E.; Creemers, G.-J.; Baars, A.; Dezentjé, V.O.; Imholz, A.L.; et al. *DPYD* Genotype-Guided Dose Individualisation of Fluoropyrimidine Therapy in Patients with Cancer: A Prospective Safety Analysis. *Lancet Oncol.* **2018**, *19*, 1459–1467. [CrossRef]
11. Longley, D.B.; Harkin, P.D.; Johnston, P.G. 5-Fluorouracil: Mechanisms of Action and Clinical Strategies. *Nat. Rev. Cancer* **2003**, *3*, 330–338. [CrossRef]
12. Birnie, G.; Kroeger, H.; Heidelberger, C. Studies of Fluorinated Pyrimidines. XVIII. The Degradation of 5-Fluoro-2′-Deoxyuridine and Related Compounds by Nucleoside Phosphorylase*. *Biochemistry* **1963**, *2*, 566–572. [CrossRef] [PubMed]
13. Diasio, R.B.; Harris, B.E. Clinical Pharmacology of 5-Fluorouracil. *Clin. Pharmacokinet.* **1989**, *16*, 215–237. [CrossRef] [PubMed]
14. Wasternack, C. Degradation of Pyrimidines and Pyrimidine Analogs—Pathways and Mutual Influences. *Pharmacol. Therap.* **1980**, *8*, 629–651. [CrossRef]

15. Sommadossi, J.; Gewirtz, D.; Diasio, R.; Aubert, C.; Cano, J.; Goldman, I. Rapid Catabolism of 5-Fluorouracil in Freshly Isolated Rat Hepatocytes as Analyzed by High Performance Liquid Chromatography. *J. Biological Chem.* **1982**, *257*, 8171–8176.
16. Traut, T.W.; Loechel, S. Pyrimidine Catabolism: Individual Characterization of the Three Sequential Enzymes with a New Assay. *Biochemistry* **1984**, *23*, 2533–2539. [CrossRef]
17. Tuchman, M.; Stoeckeler, J.S.; Kiang, D.T.; O'Dea, R.F.; Ramnaraine, M.L.; Mirkin, B.L. Familial Pyrimidinemia and Pyrimidinuria Associated with Severe Fluorouracil Toxicity. *N. Engl. J. Med.* **1985**, *313*, 245–249. [CrossRef]
18. Shiotani, T.; Weber, G. Purification and Properties of Dihydrothymine Dehydrogenase from Rat Liver. *J. Biol. Chem.* **1981**, *256*, 219–224. [PubMed]
19. Heggie, G.; Sommadossi, J.; Cross, D.; Huster, W.; Diasio, R. Clinical Pharmacokinetics of 5-Fluorouracil and Its Metabolites in Plasma, Urine, and Bile. *Cancer Res.* **1987**, *47*, 2203–2206. [PubMed]
20. Diasio, R.; Beavers, T.; Carpenter, J. Familial Deficiency of Dihydropyrimidine Dehydrogenase. Biochemical Basis for Familial Pyrimidinemia and Severe 5-Fluorouracil-Induced Toxicity. *J. Clin. Investig.* **1988**, *81*, 47–51. [CrossRef] [PubMed]
21. Harris, B.E.; Carpenter, J.T.; Diasio, R.B. Severe 5-fluorouracil Toxicity Secondary to Dihydropyrimidine Dehydrogenase Deficiency. A Potentially More Common Pharmacogenetic Syndrome. *Cancer* **1991**, *68*, 499–501. [CrossRef]
22. Houyau, P.; Gay, C.; Chatelut, E.; Canal, P.; Roché, H.; Milano, G. Severe Fluorouracil Toxicity in a Patient with Dihydropyrimidine Dehydrogenase Deficiency. *J. Natl. Cancer I.* **1993**, *85*, 1602–1603. [CrossRef]
23. Beuzeboc, P.; Pierga, J.-Y.; Stoppa-Lyonnet, D.; Etienne, M.C.; Milano, G.; Fouillait, P. Severe 5-Fluorouracil Toxicity Possibly Secondary to Dihydropyrimidine Dehydrogenase Deficiency in a Breast Cancer Patient with Osteogenesis Imperfecta. *Eur. J. Cancer* **1996**, *32*, 369–370. [CrossRef]
24. Yokota, H.; Fernandez-Salguero, P.; Furuya, H.; Lin, K.; McBride, O.; Podschun, B.; Schnackerz, K.; Gonzalez, F. cDNA Cloning and Chromosome Mapping of Human Dihydropyrimidine Dehydrogenase, an Enzyme Associated with 5-Fluorouracil Toxicity and Congenital Thymine Uraciluria. *J. Biol. Chem.* **1994**, *269*, 23192–23196. [PubMed]
25. Meinsma, R.; Fernandez-Salguero, P.; Kuilenburg, V.A.; Gennip, V.A.; Gonzalez, F. Human Polymorphism in Drug Metabolism: Mutation in the Dihydropyrimidine Dehydrogenase Gene Results in Exon Skipping and Thymine Uracilurea. *DNA Cell Biol.* **1995**, *14*, 1–6. [CrossRef]
26. Wei, X.; McLeod, H.; McMurrough, J.; Gonzalez, F.; Fernandez-Salguero, P. Molecular Basis of the Human Dihydropyrimidine Dehydrogenase Deficiency and 5-Fluorouracil Toxicity. *J. Clin. Investig.* **1996**, *98*, 610–615. [CrossRef] [PubMed]
27. Vreken, P.; Kuilenburg, V.A.; Meinsma, R.; Smit, G.; Bakker, H.; Abreu, D.R.; van Gennip, A. A Point Mutation in an Invariant Splice Donor Site Leads to Exon Skipping in Two Unrelated Dutch Patients with Dihydropyrimidine Dehydrogenase Deficiency. *J. Inherit. Metab. Dis.* **1996**, *19*, 645–654. [CrossRef] [PubMed]
28. Amstutz, U.; Henricks, L.M.; Offer, S.M.; Barbarino, J.; Schellens, J.; Swen, J.J.; Klein, T.E.; McLeod, H.L.; Caudle, K.E.; Diasio, R.B.; et al. Clinical Pharmacogenetics Implementation Consortium (CPIC) Guideline for Dihydropyrimidine Dehydrogenase Genotype and Fluoropyrimidine Dosing: 2017 Update. *Clin. Pharmacol. Ther.* **2018**, *103*, 210–216. [CrossRef]
29. Fidai, S.S.; Sharma, A.E.; Johnson, D.N.; Segal, J.P.; Lastra, R.R. Dihydropyrimidine Dehydrogenase Deficiency as a Cause of Fatal 5-Fluorouracil Toxicity. *Autopsy Case Rep.* **2018**, *8*. [CrossRef]
30. Tong, C.C.; Lam, C.W.; Lam, K.O.; Lee, V.H.; Luk, M.-Y. A Novel *DPYD* Variant Associated with Severe Toxicity of Fluoropyrimidines: Role of Pre-Emptive *DPYD* Genotype Screening. *Front. Oncol.* **2018**, *8*, 279. [CrossRef]
31. Harris, B.; Song, R.; Soong, S.; Diasio, R. Relationship between Dihydropyrimidine Dehydrogenase Activity and Plasma 5-Fluorouracil Levels with Evidence for Circadian Variation of Enzyme Activity and Plasma Drug Levels in Cancer Patients Receiving 5-Fluorouracil by Protracted Continuous Infusion. *Cancer Res.* **1990**, *50*, 197–201.
32. Petit, E.; Milano, G.; Lévi, F.; Thyss, A.; Bailleul, F.; Schneider, M. Circadian Rhythm-Varying Plasma Concentration of 5-Fluorouracil during a Five-Day Continuous Venous Infusion at a Constant Rate in Cancer Patients. *Cancer Res.* **1988**, *48*, 1676–1679.

33. Jiang, H.; Lu, J.; Ji, J. Circadian Rhythm of Dihydrouracil/Uracil Ratios in Biological Fluids: A Potential Biomarker for Dihydropyrimidine Dehydrogenase Levels. *Brit. J. Pharmacol.* **2004**, *141*, 616–623. [CrossRef]
34. Zeng, Z.; Sun, J.; Guo, L.; Li, S.; Wu, M.; Qiu, F.; Jiang, W.; Lévi, F.; Xian, L. Circadian Rhythm in Dihydropyrimidine Dehydrogenase Activity and Reduced Glutathione Content in Peripheral Blood of Nasopharyngeal Carcinoma Patients. *Chronobiol. Int.* **2009**, *2*, 741–754. [CrossRef] [PubMed]
35. Jacobs, B.A.; Deenen, M.J.; Pluim, D.; Hasselt, C.J.; Krähenbühl, M.D.; Geel, R.M.; Vries, N.; Rosing, H.; Meulendijks, D.; Burylo, A.M.; et al. Pronounced Between-subject and Circadian Variability in Thymidylate Synthase and Dihydropyrimidine Dehydrogenase Enzyme Activity in Human Volunteers. *Brit. J. Clin. Pharmacol.* **2016**, *82*, 706–716. [CrossRef]
36. Lu, Z.; Zhang, R.; Diasio, R.B. Population Characteristics of Hepatic Dihydropyrimidine Dehydrogenase Activity, a Key Metabolic Enzyme in 5-fluorouracil Chemotherapy. *Clin. Pharmacol. Ther.* **1995**, *58*, 512–522. [CrossRef]
37. Johnston, S.; Ridge, S.; Cassidy, J.; McLeod, H. Regulation of Dihydropyrimidine Dehydrogenase in Colorectal Cancer. *Clin. Cancer Res.* **1999**, *5*, 2566–2570. [PubMed]
38. Uetake, H.; Ichikawa, W.; Takechi, T.; Fukushima, M.; Nihei, Z.; Sugihara, K. Relationship between Intratumoral Dihydropyrimidine Dehydrogenase Activity and Gene Expression in Human Colorectal Cancer. *Clin. Cancer Res.* **1999**, *5*, 2836–2839.
39. Fleming, R.; Milano, G.; Thyss, A.; Etienne, M.; Renée, N.; Schneider, M.; Demard, F. Correlation between Dihydropyrimidine Dehydrogenase Activity in Peripheral Mononuclear Cells and Systemic Clearance of Fluorouracil in Cancer Patients. *Cancer Res.* **1992**, *52*, 2899–2902.
40. Chazal, M.; Etienne, M.; Renée, N.; Bourgeon, A.; Richelme, H.; Milano, G. Link between Dihydropyrimidine Dehydrogenase Activity in Peripheral Blood Mononuclear Cells and Liver. *Clin. Cancer Res.* **1996**, *2*, 507–510.
41. Etienne, M.; Lagrange, J.; Dassonville, O.; Fleming, R.; Thyss, A.; Renée, N.; Schneider, M.; Demard, F.; Milano, G. Population Study of Dihydropyrimidine Dehydrogenase in Cancer Patients. *J. Clin. Oncol.* **1994**, *12*, 2248–2253. [CrossRef]
42. Lu, Z.; Zhang, R.; Diasio, R. Dihydropyrimidine Dehydrogenase Activity in Human Peripheral Blood Mononuclear Cells and Liver: Population Characteristics, Newly Identified Deficient Patients, and Clinical Implication in 5-Fluorouracil Chemotherapy. *Cancer Res.* **1993**, *53*, 5433–5438.
43. Ridge, S.A.; Sludden, J.; Brown, O.; Robertson, L.; Wei, X.; Sapone, A.; Fernandez-Salguero, P.M.; Gonzalez, F.J.; Vreken, P.; Kuilenburg, A.B.; et al. Dihydropyrimidine Dehydrogenase Pharmacogenetics in Caucasian Subjects. *Brit. J. Clin. Pharmacol.* **1998**, *46*, 151–156. [CrossRef]
44. Sapone, A.; Gonzalez, F.; McLeod, H.; Cassidy, J.; Sludden, J.; Brown, O.; Canney, P.; Fernandez-Salguero, P.; Hardy, S.; Ridge, S.; et al. Dihydropyrimidine Dehydrogenase Pharmacogenetics in Patients with Colorectal Cancer. *Brit. J. Cancer* **1998**, *77*, 497–500. [CrossRef]
45. Guimbaud, R.; Guichard, S.; Dusseau, C.; Bertrand, V.; Aparicio, T.; Lochon, I.; Chatelut, E.; Couturier, D.; Bugat, R.; Chaussade, S.; et al. Dihydropyrimidine Dehydrogenase Activity in Normal, Inflammatory and Tumour Tissues of Colon and Liver in Humans. *Cancer Chem. Pharm.* **2000**, *45*, 477–482. [CrossRef] [PubMed]
46. Van Kuilenburg, A. Dihydropyrimidine Dehydrogenase and the Efficacy and Toxicity of 5-Fluorouracil. *Eur. J. Cancer* **2004**, *40*, 939–950. [CrossRef]
47. Ezzeldin, H.; Diasio, R. Dihydropyrimidine Dehydrogenase Deficiency, a Pharmacogenetic Syndrome Associated with Potentially Life-Threatening Toxicity Following 5-Fluorouracil Administration. *Clin. Colorectal Cancer* **2004**, *4*, 181–189. [CrossRef]
48. Meulendijks, D.; Cats, A.; Beijnen, J.H.; Schellens, J. Improving Safety of Fluoropyrimidine Chemotherapy by Individualizing Treatment Based on Dihydropyrimidine Dehydrogenase Activity—Ready for Clinical Practice? *Cancer Treat. Rev.* **2016**, *50*, 23–34. [CrossRef] [PubMed]
49. Milano, G.; Chamorey, A.-L. Clinical Pharmacokinetics of 5-Fluorouracil with Consideration of Chronopharmacokinetics. *Chronobiol. Int.* **2009**, *19*, 177–189. [CrossRef]
50. Gamelin, E.; Boisdron-Celle, M.; Larra, F.; Robert, J. A Simple Chromatographic Method for the Analysis of Pyrimidines and Their Dihydrogenated Metabolites. *J. Liq. Chrom. Related Tech.* **1997**, *20*, 3155–3172. [CrossRef]

51. Gamelin, E.; Boisdron-Celle, M.; Guérin-Meyer, V.; Delva, R.; Lortholary, A.; Genevieve, F.; Larra, F.; Ifrah, N.; Robert, J. Correlation between Uracil and Dihydrouracil Plasma Ratio, Fluorouracil (5-FU) Pharmacokinetic Parameters, and Tolerance in Patients with Advanced Colorectal Cancer: A Potential Interest for Predicting 5-FU Toxicity and Determining Optimal 5-FU Dosage. *J. Clin. Oncol.* **1999**, *17*, 1105–1110. [CrossRef]
52. Nakayama, Y.; Matsumoto, K.; Inoue, Y. Correlation between the Urinary Dihydrouracil-Uracil Ratio and the 5-FU Plasma Concentration in Patients Treated with Oral 5-FU Analogs. *Anticancer Res.* **2006**, *26*, 3983–3988.
53. Ciccolini, J.; Mercier, C.; Evrard, A.; Dahan, L.; Boyer, J.-C.; Duffaud, F.; Richard, K.; Blanquicett, C.; Milano, G.; Blesius, A.; et al. A Rapid and Inexpensive Method for Anticipating Severe Toxicity to Fluorouracil and Fluorouracil-Based Chemotherapy. *Ther. Drug Monit.* **2006**, *28*, 678–685. [CrossRef]
54. Déporte, R.; Amiand, M.; Moreau, A.; Charbonnel, C.; Campion, L. High-Performance Liquid Chromatographic Assay with UV Detection for Measurement of Dihydrouracil/Uracil Ratio in Plasma. *J. Chromatogr.* **2006**, *834*, 170–177. [CrossRef] [PubMed]
55. Mattison, L.K.; Fourie, J.; Hirao, Y.; Koga, T.; Desmond, R.A.; King, J.R.; Shimizu, T.; Diasio, R.B. The Uracil Breath Test in the Assessment of Dihydropyrimidine Dehydrogenase Activity: Pharmacokinetic Relationship between Expired 13CO_2 and Plasma [2–13C] Dihydrouracil. *Clin. Cancer Res.* **2006**, *12*, 549–555. [CrossRef]
56. Švobaitė, R.; Solassol, I.; Pinguet, F.; Ivanauskas, L.; Brès, J.; Bressolle, F.M. HPLC with UV or Mass Spectrometric Detection for Quantifying Endogenous Uracil and Dihydrouracil in Human Plasma. *Clin. Chem.* **2008**, *54*, 1463–1472. [CrossRef] [PubMed]
57. Coudoré, F.; Roche, D.; Lefeuvre, S.; Faussot, D.; Billaud, E.M.; Loriot, M.-A.; Beaune, P. Validation of an Ultra-High Performance Liquid Chromatography Tandem Mass Spectrometric Method for Quantifying Uracil and 5,6-Dihydrouracil in Human Plasma. *J. Chromat. Sci.* **2012**, *50*, 877–884. [CrossRef] [PubMed]
58. Büchel, B.; Rhyn, P.; Schürch, S.; Bühr, C.; Amstutz, U.; Largiadèr, C.R. LC-MS/MS Method for Simultaneous Analysis of Uracil, 5,6-dihydrouracil, 5-fluorouracil and 5-fluoro-5,6-dihydrouracil in Human Plasma for Therapeutic Drug Monitoring and Toxicity Prediction in Cancer Patients. *Biomed. Chromatogr.* **2013**, *27*, 7–16. [CrossRef] [PubMed]
59. Jacobs, B.; Rosing, H.; de Vries, N.; Meulendijks, D.; Henricks, L.M.; Schellens, J.; Beijnen, J.H. Development and Validation of a Rapid and Sensitive UPLC–MS/MS Method for Determination of Uracil and Dihydrouracil in Human Plasma. *J. Pharm. Biomed. Anal.* **2016**, *126*, 75–82. [CrossRef] [PubMed]
60. Meulendijks, D.; Henricks, L.M.; Jacobs, B.A.; Aliev, A.; Deenen, M.J.; de Vries, N.; Rosing, H.; van Werkhoven, E.; de Boer, A.; Beijnen, J.H.; et al. Pretreatment Serum Uracil Concentration as a Predictor of Severe and Fatal Fluoropyrimidine-Associated Toxicity. *Brit. J. Cancer* **2017**, *116*, 1415–1424. [CrossRef] [PubMed]
61. Van Staveren, M.C.; Theeuwes-Oonk, B.; Guchelaar, H.; van Kuilenburg, A.B.; Maring, J. Pharmacokinetics of Orally Administered Uracil in Healthy Volunteers and in DPD-Deficient Patients, a Possible Tool for Screening of DPD Deficiency. *Cancer Chemoth. Pharm.* **2011**, *68*, 1611–1617. [CrossRef]
62. Grisolia, S.; Cardoso, S.S. The Purification and Properties of Hydropyrimidine Dehydrogenase. *Biochim. Biophys. Acta* **1957**, *25*, 430–431. [CrossRef]
63. Kristensen, M.; Pedersen, P.; Mejer, J. The Value of Dihydrouracil/Uracil Plasma Ratios in Predicting 5-Fluorouracil-Related Toxicity in Colorectal Cancer Patients. *J. Int. Med. Res.* **2010**, *38*, 1313–1323. [CrossRef]
64. Boisdron-Celle, M.; Remaud, G.; Traore, S.; Poirier, A.L.; Gamelin, L.; Morel, A.; Gamelin, E. 5-Fluorouracil-Related Severe Toxicity: A Comparison of Different Methods for the Pretherapeutic Detection of Dihydropyrimidine Dehydrogenase Deficiency. *Cancer Lett.* **2007**, *249*, 271–282. [CrossRef] [PubMed]
65. Boisdron-Celle, M.; Capitain, O.; Faroux, R.; Borg, C.; Metges, J.; Galais, M.; Kaassis, M.; Bennouna, J.; Bouhier-Leporrier, K.; Francois, E.; et al. Prevention of 5-Fluorouracil-Induced Early Severe Toxicity by Pre-Therapeutic Dihydropyrimidine Dehydrogenase Deficiency Screening: Assessment of a Multiparametric Approach. *Sem. Oncol.* **2017**, *44*. [CrossRef] [PubMed]
66. *DPYD*[gene]-ClinVar-NCBI. Available online: www.ncbi.nlm.nih.gov/clinvar/?term=DPYD%5Bgene%5D (accessed on 22 March 2019).
67. Offer, S.; Wegner, N.; Fossum, C.; Wang, K.; Diasio, R. Phenotypic Profiling of *DPYD* Variations Relevant to 5-Fluorouracil Sensitivity Using Real-Time Cellular Analysis and In Vitro Measurement of Enzyme Activity. *Cancer Res.* **2013**, *17*, 1958–1968. [CrossRef] [PubMed]

68. Offer, S.; Fossum, C.; Wegner, N.; Stuflesser, A.; Butterfield, G.; Diasio, R. Comparative Funcational Analysis of *DPYD* Variants of Potential Clinical Relevance to Dihydropyrimidine Dehydrogenase Activity. *Cancer Res.* **2014**, *74*, 2545–2554. [CrossRef]
69. Boige, V.; Vincent, M.; Alexandre, P.; Tejpar, S.; Landolfi, S.; Malicot, K.; Greil, R.; Cuyle, P.; Yilmaz, M.; Faroux, R.; et al. *DPYD* Genotyping to Predict Adverse Events Following Treatment With Flourouracil-Based Adjuvant Chemotherapy in Patients With Stage III Colon Cancer: A Secondary Analysis of the PETACC-8 Randomized Clinical Trial. *JAMA Oncol.* **2016**, *2*, 655–661. [CrossRef]
70. Braun, M.S.; Richman, S.D.; Thompson, L.; Daly, C.L.; Meade, A.M.; Adlard, J.W.; Allan, J.M.; Parmar, M.; Quirke, P.; Seymour, M.T. Association of Molecular Markers with Toxicity Outcomes in a Randomized Trial of Chemotherapy for Advanced Colorectal Cancer: The FOCUS Trial. *J. Clin. Oncol.* **2009**, *27*, 5519–5528. [CrossRef] [PubMed]
71. Lee, K.-H.; Chang, H.; Han, S.-W.; Oh, D.-Y.; Im, S.-A.; Bang, Y.-J.; Kim, S.; Lee, K.-W.; Kim, J.; Hong, Y.; et al. Pharmacogenetic Analysis of Adjuvant FOLFOX for Korean Patients with Colon Cancer. *Cancer Chem. Pharm.* **2013**, *71*, 843–851. [CrossRef]
72. Lee, A.M.; Shi, Q.; Pavey, E.; Alberts, S.R.; Sargent, D.J.; Sinicrope, F.A.; Berenberg, J.L.; Goldberg, R.M.; Diasio, R.B. *DPYD* Variants as Predictors of 5-Fluorouracil Toxicity in Adjuvant Colon Cancer Treatment (NCCTG N0147). *J. Nat. Cancer I.* **2014**, *106*. [CrossRef]
73. Lee, A.M.; Shi, Q.; Alberts, S.R.; Sargent, D.J.; Sinicrope, F.A.; Berenberg, J.L.; Grothey, A.; Polite, B.; Chan, E.; Gill, S.; et al. Association between *DPYD* c.1129–5923 C>G/HapB3 and Severe Toxicity to 5-Fluorouracil-Based Chemotherapy in Stage III Colon Cancer Patients. *Pharmacogenet. Genom.* **2016**, *26*, 133–137. [CrossRef]
74. Deenen, M.J.; Tol, J.; Burylo, A.M.; Doodeman, V.D.; de Boer, A.; Vincent, A.; Guchelaar, H.-J.; Smits, P.; Beijnen, J.H.; Punt, C.; et al. Relationship between Single Nucleotide Polymorphisms and Haplotypes in *DPYD* and Toxicity and Efficacy of Capecitabine in Advanced Colorectal Cancer. *Clin. Cancer Res.* **2011**, *17*, 3455–3468. [CrossRef]
75. Schwab, M.; Zanger, U.M.; Marx, C.; Schaeffeler, E.; Klein, K.; Dippon, J.; Kerb, R.; Blievernicht, J.; Fischer, J.; Hofmann, U.; et al. Role of Genetic and Nongenetic Factors for Fluorouracil Treatment-Related Severe Toxicity: A Prospective Clinical Trial by the German 5-FU Toxicity Study Group. *J. Clin. Oncol.* **2008**, *26*, 2131–2138. [CrossRef] [PubMed]
76. Hiratsuka, M.; Yamashita, H.; Akai, F.; Hosono, H.; Hishinuma, E.; Hirasawa, N.; Mori, T. Genetic Polymorphisms of Dihydropyrimidinase in a Japanese Patient with Capecitabine-Induced Toxicity. *PLoS ONE* **2015**, *10*. [CrossRef] [PubMed]
77. Terrazzino, S.; Cargnin, S.; Re, M.; Danesi, R.; Canonico, P.; Genazzani, A.A. *DPYD* IVS14+1G>A and 2846A>T Genotyping for the Prediction of Severe Fluoropyrimidine-Related Toxicity: A Meta-Analysis. *Pharmacogenomics* **2013**, *14*. [CrossRef] [PubMed]
78. Rosmarin, D.; Palles, C.; Church, D.; Domingo, E.; Jones, A.; Johnstone, E.; Wang, H.; Love, S.; Julier, P.; Scudder, C.; et al. Genetic Markers of Toxicity From Capecitabine and Other Fluorouracil-Based Regimens: Investigation in the QUASAR2 Study, Systematic Review, and Meta-Analysis. *J. Clin. Oncol.* **2014**, *32*, 1031–1039. [CrossRef] [PubMed]
79. Meulendijks, D.; Henricks, L.M.; Sonke, G.S.; Deenen, M.J.; Froehlich, T.K.; Amstutz, U.; Largiadèr, C.R.; Jennings, B.A.; Marinaki, A.M.; Sanderson, J.D.; et al. Clinical Relevance of *DPYD* Variants c.1679T>G, c.1236G>A/HapB3, and c.1601G>A as Predictors of Severe Fluoropyrimidine-Associated Toxicity: A Systematic Review and Meta-Analysis of Individual Patient Data. *Lancet Oncol.* **2015**, *16*, 1639–1650. [CrossRef]
80. Swen, J.; Nijenhuis, M.; Boer, A.; Grandia, L.; der Zee, M.A.; Mulder, H.; Rongen, G.; Schaik, R.; Schalekamp, T.; Touw, D.; et al. Pharmacogenetics: From Bench to Byte-An Update of Guidelines. *Clin. Pharmacol. Ther.* **2011**, *89*, 662–673. [CrossRef]
81. Caudle, K.; Thorn, C.; Klein, T.; Swen, J.; McLeod, H.; Diasio, R.; Schwab, M. Clinical Pharmacogenetics Implementation Consortium Guidelines for Dihydropyrimidine Dehydrogenase Genotype and Fluoropyrimidine Dosing. *Clin. Pharmacol. Ther.* **2013**, *94*, 640–645. [CrossRef]
82. Van kuilenbrg, A.B.; Dobritzsch, D.; Meinsma, R.; Haasjes, J.; Waterham, H.R.; Nowaczyk, M.J.; Maropoulos, G.D.; Guido, H.E.I.N.; Kalhoff, H.; Baaske, H.; et al. Novel disease-causing mutations in the dihydropyrimidine dehydrogenase gene interpreted by analysis of the three-dimensional protein structure. *Biochem. J.* **2002**, *364*, 157–163. [CrossRef]

83. Salgueiro, N.; Veiga, I.; Fragoso, M.; Sousa, O.; Costa, N.; Pellon, M.L.; Sanches, E.; dos Santos, J.G.; Teixeira, M.R.; Castedo, S. Mutations in exon 14 of dihydropyrimidine dehydrogenase and 5-Fluorouracil toxicity in Portuguese colorectal cancer patients. *Genet. Med.* **2004**, *6*, 102–107. [CrossRef]
84. Toffoli, G.; Giodini, L.; Buonadonna, A.; Berretta, M.; De Paoli, A.; Scalone, S.; Miolo, G.; Mini, E.; Nobili, S.; Lonardi, S.; et al. Clinical validity of a *DPYD*-based pharmacogenetic test to predict severe toxicity to fluoropyrimidines. *Int. J. Cancer* **2015**, *137*, 2971–2980. [CrossRef]
85. Collie-Duguid, E.S.R.; Etienne, M.C.; Milano, G.; McLeod, H.L. Known variant *DPYD* alleles do not explain DPD deficiency in cancer patients. *Pharmacogenet. Genomics* **2000**, *10*, 217–223. [CrossRef]
86. Van Kuilenburg, A.B.; Meijer, J.; Tanck, M.W.; Dobritzsch, D.; Zoetekouw, L.; Dekkers, L.L.; Roelofsen, J.; Meinsma, R.; Wymenga, M.; Kulik, W.; et al. Phenotypic and clinical implications of variants in the dihydropyrimidine dehydrogenase gene. *BBA Mol. Basis Dis.* **2016**, *1862*, 754–762. [CrossRef]
87. Amstutz, U.; Farese, S.; Aebi, S.; Largiadèr, C.R. Dihydropyrimidine dehydrogenase gene variation and severe 5-fluorouracil toxicity: a haplotype assessment. *Pharmacogenomics* **2009**, *10*, 931–944. [CrossRef] [PubMed]
88. Sistonen, J.; Büchel, B.; Froehlich, T.K.; Kummer, D.; Fontana, S.; Joerger, M.; van Kuilenburg, A.B.; Larqiader, C.R. Predicting 5-fluorouracil toxicity: DPD genotype and 5, 6-dihydrouracil: uracil ratio. *Pharmacogenomics* **2014**, *15*, 1653–1666. [CrossRef]
89. Nie, Q.; Shrestha, S.; Tapper, E.E.; Trogstad-Isaacson, C.S.; Bouchonville, K.J.; Lee, A.M.; Wu, R.; Jerde, C.R.; Wang, Z.; Kubica, P.A.; et al. Quantitative contribution of rs75017182 to dihydropyrimidine dehydrogenase mRNA splicing and enzyme activity. *CPT* **2017**, *102*, 662–670. [CrossRef]
90. Henricks, L.; Lunenburg, C.; de Man, F.; Meulendijks, D.; Frederix, G.; Kienhuis, E.; Creemers, G.; Baars, A.; Dezentjé, V.; Imholz, A.; et al. A Cost Analysis of Upfront *DPYD* Genotype–Guided Dose Individualisation in Fluoropyrimidine-Based Anticancer Therapy. *Eur. J. Cancer* **2019**, *107*, 60–67. [CrossRef]
91. Cutsem, V.; Cervantes, A.; Adam, R.; Sobrero, A.; Krieken, V.; Aderka, D.; Aguilar, A.; Bardelli, A.; Benson, A.; Bodoky, G.; et al. ESMO Consensus Guidelines for the Management of Patients with Metastatic Colorectal Cancer. *Ann. Oncol.* **2016**, *27*, 1386–1422. [CrossRef]
92. Milano, G. DPD Testing Must Remain a Recommended Option, but Not a Recommended Routine Test. *Annu. Oncol.* **2017**, *28*, 1399. [CrossRef]
93. Lunenburg, C.; Henricks, L.M.; Dreussi, E.; Peters, F.P.; Fiocco, M.; Meulendijks, D.; Toffoli, G.; Guchelaar, H.-J.; Swen, J.J.; Cecchin, E.; et al. Standard Fluoropyrimidine Dosages in Chemoradiation Therapy Result in an Increased Risk of Severe Toxicity in *DPYD* Variant Allele Carriers. *Eur. J. Cancer* **2018**, *104*, 210–218. [CrossRef] [PubMed]
94. Henricks, L.M.; Merendonk, L.N.; Meulendijks, D.; Deenen, M.J.; Beijnen, J.H.; Boer, A.; Cats, A.; Schellens, J. Effectiveness and Safety of Reduced-dose Fluoropyrimidine Therapy in Patients Carrying the *DPYD**2A Variant: A Matched Pair Analysis. *Int. J. Cancer* **2019**, *144*, 2347–2354. [CrossRef] [PubMed]
95. Coenen, M.; Paulussen, A.; Breuer, M.; Lindhout, M.; Tserpelis, D.; Steyls, A.; Bierau, J.; van den Bosch, B. Evolution of Dihydropyrimidine Dehydrogenase Diagnostic Testing in a Single Center during an 8-Year Period of Time. *Curr. Ther. Res.* **2019**, *90*. [CrossRef] [PubMed]
96. Loriot, M.-A.; Ciccolini, J.; Thomas, F.; Barin-Le-Guellec, C.; Royer, B.; Milano, G.; Picard, N.; Becquemont, L.; Verstuyft, C.; Narjoz, C.; et al. Dépistage Du Déficit En Dihydropyrimidine Deshydrogénase (DPD) et Sécurisation Des Chimiothérapies à Base de Fluoropyrimidines: Mise Au Point et Recommandations Nationales Du GPCO-Unicancer et Du RNPGx. *Bull. Cancer* **2018**, *105*, 397–407. [CrossRef]
97. Hillcoat, B.; McCulloch, P.; Figueredo, A.; Ehsan, M.; Rosenfeld, J. Clinical Response and Plasma Levels of 5-Fluorouracil in Patients with Colonic Cancer Treated by Drug Infusion. *Brit. J. Cancer* **1978**, *38*, 719–724. [CrossRef] [PubMed]
98. Thyss, A.; Milano, G.; Renée, N.; Vallicioni, J.; Schneider, M.; Demard, F. Clinical Pharmacokinetic Study of 5-FU in Continuous 5-Day Infusions for Head and Neck Cancer. *Cancer Chemother. Pharm.* **1986**, *16*, 64–66. [CrossRef]
99. Santini, J.; Milano, G.; Thyss, A.; Renee, N.; Viens, P.; Ayela, P.; Schneider, M.; Demard, F. 5-FU Therapeutic Monitoring with Dose Adjustment Leads to an Improved Therapeutic Index in Head and Neck Cancer. *Brit. J. Cancer* **1989**, *59*, 287–290. [CrossRef]

100. Gamelin, E.C.; Danquechin-Dorval, E.M.; Dumesnil, Y.F.; Maillart, P.J.; Goudier, M.; Burtin, P.C.; Delva, R.G.; Lortholary, A.H.; Gesta, P.H.; Larra, F.G. Relationship between 5-fluorouracil (5-FU) Dose Intensity and Therapeutic Response in Patients with Advanced Colorectal Cancer Receiving Infusional Therapy Containing 5-FU. *Cancer* **1996**, *77*, 441–451. [CrossRef]
101. Gamelin, E.; Boisdron-Celle, M.; Delva, R.; Regimbeau, C.; Cailleux, P.E.; Alleaume, C.; Maillet, M.L.; Goudier, M.J.; Sire, M.; Person-Joly, M.C.; et al. Long-Term Weekly Treatment of Colorectal Metastatic Cancer with Fluorouracil and Leucovorin: Results of a Multicentric Prospective Trial of Fluorouracil Dosage Optimization by Pharmacokinetic Monitoring in 152 Patients. *J. Clin. Oncol.* **1998**, *16*, 1470–1478. [CrossRef]
102. Fety, R.; Rolland, F.; Barberi-Heyob, M.; Hardouin, A.; Campion, L.; Conroy, T.; Merlin, J.; Riviere, A.; Perrocheau, G.; Etienne, M.C.; et al. Clinical Impact of Pharmacokinetically-Guided Dose Adaptation of 5-Fluorouracil: Results from a Multicentric Randomized Trial in Patients with Locally Advanced Head and Neck Carcinomas. *Clin. Cancer Res.* **1998**, *4*, 2039–2045.
103. Gamelin, E.; Delva, R.; Jacob, J.; Merrouche, Y.; Raoul, J.; Peset, D.; Dorval, E.; Piot, G.; Morel, A.; Boisdron-Celle, M. Individual Fluorouracil Dose Adjustment Base on Pharmacokinetic Follow-Up Compared with Conventional Dosage: Results of a Multicenter Randomized Trial of Patients with Metastatic Colorectal Cancer. *J. Clin. Oncol.* **2008**, *26*, 2099–2105. [CrossRef]
104. Lee, J.J.; Beumer, J.H.; Chu, E. Therapeutic Drug Monitoring of 5-Fluorouracil. *Cancer Chemother. Pharm.* **2016**, *78*, 447–464. [CrossRef] [PubMed]
105. Kaldate, R.; Haregewoin, A.; Grier, C.; Hamilton, S.; McLeod, H. Modeling the 5-Fluorouracil Area Under the Curve Versus Dose Relationship to Develop a Pharmacokinetic Dosing Algorithm for Colorectal Cancer Patients Receiving FOLFOX6. *Oncologist* **2012**, *17*, 296–302. [CrossRef] [PubMed]
106. Fang, L.; Xin, W.; Ding, H.; Zhang, Y.; Zhong, L.; Luo, H.; Li, J.; Yang, Y.; Huang, P. Pharmacokinetically Guided Algorithm of 5-Fluorouracil Dosing, a Reliable Strategy of Precision Chemotherapy for Solid Tumors: A Meta-Analysis. *Sci. Rep.* **2016**, *6*, 25913. [CrossRef]
107. Patel, J.N.; O'Neil, B.H.; Deal, A.M.; Ibrahim, J.G.; Sherrill, G.B.; Olajide, O.A.; Atluri, P.M.; Inzerillo, J.J.; Chay, C.H.; McLeod, H.L.; et al. A Community-Based Multicenter Trial of Pharmacokinetically Guided 5-Fluorouracil Dosing for Personalized Colorectal Cancer Therapy. *Oncologist* **2014**, *19*, 959–965. [CrossRef] [PubMed]
108. Goldstein, D.A.; Chen, Q.; Ayer, T.; Howard, D.H.; Lipscomb, J.; Harvey, D.R.; El-Rayes, B.F.; Flowers, C.R. Cost Effectiveness Analysis of Pharmacokinetically-Guided 5-Fluorouracil in FOLFOX Chemotherapy for Metastatic Colorectal Cancer. *Clin. Colorectal Cancer* **2014**, *13*, 219–225. [CrossRef] [PubMed]
109. Beumer, J.; Chu, E.; Allegra, C.; Tanigawara, Y.; Milano, G.; Diasio, R.; Kim, T.; Mathijssen, R.; Zhang, L.; Arnold, D.; et al. Therapeutic Drug Monitoring in Oncology: International Association of Therapeutic Drug Monitoring and Clinical Toxicology Recommendations for 5-Fluorouracil Therapy. *Clin. Pharm. Ther.* **2018**, *105*, 598–613. [CrossRef]
110. Haagsma, E.B.; Hagens, V.E.; Schaapveld, M.; van den Berg, A.P.; de Vries, E.; Klompmaker, I.J.; Slooff, M.; Jansen, P. Increased Cancer Risk after Liver Transplantation: A Population-Based Study. *J. Hepatol.* **2001**, *34*, 84–91. [CrossRef]
111. Mukthinuthalapati, P.; Gotur, R.; Ghabril, M. Incidence, Risk Factors and Outcomes of de Novo Malignancies Post Liver Transplantation. *World J. Hepatol.* **2016**, *8*, 533–544. [CrossRef]
112. Nishihori, T.; Strazzabosco, M.; Saif, M. Incidence and Management of Colorectal Cancer in Liver Transplant Recipients. *Clin. Colorectal Cancer* **2008**, *7*, 260–266. [CrossRef]
113. Karlsen, T.H.; Folseraas, T.; Thorburn, D.; Vesterhus, M. Primary Sclerosing Cholangitis-a Comprehensive Review. *J. Hepatol.* **2017**, *67*, 1298–1323. [CrossRef]
114. Palmela, C.; Peerani, F.; Castaneda, D.; Torres, J.; Itzkowitz, S.H. Inflammatory Bowel Disease and Primary Sclerosing Cholangitis: A Review of the Phenotype and Associated Specific Features. *Gut Liver* **2018**, *12*, 17–29. [CrossRef]
115. Bonato, G.; Cristoferi, L.; Strazzabosco, M.; Fabris, L. Malignancies in Primary Sclerosing Cholangitis—A Continuing Threat. *Digest. Dis.* **2015**, *33*, 140–148. [CrossRef]
116. Ryan, D.; Hong, T.; Bardeesy, N. Pancreatic Adenocarcinoma. *N. Engl. J. Med.* **2014**, *371*, 1039–1049. [CrossRef]

117. Suker, M.; Beurmer, B.; Sadot, E.; Marthey, L.; Faris, J.; Mellon, E.; El-Rayes, B.; Wang-Gillam, A.; Lacy, J.; Hhosein, P.J.; et al. FOLFIRINOX for Locally Advanced Pancreatic Cancer: A Systematic Review and Patient-Level Meta-Analysis. *Lancet Oncol.* **2016**, *17*, 801–810. [CrossRef]
118. Zhan, H.; Xu, J.; Wu, D.; Wu, Z.; Wang, L.; Hu, S.; Zhang, G. Neoadjuvant Therapy in Pancreatic Cancer: A Systematic Review and Meta-Analysis of Prospective Studies. *Cancer Med.* **2017**, *6*, 1201–1219. [CrossRef]
119. Olthoff, K.; Rosove, M.; Shackleton, C.; Imagawa, D.; Farmer, D. Adjuvant Chemotherapy Improves Survival After Liver Trasplantation for Hepatcellular Carcinoma. *Ann. Surg.* **1995**, *221*, 734–743. [CrossRef]
120. Zhang, Q.; Chen, H.; Li, Q.; Zang, Y.; Chen, X.; Zou, W.; Wang, L.; Shen, Z. Combination Adjuvant Chemotherapy with Oxaliplating and Leucovorin after Liver Transplantation for Hepatocellulat Carcinoma: A Preliminary Open-Label Study. *Invet. New. Drugs* **2011**, *29*, 1360–1369. [CrossRef]
121. Coriat, R.; Mir, O.; Cessot, A.; Brezault, C.; Ropert, S.; Durand, J.; Cacheux, W.; Chaussade, S.; Goldwasser, F. Feasibility of Oxaliplatin, 5-Fluorouracil and Leucovorin(FOLFOX-4) in Cirrhotic or Liver Transplant Patients: Experience in a Cohort of Advanced Hepatocellularcarcinoma Patients. *Investig. New Drugs* **2012**, *30*, 376–381. [CrossRef]
122. Raza, A.; Sood, G. Hepatocellular Carcinoma Review: Current Treatment, and Evidence Based Medicine. *World J. Gastro.* **2014**, *20*, 4115–4127. [CrossRef]
123. Kew, M. Hepatocellular Carcinoma: Epidemiology and Risk Factors. *J. Hepat. Carcinoma* **2014**, *1*, 115–125. [CrossRef] [PubMed]
124. Tan, H.; Fiel, M.; Martin, J.; Schiano, T. Graft Rejection Occuring in Post-Liver Transplant Patients Receiving Cytotoxic Chemotherapy: A Case Series. *Liver Transplant.* **2009**, *15*, 634–639. [CrossRef] [PubMed]
125. Zhu, L.; Jiang, W.; Pan, C.; Liu, Y.; Thian, Y. Liver Injury Possibly Related to Drug Interaction after Liver Transplant: A Case Report. *Clin. Pharm. Ther.* **2014**, *39*, 439–441. [CrossRef] [PubMed]

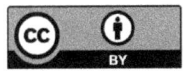

© 2019 by the authors. Licensee MDPI, Basel, Switzerland. This article is an open access article distributed under the terms and conditions of the Creative Commons Attribution (CC BY) license (http://creativecommons.org/licenses/by/4.0/).

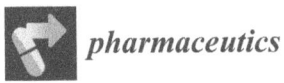

Article

Impact of *GSTA1* Polymorphisms on Busulfan Oral Clearance in Adult Patients Undergoing Hematopoietic Stem Cell Transplantation

Veronique Michaud [1,2], My Tran [3], Benoit Pronovost [1], Philippe Bouchard [1,4], Sarah Bilodeau [1,4], Karine Alain [1,4], Barbara Vadnais [1,4], Martin Franco [1,4], François Bélanger [2] and Jacques Turgeon [1,2,*]

1. Faculty of Pharmacy, Université de Montréal, Montreal, QC H3C 3J7, Canada
2. CRCHUM, Centre de Recherche du Centre Hospitalier de l'Université de Montréal, Montreal, QC H2X 0A9, Canada
3. College of Pharmacy, Lake Nona Campus, University of Florida, Orlando, FL 32827, USA
4. Hôpital Maisonneuve-Rosemont, Montreal, QC H1T 2M4, Canada
* Correspondence: jturgeon@trhc.com; Tel.: +01-856-938-8793

Received: 9 July 2019; Accepted: 18 August 2019; Published: 1 September 2019

Abstract: Background: Busulfan pharmacokinetics exhibit large inter-subject variability. Our objective was to evaluate the influence of glutathione S-transferase A1 (*GSTA1*) gene variants on busulfan oral clearance (CLo) in a population of patients undergoing hematopoietic stem cell transplantation. Methods: This is a quasi-experimental retrospective study in adult patients ($n = 87$ included in the final analyses) receiving oral busulfan. Pharmacokinetics data (area under the plasma concentration-time curve (AUC) determined from 10 blood samples) were retrieved from patients' files and *GSTA1* *A and *B allele polymorphisms determined from banked DNA samples. Three different limited sampling methods (LSM) using four blood samples were also compared. Results: Carriers of *GSTA1*B* exhibited lower busulfan CLo than patients with an *A/*A genotype ($p < 0.002$): Busulfan CLo was 166 ± 31, 187 ± 37 vs. 207 ± 47 mL/min for *GSTA1*B/*B*, *A/*B* and *A/*A* genotypes, respectively. Similar results were obtained with the tested LSMs. Using the standard AUC method, distribution of patients above the therapeutic range after the first dose was 29% for *GSTA1*A/*A*, 50% for *A/*B*, and 65% for *B/*B*. The LSMs correctly identified ≥91% of patients with an AUC above the therapeutic range. The misclassified patients had a mean difference less than 5% in their AUCs. Conclusion: Patients carrying *GSTA1* loss of function **B* allele were at increased risk of overdosing on their initial busulfan oral dose. Genetic polymorphisms associated with *GSTA1* explain a significant part of busulfan CLo variability which could be captured by LSM strategies.

Keywords: busulfan; glutathione S-transferase; genetic polymorphism; limited sampling strategy; pharmacokinetics

1. Introduction

In current hematopoietic stem cell transplantation (HSCT) practices, busulfan is a commonly used alkylating agent. When combined with other drugs, busulfan exhibits a beneficial immunosuppressive effect [1]. The drug has a very narrow therapeutic index which requires close therapeutic monitoring. Low concentrations of busulfan can result in an increased risk of graft failure and recurrence of the disease whereas high concentrations of busulfan can result in an increased risk of hepatic toxicity [2,3]. Current therapeutic monitoring methods of the drug involve taking numerous (often up to 10) blood samples to calculate patient's plasma concentration vs. time area under the curve (AUC) [4]. However, we and others have demonstrated the value of limited sampling strategies to estimate mean busulfan plasma concentration and compute required busulfan doses in these leukemic patients [5–9].

The glutathione S-transferase enzymes (GSTs) are important Phase II biotransformation enzymes that catalyze the conjugation of many hydrophobic and electrophilic compounds with reduced glutathione [10,11]. Based on their biochemical, immunologic, and structural properties, soluble GSTs (including cytosolic and mitochondrial forms) are divided into several classes; alpha, mu, kappa (mitochondrial), theta, pi, omega, and zeta [10,11]. The GST alpha 1 (A1) isoform is mainly expressed in the liver, intestine, kidneys and endocrine tissues and contributes to the metabolism of several anticancer drugs as well as steroids and products of lipid degradation [12,13]. The *GSTA1* gene has been mapped to the GST-alpha gene cluster on chromosome 6p12, it is approximately 12 kb long and contains seven exons [14]. *GSTA1* expression is influenced by a genetic polymorphism that consists of two alleles, *GSTA1*A* and *GSTA1*B*, containing three linked base substitutions in the proximal promoter, at positions −567, −69, and −52 [14,15]. The G-to-A change at position −52 appears to be responsible for the differential promoter activities of *GSTA1*A* and *GSTA1*B*, expression of *GSTA1*A* being greater than *GSTA1*B*.

Busulfan pharmacokinetics properties are highly variable among patients and dosing regimens are affected by patients' characteristics such as body weight, age and genotype [16]. For instance, busulfan pharmacokinetics in children differs largely from that observed in adults as clearance decreases with age even when expressed relative to body weight or body surface area [17]. Notably, busulfan is a lipophilic molecule with highly variable absorption and bioavailability [18]. The drug is highly protein bound and extensively metabolized in the liver with less than 2% being excreted unchanged in the urine [19,20]. Busulfan is mainly metabolized through conjugation with glutathione by the major hepatic isoform *GSTA1*. In vitro experiments showed that two other isoenzymes, *GSTM1* and *GSTP1*, contribute to a lesser extent in the formation of busulfan glutathione conjugates (46% and 18% of *GSTA1* busulfan activity, respectively) [19]. At this time, the relevance of *GSTA1* polymorphisms on busulfan pharmacokinetics in adults, following oral administration, has been suggested but not clearly established [16,21–25].

The primary objective of our study was to investigate the influence of *GSTA1* gene variants on busulfan oral clearance in adult patients. Our secondary objective was to combine use of genetic information and AUCs calculated from various limited sampling models (LSM) to characterize the predictive value of these joint strategies for required oral busulfan dose.

2. Methods

This is a quasi-experimental retrospective study. De-identified pharmacokinetic data generated in the context of a standard of care procedure was collected from adult patients who underwent HSCT preparation at Maisonneuve-Rosemont hospital over a 4-year period. The research protocol was approved by the ethics committee of Maisonneuve-Rosemont hospital (No. 06068; 5 October 2006).

2.1. Clinical Study Design

Adult patients ($n = 119$) aged 18 years and older receiving an oral dose of busulfan 4 mg/kg/d (using ideal body weight) divided into 4 doses per day for 4 days (total of 16 doses) were included in this study. Patients were excluded if they vomited in the hour following administration of the first dose. Patients who vomited and who required the administration of additional busulfan tablets were also excluded. Patients were also excluded if a complete pharmacokinetic profile could not be generated or if a DNA sample for genotype determination could not be obtained (e.g., patient's refusal to participate in Maisonneuve-Rosemont DNA banking for research purposes). A total of 97 pharmacokinetic profiles were obtained following the first administration of busulfan or after the second dose for 3 patients (therapeutic monitoring could not be performed on the first dose and standard dose was administered on first and second dose). Standard therapeutic drug monitoring consisted of obtaining 10 blood samples drawn at 0, 20, 40, 60, 90, 120, 180, 240, 300 and 360 min following the first busulfan dose on day one. Additional therapeutic drug monitoring was performed on subsequent doses in patients for whom the dose of busulfan was modified based on their pharmacokinetic profile (target AUC at Maisonneuve-Rosemont hospital = 1150–1450 µmol·min/L; 283, 245–357, 140 ng·min/mL).

2.2. Pharmacokinetic Profile Determination

Pharmacokinetic profiles were obtained by reviewing medical charts. Busulfan plasma levels were determined by a validated HPLC assay with UV detection [26]. The drug concentration–time data were analyzed by standard noncompartmental methods using WinNonLin® 10.0 software (Certara, Mountain View, CA, USA) to determine $AUC_{0\to\infty}$ (considered as the reference AUC). Apparent oral clearance (CLo) of busulfan was calculated as $CL/F = Dose_{(oral)}/AUC_{0\to\infty\,(oral)}$.

2.3. Genotyping Procedure

GSTA A1 C<-69>T polymorphism was determined by polymerase chain reaction-restriction fragment length polymorphism as described by Kusama et al. with minor modifications. [24] A 821 bp fragment in the promoter region of the *GSTA1* gene was amplified with a forward primer (F: 5'-CCC TAC ATG GTA TAG GTG AAA T-3') and reverse primer (R: 5'-GTG CTA AGG ACA CAT ATT AGC-3'). PCR reactions were performed in a PTC-100 Thermal Cycler (MJ Research Inc., Watertown, MA, USA) under the following conditions: an initial 5 min denaturation step at 95 °C, followed by 35 cycles of 1 min for each step i.e., denaturation at 96 °C, annealing at 63 °C and extension at 72 °C, and a final extension step at 72 °C for 5 min. PCR products were digested with *Hinf*I for 3–4 h at 37 °C and separated by electrophoresis (100 V, 45 min) on a 2% agarose/Synergel.

2.4. Validation Cohort

Genotyping procedures for *GSTA1* were also performed in random samples (*n* = 116) obtained from a genetic bank constituted of isolated DNA samples provided by a group of individuals (18–25 years old) without known cardiovascular diseases. These analyses were performed to establish *GSTA1* allele frequencies in "young heathy" adults. Consent was obtained from each individual prior to participation in this DNA banking initiative.

2.5. Comparison of the Standard Sampling Strategy to LSMs

We compared results of the standard sampling model to LSMs. From our previous paper, we have determined that the Bullock 4 limited sampling model as well as the New 4.2 and the New 4.3 LSM would be ideal for this study [5,6]. The Bullock 4 LSM requires blood samples at 0.5, 1, 4, and 6 h after the first dose whereas the New 4.2 LSM require blood samples at 1, 1.5, 3, and 6 h after the first dose while New 4.3 LSM requires blood samples at 1, 2, 4 and 6 h post-dose.

2.6. Statistical Analyses

Data are expressed as mean ± SD. The AUCs and oral clearance of busulfan were compared across the genotype groups of *GSTA1* using non-parametric tests. Tukey correction was used to determine the *p* values for multiple comparisons. The allele and genotype frequencies, and Hardy-Weinberg equilibrium were analyzed. Statistical analyses were performed using GraphPad v7.05 (GraphPad Software, Inc., San Diego, CA, USA).

3. Results

Over the four-year period of our study, 119 patients received oral busulfan. Therapeutic monitoring was performed on the first (or second dose, *n* = 3) of busulfan. A total of 100 pharmacokinetic profiles were obtained from those patients' medical charts. Genetic analyses were performed in 89 patients of which two patients were excluded (DNA quality). The characteristics of the 87 patients included in our final analysis are presented in Table 1. Fifty-five percent (55%) of these patients were male. Mean age was 48.3 ± 9.7 (range 25–65) years, adjusted body weight was 65.2 ± 10 (range 46–88) kg, and their lean body weight was 63.3 ± 9.6 (44–84) kg. Acetaminophen, which could decrease glutathione reserve, was co-administered in 23 patients. Antifungals such as voriconazole and fluconazole but not itraconazole (which has been associated with a decrease in busulfan clearance) were co-administered in six patients ($n = 1$ and 5, respectively). The mean initial dose of busulfan administered was 65 mg and the mean population AUC was 358,066 ng·min/mL.

Table 1. Patient demographics.

Variable	GSTA1 Genotype Groups			p-Value
	*A*A	*A*B	*B*B	
Age: Years ± SD (range)	50 ± 11 (27–65)	48 ± 9 (27–63)	48 ± 10 (25–60)	0.8
Gender: Male/female (% male)	13/11 (54)	26/14 (65)	9/14 (39)	0.4
Weight (Kg)				
Real Body Weight	74 ± 11	73 ± 15	76 ± 19	0.8
Adjusted Ideal Body Weight	65 ± 9	66 ± 11	64 ± 11	0.7
Lean Body Weight	64 ± 9	64 ± 10	61 ± 10	0.3
Bilirubin (U/L)	11 ± 6	14 ± 10	10 ± 5	0.2
AST (U/L)	22 ± 10	24 ± 9	22 ± 11	0.7
ALT (U/L)	27 ± 22	34 ± 23	33 ± 34	0.5
Albumin (g/L)	41 ± 4	42 ± 3	43 ± 5	0.3
Alkaline Phosphatase (U/L)	95 ± 38	86 ± 36*	81 ± 23	0.01
LDH (U/L)	280 ± 285*	166 ± 59	169 ± 43	0.01
Previously received chemotherapy (%)	22 (92)	35 (88)	19 (83)	0.2
Previously received radiotherapy (%)	3 (13)	4 (10)	2 (13)	0.8
Number of patients taking Acetaminophen (%)	9 (37)	8 (20)	6 (26)	0.02
Number of patients taking Antifungal Drugs (%)	2 (8)	3 (7)	1 (4)	0.4
First dose administered (mg)	65 ± 8	66 ± 12	65 ± 14	0.9

* Tukey's multiple comparison analysis, the group (*) was statistically different vs. the 2 other genotype groups.

The genotype frequencies found in our cohort were 27.5% ($n = 24$), 45.9% ($n = 40$), and 26.4% ($n = 23$) for the GSTA1*A/*A, *A/*B, and *B/*B groups, respectively. These frequencies were in Hardy-Weinberg equilibrium but differ from the distribution of alleles observed in our validation cohort (Table 2); more patients presented with a *B*B genotype (26.4%) compared to young healthy subjects (20%). Demographic data among GSTA1 genotype groups are presented in Table 1. There was no significant difference observed in most of these parameters among the groups except for alkaline phosphatase (APL) and lactate dehydrogenase (LDH) levels. The difference observed for the LDH results can be explained by outlier values for two individuals in the GSTA1*A*A group. A higher proportion of patients receiving acetaminophen was found in the GSTA1*A*A group. However, there was no statistically significant difference in measured AUC or in the apparent oral clearance of busulfan between acetaminophen users and non-users ($p = 0.6$).

Table 2. GSTA1 genotype frequencies.

Patients/Cohort	n	GSTA1 Genotypes % (n)		
		*A*A	*A*B	*B*B
Adult patients treated at HRM (study population)	87	27.6% (24)	46% (40)	26.4% (23)
Healthy man subjects (validation cohort)	116	31% (36)	49% (57)	20% (23)

Pharmacokinetic profiles obtained from patients demonstrated that 33/87 (38%) patients reached therapeutic range on the first dose: 12 patients were exhibiting subtherapeutic levels while 42 patients were having supratherapeutic levels. Figure 1 illustrates that higher AUCs were observed in patients with a GSTA1*B*B genotype (395,562 ± 77,083 ng/mL/min) compared to GSTA1*A/*B (357,062 ± 53,100 ng/mL/min) and GSTA1*A/*A patients (323,691 ± 65,906 ng/mL/min; $p < 0.001$). Hence, carriers of GSTA1*B ($n = 64$) were significantly associated with lower busulfan CLo compared to wild-type GSTA1*A: 179 ± 36 vs. 207 ± 47 mL/min ($p = 0.003$). Busulfan CLo among the three genotype groups are illustrated in Figure 2: 166 ± 31, 187 ± 40 and 207 ± 47 mL/min, for GSTA1*B/*B, *A/*B and *A/*A, respectively.

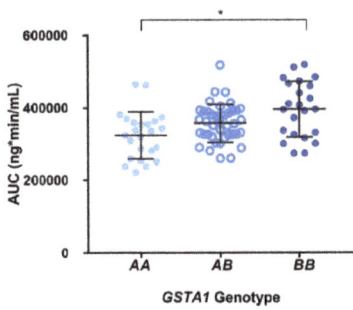

Figure 1. Busulfan plasma concentrations ($AUC_{0-\infty}$) measured after administration of the initial oral 1 mg/kg dose (1 mg/kg/day, four times a day, for 4 days) observed among the individual GSTA1 genotypes for 89 patients enrolled in this study.

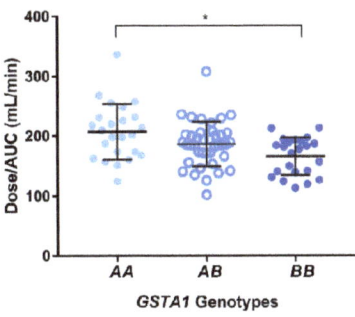

Figure 2. Oral clearance of busulfan calculated after administration of the initial oral dose as a function of patients ($n = 89$) GSTA1 genotypes.

Using the standard AUC method, distribution of patients (%) above the therapeutic range after the first dose was 29% for GSTA1*A/*A, 50% for *A/*B and 65% for *B/*B (Figure 3). Patients with a GSTA1*A/*A genotype were more likely to have achieved therapeutic levels (overall 42%) after the first dose of treatment compared to subjects with a GSTA1*B/*B genotype (26%).

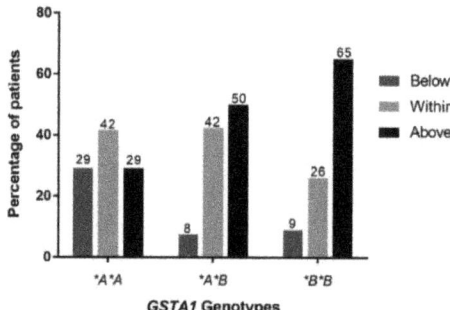

Figure 3. Distribution of patients with an AUC below, within and above the therapeutic range after the initial oral dose of busulfan for each *GSTA1* genotype.

The LSMs correctly associated 91% of patients with their therapeutic level category. In our final patients' cohort ($n = 87$), percent of patients with busulfan mean concentrations in the therapeutic range were 38%, 37%, 38% and 41% for the standard model (AUC with 10 time points), Bullock 4 model, New 4.2 and New 4.3 models, respectively (Supplemental Figure S1). Patients with busulfan mean concentrations above the therapeutic range were 48%, 47%, 44% and 44% for the standard model, Bullock 4 model, New 4.2 and New 4.3 models, respectively. The misclassified patients had a mean difference less than 5% (±4.8%, range AUC_{ref}/AUC_{LSM} 0.89–1.05) in their AUCs. The proportion of patients and their corresponding therapeutic levels using LSMs is illustrated in Figure 4 for the three *GSTA1* genotype groups. The LSMs correctly identified busulfan's AUC above the therapeutic range for individuals carrying *GSTA1*B*B* genotype for 15/15 (100%) using the Bullock 4 model and for 14/15 using New 4.2 and New 4.3 models. The only misclassified patient had a difference of 6% in the estimated AUCs compared to the standard AUC determination model.

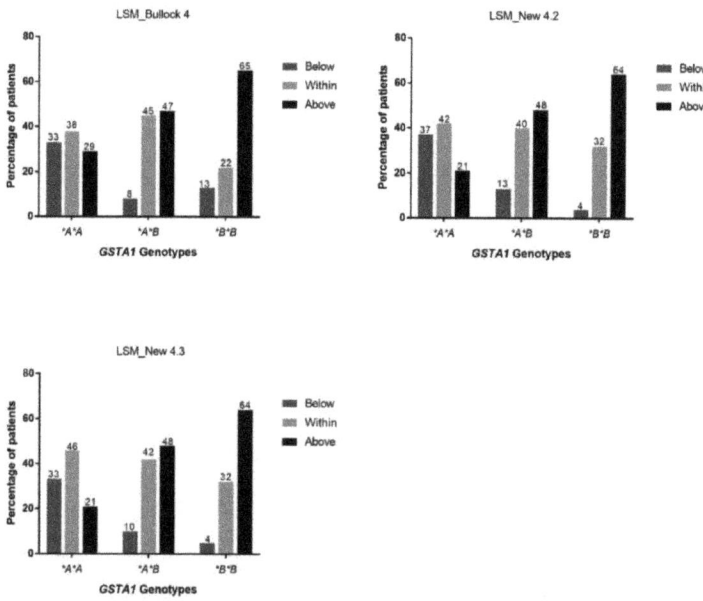

Figure 4. Distribution of patients with an AUC below, within and above the therapeutic range according to their GSTA1 genotype after the first dose of busulfan using 3 limited sampling methods (LSMs) based on 4 blood samples: Bullock 4, New 4.2 and New 4.3.

4. Discussion

In this study, we demonstrated that the administration of an initial standard oral dose of busulfan (1 mg/kg of a 4 mg/kg/day regimen) to patients with a *GSTA1*B*B* genotype was associated with higher plasma concentrations of busulfan and consequently, with lower estimated oral clearance of the drug. More patients with a *GSTA1*B*B* genotype were exhibiting mean plasma concentrations above the targeted therapeutic range for busulfan after the initial dose which could predispose them to increased toxicity from the drug. We also demonstrated that patients from the various *GSTA1* genotypes could be efficiently classified for their therapeutic level status by limited sampling strategies using four blood samples instead of 10.

Busulfan pharmacokinetics has been the subject of intense research due to important inter-subject variability and its narrow therapeutic index [2,3,16]. Clinical consequences of inappropriate dosing are well established with significant loss of efficacy in patients with sub-therapeutic levels and toxicity in patients with supra-therapeutic levels of the drug [2]. Various determinants of busulfan pharmacokinetics have been identified including weight, age and genetics. Dosing based on lean body weight and dose adjustment with age are well established [17]. However, the role of genetic polymorphisms still remains to be confirmed.

In the early 1960s, it was established that busulfan spontaneously reacts with glutathione and that conjugation with glutathione is the primary route of elimination [27,28]. Studies conducted with various purified human liver GST isoforms established that the highest busulfan-conjugating activity was observed with GSTA1 [19]. Genetic studies described the genomic organization of the human *GST* gene cluster and characterized the functional activity of genetic polymorphisms in the *GSTA1* promoter region [14,15]. From these studies, hypotheses were generated suggesting that decreased functional activity associated with the *GSTA1*B* allele would result in a decreased clearance of busulfan.

In 2006, Kusama et al., investigated for the first time the role of *GSTA1* polymorphisms on busulfan pharmacokinetics in a series of 12 patients [24]. Their results demonstrated that the heterozygous group (*GSTA1*A*B*; $n = 3$) had lower oral clearance, prolonged elimination half-life and higher plasma levels than the wildtype individuals (*GSTA1*A/*A*; $n = 9$). One year later, Kim et al. reported on the first association between *GSTA1* polymorphisms and response to busulfan therapy. [29] To date, very few studies have reexamined the role of *GSTA1* polymorphisms on busulfan pharmacokinetics after oral administration in adult patients. The study by Abbasi et al. reported on a decrease in busulfan clearance in their *GSTA1*B*B* patients' group treated with oral busulfan while Bremer et al. reported on increased averaged concentration and steady-state (Css) in *GSTA1*B*B* patients [21,25]. The magnitude of changes in busulfan oral clearance observed in our study (20%) in patients with a *GSTA1*B/*B* genotype compared to *GST*A/*A* patients agrees with these results.

The role of *GSTA1* polymorphisms in adults and in children as well as the impact of polymorphisms on other GST isoforms (*GSTM1* or *GSTP1*) on busulfan disposition, effects or toxicity are still controversial [16,21–23,25,30–39]. For instance, Rocha et al. established an association between *GSTP1* and chronic graft vs. host disease but Goekkurt et al. did not observe any correlation between various GST polymorphisms and liver toxicity [30,33]. Following intravenous administration, ten Brink et al., Kim et al. and Choi et al., found a decrease in busulfan clearance ranging from about 12–15% in expresser of the *GSTA1*B* allele while Abbasi et al. found no association [16,23,25,40].

One important observation of our study was that 2/3 of the patients with a *GSTA1*B*B* genotype had mean plasma levels above the upper limit of the therapeutic range (357,140 ng·min/mL) after the first oral dose of busulfan (442,711 ± 46,830 ng·min/mL). A 23% decrease in their subsequent oral doses was required to achieve therapeutic levels. Similar results were observed by Abbasi et al. in their *GSTA1*B*B* patients where a 20% decrease in dose was required between Dose 1 and 5 in order to achieve therapeutic levels [25].

The frequency of the *GSTA1*B*B* observed in our validation healthy subject cohort (20%) was almost identical to the one observed in two other Caucasian populations (20 and 20.8%, respectively) [41,42]. In our adult study cohort receiving busulfan, the *B variant was found in slightly higher frequency

(26% for the *B*B genotype). An increased frequency of GSTA1*B*B expressers was also observed in other Caucasian patients' population [15,43,44]. The significance of these observations would need to be confirmed in larger studies.

Finally, we have reported previously on the value of limited sampling strategies (four blood samples) to estimate mean plasma levels of patients undergoing treatment with oral busulfan [5]. This type of approach is of great relevance in sparing blood in patients with leukemia or other blood-related diseases. Bullock et al. also reported very similar results using slightly different time points (4) to calculate AUC [6].

5. Conclusions

Our study suggests that genetic polymorphisms associated with GSTA1 explain a significant part of the variability observed for busulfan pharmacokinetics. Our data support the utility of busulfan LSMs strategy clinically and for the interpretation of pharmacogenetics results.

Supplementary Materials: The following are available online at http://www.mdpi.com/1999-4923/11/9/440/s1, Figure S1. Percentage of patients with an AUC below, within and above the therapeutic range after the initial oral dose of busulfan using the refence AUC vs. 3 limited sampling methods (LSMs) based on 4 blood samples: Bullock 4, New 4.2 and New 4.3.

Author Contributions: Conceptualization, V.M., B.V., M.F. and J.T.; data collection, P.B., S.B. and K.A.; methodology development and validation, F.B. and B.P.; data analysis, M.T., P.B., S.B., K.A. and V.M.; writing—original draft preparation, M.T., V.M.; writing—review and editing, V.M. and J.T.; visualization, V.M.; supervision, V.M project administration, V.M. and J.T.; funding acquisition, V.M. and J.T.

Funding: Supported by internal funding obtained from the University of Montreal. Veronique Michaud was the recipient of a research scholarship from Fonds de Recherche du Québec-Santé (FRQS) in partnership with the Institut National d'Excellence en Santé et en Services Sociaux (INESSS).

Conflicts of Interest: The authors declare no conflict of interest.

References

1. Ben-Barouch, S.; Cohen, O.; Vidal, L.; Avivi, I.; Ram, R. Busulfan fludarabine vs busulfan cyclophosphamide as a preparative regimen before allogeneic hematopoietic cell transplantation: Systematic review and meta-analysis. *Bone Marrow Transpl.* **2016**, *51*, 232–240. [CrossRef] [PubMed]
2. Krivoy, N.; Hoffer, E.; Lurie, Y.; Bentur, Y.; Rowe, J.M. Busulfan use in hematopoietic stem cell transplantation: Pharmacology, dose adjustment, safety and efficacy in adults and children. *Curr. Drug Saf.* **2008**, *3*, 60–66. [CrossRef] [PubMed]
3. Russell, J.A.; Kangarloo, S.B. Therapeutic drug monitoring of busulfan in transplantation. *Curr. Pharm. Des.* **2008**, *14*, 1936–1949. [CrossRef] [PubMed]
4. Schuler, U.; Schroer, S.; Kuhnle, A.; Blanz, J.; Mewes, K.; Kumbier, I.; Proksch, B.; Zeller, K.P.; Ehninger, G. Busulfan pharmacokinetics in bone marrow transplant patients: Is drug monitoring warranted? *Bone Marrow Transpl.* **1994**, *14*, 759–765.
5. Bouchard, P.; Bilodeau, S.; Alain, K.; Vadnais, B.; Franco, M.; Turgeon, J.; Michaud, V. Evaluation of Limited Sampling Methods for Oral Busulfan Pharmacokinetic Monitoring in Adult Patients Undergoing Hematopoietic Stem Cell Transplantation. *Ther. Drug Monit.* **2016**, *38*, 414–418. [CrossRef]
6. Bullock, J.M.; Smith, P.F.; Booker, B.M.; Loughner, J.; Capozzi, D.; McCarthy, P.L., Jr.; Shaw, L.M. Development of a pharmacokinetic and Bayesian optimal sampling model for individualization of oral busulfan in hematopoietic stem cell transplantation. *Ther. Drug Monit.* **2006**, *28*, 62–66. [CrossRef] [PubMed]
7. Chattergoon, D.S.; Saunders, E.F.; Klein, J.; Calderwood, S.; Doyle, J.; Freedman, M.H.; Koren, G. An improved limited sampling method for individualised busulphan dosing in bone marrow transplantation in children. *Bone Marrow Transpl.* **1997**, *20*, 347–354. [CrossRef]
8. Hassan, M.; Fasth, A.; Gerritsen, B.; Haraldsson, A.; Syruckova, Z.; van den Berg, H.; Sandstrom, M.; Karlsson, M.; Kumlien, S.; Vossen, J. Busulphan kinetics and limited sampling model in children with leukemia and inherited disorders. *Bone Marrow Transpl.* **1996**, *18*, 843–850.

9. Balasubramanian, P.; Chandy, M.; Krishnamoorthy, R.; Srivastava, A. Evaluation of existing limited sampling models for busulfan kinetics in children with beta thalassaemia major undergoing bone marrow transplantation. *Bone Marrow Transpl.* **2001**, *28*, 821–825. [CrossRef]
10. Allocati, N.; Masulli, M.; Di Ilio, C.; Federici, L. Glutathione transferases: Substrates, inihibitors and pro-drugs in cancer and neurodegenerative diseases. *Oncogenesis* **2018**, *7*, 8. [CrossRef]
11. Nissar, S.; Sameer, A.; Chowdri, N.; Rashid, F. Glutathione S Transferases: Biochemistry, Polymorphism and Role in Colorectal Carcinogenesis. *J. Carcinog. Mutagenesis* **2017**, *8*, 286. [CrossRef]
12. Coles, B.F.; Kadlubar, F.F. Human alpha class glutathione S-transferases: Genetic polymorphism, expression, and susceptibility to disease. *Methods Enzymol.* **2005**, *401*, 9–42. [PubMed]
13. Available online: https://www.proteinatlas.org/ENSG00000243955-GSTA1/tissue (accessed on 8 July 2019).
14. Morel, F.; Rauch, C.; Coles, B.; Le Ferrec, E.; Guillouzo, A. The human glutathione transferase alpha locus: Genomic organization of the gene cluster and functional characterization of the genetic polymorphism in the hGSTA1 promoter. *Pharmacogenetics* **2002**, *12*, 277–286. [CrossRef] [PubMed]
15. Coles, B.F.; Morel, F.; Rauch, C.; Huber, W.W.; Yang, M.; Teitel, C.H.; Green, B.; Lang, N.P.; Kadlubar, F.F. Effect of polymorphism in the human glutathione S-transferase A1 promoter on hepatic GSTA1 and GSTA2 expression. *Pharmacogenetics* **2001**, *11*, 663–669. [CrossRef] [PubMed]
16. Choi, B.; Kim, M.G.; Han, N.; Kim, T.; Ji, E.; Park, S.; Kim, I.W.; Oh, J.M. Population pharmacokinetics and pharmacodynamics of busulfan with GSTA1 polymorphisms in patients undergoing allogeneic hematopoietic stem cell transplantation. *Pharmacogenomics* **2015**, *16*, 1585–1594. [CrossRef] [PubMed]
17. Hoffer, E.; Akria, L.; Tabak, A.; Scherb, I.; Rowe, J.M.; Krivoy, N. A simple approximation for busulfan dose adjustment in adult patients undergoing bone marrow transplantation. *Ther. Drug Monit.* **2004**, *26*, 331–335. [CrossRef]
18. Sjoo, F.; El-Serafi, I.; Enestig, J.; Mattsson, J.; Liwing, J.; Hassan, M. Comparison of algorithms for oral busulphan area under the concentration-time curve limited sampling estimate. *Clin. Drug Investig.* **2014**, *34*, 43–52. [CrossRef] [PubMed]
19. Czerwinski, M.; Gibbs, J.P.; Slattery, J.T. Busulfan conjugation by glutathione S-transferases alpha, mu, and pi. *Drug Metab. Dispos.* **1996**, *24*, 1015–1019.
20. Wu, X.; Xie, H.; Lin, W.; Yang, T.; Li, N.; Lin, S.; Yuan, X.; Ren, J.; Li, X.; Huang, X. Population pharmacokinetics analysis of intravenous busulfan in Chinese patients undergoing hematopoietic stem cell transplantation. *Clin. Exp. Pharmacol. Physiol.* **2017**, *44*, 529–538. [CrossRef]
21. Bremer, S.; Floisand, Y.; Brinch, L.; Gedde-Dahl, T.; Bergan, S. Glutathione Transferase Gene Variants Influence Busulfan Pharmacokinetics and Outcome After Myeloablative Conditioning. *Ther. Drug Monit.* **2015**, *37*, 493–500. [CrossRef]
22. Ten Brink, M.H.; Swen, J.J.; Bohringer, S.; Wessels, J.A.; van der Straaten, T.; Marijt, E.W.; von dem Borne, P.A.; Zwaveling, J.; Guchelaar, H.J. Exploratory analysis of 1936 SNPs in ADME genes for association with busulfan clearance in adult hematopoietic stem cell recipients. *Pharm. Genom.* **2013**, *23*, 675–683. [CrossRef] [PubMed]
23. Ten Brink, M.H.; Wessels, J.A.; den Hartigh, J.; van der Straaten, T.; von dem Borne, P.A.; Guchelaar, H.J.; Zwaveling, J. Effect of genetic polymorphisms in genes encoding GST isoenzymes on BU pharmacokinetics in adult patients undergoing hematopoietic SCT. *Bone Marrow Transpl.* **2012**, *47*, 190–195. [CrossRef] [PubMed]
24. Kusama, M.; Kubota, T.; Matsukura, Y.; Matsuno, K.; Ogawa, S.; Kanda, Y.; Iga, T. Influence of glutathione S-transferase A1 polymorphism on the pharmacokinetics of busulfan. *Clin. Chim. Acta* **2006**, *368*, 93–98. [CrossRef] [PubMed]
25. Abbasi, N.; Vadnais, B.; Knutson, J.A.; Blough, D.K.; Kelly, E.J.; O'Donnell, P.V.; Deeg, H.J.; Pawlikowski, M.A.; Ho, R.J.; McCune, J.S. Pharmacogenetics of intravenous and oral busulfan in hematopoietic cell transplant recipients. *J. Clin. Pharmacol.* **2011**, *51*, 1429–1438. [CrossRef] [PubMed]
26. Rifai, N.; Sakamoto, M.; Lafi, M.; Guinan, E. Measurement of plasma busulfan concentration by high-performance liquid chromatography with ultraviolet detection. *Ther. Drug Monit.* **1997**, *19*, 169–174. [CrossRef] [PubMed]
27. Roberts, J.J.; Warwick, G.P. The mode of action of alkylating agents. II. Studies of the metabolism of myleran. The reaction of myleran with some naturally occurring thiols in vitro. *Biochem. Pharmacol.* **1961**, *6*, 205–216. [CrossRef]

28. Roberts, J.J.; Warwick, G.P. The mode of action of alkylating agents—III: The formation of 3-hydroxytetrahydrothiophene-1:1-dioxide from 1:4-dimethanesulphonyloxybutane (Myleran), S-β-l-alanyltetrahydrothiophenium mesylate, tetrahydro-thiophene and tetrahydrothiophene-1:1-dioxide in the rat, rabbit and mouse. *Biochem. Pharmacol.* **1961**, *6*, 217–220.
29. Kim, I.; Keam, B.; Lee, K.H.; Kim, J.H.; Oh, S.Y.; Ra, E.K.; Yoon, S.S.; Park, S.S.; Kim, C.S.; Park, S.; et al. Glutathione S-transferase A1 polymorphisms and acute graft-vs.-host disease in HLA-matched sibling allogeneic hematopoietic stem cell transplantation. *Clin. Transpl.* **2007**, *21*, 207–213. [CrossRef] [PubMed]
30. Goekkurt, E.; Stoehlmacher, J.; Stueber, C.; Wolschke, C.; Eiermann, T.; Iacobelli, S.; Zander, A.R.; Ehninger, G.; Kroger, N. Pharmacogenetic analysis of liver toxicity after busulfan/cyclophosphamide-based allogeneic hematopoietic stem cell transplantation. *Anticancer Res.* **2007**, *27*, 4377–4380. [PubMed]
31. Johnson, L.; Orchard, P.J.; Baker, K.S.; Brundage, R.; Cao, Q.; Wang, X.; Langer, E.; Farag-El Maasah, S.; Ross, J.A.; Remmel, R.; et al. Glutathione S-transferase A1 genetic variants reduce busulfan clearance in children undergoing hematopoietic cell transplantation. *J. Clin. Pharmacol.* **2008**, *48*, 1052–1062. [CrossRef]
32. Zwaveling, J.; Press, R.R.; Bredius, R.G.; van Derstraaten, T.R.; den Hartigh, J.; Bartelink, I.H.; Boelens, J.J.; Guchelaar, H.J. Glutathione S-transferase polymorphisms are not associated with population pharmacokinetic parameters of busulfan in pediatric patients. *Ther. Drug Monit.* **2008**, *30*, 504–510. [CrossRef] [PubMed]
33. Rocha, V.; Porcher, R.; Fernandes, J.F.; Filion, A.; Bittencourt, H.; Silva, W., Jr.; Vilela, G.; Zanette, D.L.; Ferry, C.; Larghero, J.; et al. Association of drug metabolism gene polymorphisms with toxicities, graft-versus-host disease and survival after HLA-identical sibling hematopoietic stem cell transplantation for patients with leukemia. *Leukemia* **2009**, *23*, 545–556. [CrossRef] [PubMed]
34. Elhasid, R.; Krivoy, N.; Rowe, J.M.; Sprecher, E.; Adler, L.; Elkin, H.; Efrati, E. Influence of glutathione S-transferase A1, P1, M1, T1 polymorphisms on oral busulfan pharmacokinetics in children with congenital hemoglobinopathies undergoing hematopoietic stem cell transplantation. *Pediatr. Blood Cancer* **2010**, *55*, 1172–1179. [CrossRef] [PubMed]
35. Krivoy, N.; Zuckerman, T.; Elkin, H.; Froymovich, L.; Rowe, J.M.; Efrati, E. Pharmacokinetic and pharmacogenetic analysis of oral busulfan in stem cell transplantation: Prediction of poor drug metabolism to prevent drug toxicity. *Curr. Drug Saf.* **2012**, *7*, 211–217. [CrossRef] [PubMed]
36. Ten Brink, M.H.; van Bavel, T.; Swen, J.J.; van der Straaten, T.; Bredius, R.G.; Lankester, A.C.; Zwaveling, J.; Guchelaar, H.J. Effect of genetic variants GSTA1 and CYP39A1 and age on busulfan clearance in pediatric patients undergoing hematopoietic stem cell transplantation. *Pharmacogenomics* **2013**, *14*, 1683–1690. [CrossRef] [PubMed]
37. Ansari, M.; Rezgui, M.A.; Theoret, Y.; Uppugunduri, C.R.; Mezziani, S.; Vachon, M.F.; Desjean, C.; Rousseau, J.; Labuda, M.; Przybyla, C.; et al. Glutathione S-transferase gene variations influence BU pharmacokinetics and outcome of hematopoietic SCT in pediatric patients. *Bone Marrow Transpl.* **2013**, *48*, 939–946. [CrossRef]
38. Yin, J.; Xiao, Y.; Zheng, H.; Zhang, Y.C. Once-daily i.v. BU-based conditioning regimen before allogeneic hematopoietic SCT: A study of influence of GST gene polymorphisms on BU pharmacokinetics and clinical outcomes in Chinese patients. *Bone Marrow Transpl.* **2015**, *50*, 696–705. [CrossRef]
39. Huezo-Diaz Curtis, P.; Uppugunduri, C.R.S.; Muthukumaran, J.; Rezgui, M.A.; Peters, C.; Bader, P.; Duval, M.; Bittencourt, H.; Krajinovic, M.; Ansari, M. Association of CTH variant with sinusoidal obstruction syndrome in children receiving intravenous busulfan and cyclophosphamide before hematopoietic stem cell transplantation. *Pharm. J.* **2018**, *18*, 64–69. [CrossRef]
40. Kim, S.D.; Lee, J.H.; Hur, E.H.; Lee, J.H.; Kim, D.Y.; Lim, S.N.; Choi, Y.; Lim, H.S.; Bae, K.S.; Noh, G.J.; et al. Influence of GST gene polymorphisms on the clearance of intravenous busulfan in adult patients undergoing hematopoietic cell transplantation. *Biol. Blood Marrow Transpl.* **2011**, *17*, 1222–1230. [CrossRef]
41. Skrzypczak-Zielinska, M.; Zakerska-Banaszak, O.; Tamowicz, B.; Sobieraj, I.; Drweska-Matelska, N.; Szalata, M.; Slomski, R.; Mikstacki, A. Polymorphisms and allele frequencies of glutathione S-transferases A1 and P1 genes in the Polish population. *Genet. Mol. Res.* **2015**, *14*, 2850–2859. [CrossRef]
42. Bredschneider, M.; Klein, K.; Murdter, T.E.; Marx, C.; Eichelbaum, M.; Nussler, A.K.; Neuhaus, P.; Zanger, U.M.; Schwab, M. Genetic polymorphisms of glutathione S-transferase A1, the major glutathione S-transferase in human liver: Consequences for enzyme expression and busulfan conjugation. *Clin. Pharmacol. Ther.* **2002**, *71*, 479–487. [CrossRef] [PubMed]

43. Suvakov, S.; Damjanovic, T.; Stefanovic, A.; Pekmezovic, T.; Savic-Radojevic, A.; Pljesa-Ercegovac, M.; Matic, M.; Djukic, T.; Coric, V.; Jakovljevic, J.; et al. Glutathione S-transferase A1, M1, P1 and T1 null or low-activity genotypes are associated with enhanced oxidative damage among haemodialysis patients. *Nephrol. Dial. Transpl.* **2013**, *28*, 202–212. [CrossRef] [PubMed]
44. Spalletta, G.; Piras, F.; Gravina, P.; Bello, M.L.; Bernardini, S.; Caltagirone, C. Glutathione S-transferase alpha 1 risk polymorphism and increased bilateral thalamus mean diffusivity in schizophrenia. *Psychiatry Res.* **2012**, *203*, 180–183. [CrossRef] [PubMed]

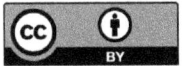

© 2019 by the authors. Licensee MDPI, Basel, Switzerland. This article is an open access article distributed under the terms and conditions of the Creative Commons Attribution (CC BY) license (http://creativecommons.org/licenses/by/4.0/).

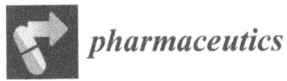

Review

Can Implementation of Genetics and Pharmacogenomics Improve Treatment of Chronic Low Back Pain?

Vladislav Suntsov [1], Filip Jovanovic [1], Emilija Knezevic [1], Kenneth D. Candido [1,2,3] and Nebojsa Nick Knezevic [1,2,3,*]

1. Department of Anesthesiology, Advocate Illinois Masonic Medical Center, 836 W. Wellington Ave. Suite 4815, Chicago, IL 60657, USA; vladislav.suntsov@aah.org (V.S.); drfilipjovanovic91@gmail.com (F.J.); ekneze2@illinois.edu (E.K.); kenneth.candido@aah.org (K.D.C.)
2. Department of Anesthesiology, University of Illinois, Chicago, IL 60612, USA
3. Department of Surgery, University of Illinois, Chicago, IL 60612, USA
* Correspondence: nebojsa@uic.edu; Tel.: +1-773-296-5619; Fax: +1-773-296-5362

Received: 11 August 2020; Accepted: 14 September 2020; Published: 21 September 2020

Abstract: Etiology of back pain is multifactorial and not completely understood, and for the majority of people who suffer from chronic low back pain (cLBP), the precise cause cannot be determined. We know that back pain is somewhat heritable, chronic pain more so than acute. The aim of this review is to compile the genes identified by numerous genetic association studies of chronic pain conditions, focusing on cLBP specifically. Higher-order neurologic processes involved in pain maintenance and generation may explain genetic contributions and functional predisposition to formation of cLBP that does not involve spine pathology. Several genes have been identified in genetic association studies of cLBP and roughly, these genes could be grouped into several categories, coding for: receptors, enzymes, cytokines and related molecules, and transcription factors. Treatment of cLBP should be multimodal. In this review, we discuss how an individual's genotype could affect their response to therapy, as well as how genetic polymorphisms in CYP450 and other enzymes are crucial for affecting the metabolic profile of drugs used for the treatment of cLBP. Implementation of gene-focused pharmacotherapy has the potential to deliver select, more efficacious drugs and avoid unnecessary, polypharmacy-related adverse events in many painful conditions, including cLBP.

Keywords: chronic low back pain (cLBP); genetics; pharmacogenomics; personalized treatment; polymorphism; CYP450

---

1. Introduction

Low back pain (LBP) is an extremely common problem affecting 80% of individuals at some point in their lifetime. It is the fifth most common motive for all physician visits. A lifetime prevalence of LBP was found to be about 40% worldwide [1]. In the United States (US), LBP and related costs are escalating [1], along with many modalities and their application in managing this problem. Five to ten percent of patients will develop constant back pain. Chronic low back pain (cLBP) has a strong impact on society. The US Burden of Disease Collaborators have shown that in 1990 and 2010, LBP was a disability that persistently affected people for the longest amount of time.

From the 1990s to 2000s, healthcare costs for adults with spinal problems continuously increased, with a rough estimate of 6000 USD per person with cLBP in 2005, totaling 102 billion USD [2]. In the US, adults suffering from cLBP were found to make more frequent healthcare visits usually covered by government-sponsored health insurance plans and to be more socioeconomically disadvantaged [2].

The etiology of back pain is multifaceted and not completely understood. We know that back pain is somewhat heritable, chronic pain more so than acute. In as many as 80% of people suffering from cLBP, the precise cause cannot be determined. Despite cLBP often being connected to anatomic perturbations such as herniation or degeneration of the intervertebral disc (IVD), these physical findings have a weak association with cLBP [3,4] and account for only a fraction (7–23%) of the genetic influence on back pain [5]. Conversely, objective findings such as degenerative findings on imaging often do not translate into chronicity of LBP. Higher-order neurologic processes involved in pain maintenance and generation may explain genetic contributions and functional predisposition to the development of cLBP that does not involve spine pathology [6–8].

Several genes have been identified in genetic association studies of chronic pain conditions. The results of the mentioned studies suggest a pathophysiology based on disruption of tissue remodeling, with abundant pro-inflammatory signaling leading to pain [9]. In the following review, we compiled the genes identified by numerous genetic association studies with chronic pain conditions, focusing on LBP specifically. Roughly, these genes group into several categories, coding for: receptors, enzymes, cytokines and related molecules, opioid receptor ligands, and transcription factors.

2. Materials and Methods

We reviewed genetic association studies by conducting a keyword search on the PubMed database. The search keywords included: "chronic back pain", "low back pain" combined with "genetics", "genetic association", "variant", or "polymorphism". Publications were screened by title and abstract. If the screening presented incomplete information, the text and tables/figures of the relevant publication were read and examined. We excluded reviews and publications that reported equivalent results from the same cohort. Barring several large populations studies, the bulk of the studies conducted presently have been done on modest population samples containing fewer than 1000 individuals.

3. Genes of Interest

3.1. Receptors

3.1.1. OPRM1 (Opioid Receptor Mu 1)

OPRM1 is a gene coding for the mu (µ) opioid receptor, which is the primary target of opioid analgesics as well as endogenous opioid peptides (e.g., beta-endorphin and enkephalins). The mu-opioid receptor also has an important role in modulation of the dopamine system and subsequently, dependence on drugs of abuse, e.g., as nicotine, cocaine, and alcohol. Hasvik et al. [10] explored the relationship between the OPRM1 genotype and subjective health complaints (SHC) in patients with disc herniation and radicular pain. The Subjective Health Complaints Inventory was used as the primary outcome. The inventory includes 27 prevalent complaints experienced in the month prior and rated on a scale from 'not at all' (0) to 'severe' (3) [10]. Twenty-three out of 118 patients carried the OPRM1 G-allele. Single nucleotide polymorphism (SNP) genotyping was performed on the OPRM1 A118G. Females that carried the G-allele reported a decrease in pain at the one-year follow-up. When asked for pain scores and pain duration, female carriers had consistently more health complaints than male carriers throughout the study. Thus, the study surmised that in patients with radicular pain, SHCs are associated with sex, as seen through OPRM1 A118G polymorphism interaction [10]. Although it was formerly thought that the increased SHC was secondary to pain, these results suggested it might be more significant [11]. The interaction between sex and the OPRM1 polymorphism observed in this study confirms earlier findings. Reports state that µ-opioid receptor binding potential could be greater in women and with increasing age [12]. One study demonstrated region-specific divergence in levels of OPRM1 between individuals with AA and G alleles [13]. The *OPRM1* genotype may impart sensitivity to pro-inflammatory, immune, and stress responses [14], and sensitivity to social rejection [15]. Acute and chronic stress affects µ-opioid receptors in GABAergic neurons differently in male and female rats [16]. This occurs by a mechanism that is not understood.

3.1.2. HTR2A (5-Hydroxytryptamine Receptor 2A)

Research has shown the associations between being susceptible to chronic pain conditions (e.g., chronic widespread pain and fibromyalgia) and serotonin receptor 2A (HTR2A) gene polymorphisms [17]. HTR2A gene polymorphisms rs6311 and rs6313 were found to be associated with higher disability, as measured by ODI (Oswestry Disability index) [18]. Polymorphism rs6311 (1438 A/G) was associated with chronic LBP, but patients with genotypes AA and AG had greater ODI scores [18]. Likewise, patients with TT or TC genotypes in rs6313 (102 T/C) polymorphism had higher ODI scores, but these genotypes were not associated with cLBP [18]. In an animal model, injection of exogenous 5-HT to the nerve root caused pain-associated findings, thus illustrating the role 5-HT plays in the initial biochemical pathogenesis of sciatic pain [19]. Moreover, selective serotonin reuptake inhibitors (SSRIs) have seen successful use in the treatment of cLBP. In a 2003 study by Kanayama et al., 300 mg of sarpogrelate hydrochloride, which is a selective 5-HT(2A) receptor blocker, was given orally for two weeks to 44 patients with symptomatic lumbar disc herniation. Visual analog scale (VAS) of LBP, numbness, and sciatic pain significantly improved post treatment with the serotonin receptor blocker, with >50% pain relief in 23 patients, 25–50% relief in five patients, and <25% relief in 16 patients. The effects of the 5HT2A receptor blocker saw more favorable response in patients with uncontained disc herniation than in patients with contained disc herniation [20].

3.1.3. DCC (Deleted in Colorectal Carcinoma)

Another significant CBP-associated gene variant is the lead SNP rs4384683, an intronic variant in the gene DCC (deleted in colorectal carcinoma) [21]. Netrin-1 is an axonal guidance molecule, and as such, participates in the development of cortical and spinal commissural neurons. DCC encodes the protein that serves as a receptor for Netrin-1 [22]. DCC–Netrin-1 interactions are a well-studied axonal guidance mechanism that affects angiogenesis and are vital during development and adulthood [23,24]. Compared to healthy human IVDs, expression of both these genes is greater in degraded discs. They are also found less frequently in the annulus fibrosus than in the nucleus pulposus [25]. Neurovascular ingrowth into the IVD may be mediated by netrin-1 and DCC, which is a mechanism that has long been implicated in chronic discogenic back pain [25,26]. Given the phenotypic correlation between CBP and depression [27], the correlation between CBP and DCC (depressive symptoms associated with cross phenotype of rs4384683) could also be explained by pleiotropy [21]. In animal models of mechanical allodynia, interactions of Netrin1/DCC have been found to impact pain processing in the spinal cord [23]. In accord, these data suggest numerous possible causes for the relationship between CBP and DCC, including the involvement of mood and/or nociceptive pathways [21]. rs4384683 in the DCC gene was also associated with depressive symptoms [28] with the same trend i.e., the A allele was associated with lower risk of CBP.

3.1.4. ESR (Estrogen Receptor 1)

Roh et al. [29] examined the relationship between estrogen receptor (ER) alpha (α) (ERα) polymorphisms and degenerative spondylolisthesis (DS) patients. A strong association was found between XbaI polymorphism and the VAS score of back pain. Subjects with AG and AA genotypes had significantly lower back pain ($p < 0.05$) VAS scores than did patients with a GG genotype. Identification of the CG haplotype with PvuII and XbaI polymorphism analysis in patients with back pain showed increased pain intensity on the VAS scale. ERα, a steroid hormone nuclear receptor, transactivates estrogen-responsive elements. Estrogen receptors are classified as ERα or ER beta (β), based on the mode of alternate gene splicing. The two receptors are significant regulators of skeletal maturation and growth [30,31]. The relationship between ERα and osteoarthritis has been recognized in a number of studies [32]. Thus, a gene in any part of the estrogen endocrine pathway is of interest to research in the pathogenesis of degenerative spondylolisthesis and broader implications for LBP.

3.1.5. CNR2 (Cannabinoid Receptor 2)

The CNR2 receptor system is dynamically involved in pain processing. The current hypothesis is that following pain induction, the functional upregulation of spinal CNR2 protein and mRNA seems to contribute an important countermeasure to the formation of central sensitization. This is corroborated by the exacerbation of allodynia at the painful site, and the novel manifestation of allodynia in the control site in mice with genetically deleted $Cnr2$ ($Cnr2^{-/-}$) [33]. In a study by Ramesh et al., CNR2 mRNA expression was increased among patients with both acute and chronic LBP at baseline compared to healthy controls [34].

3.1.6. ADRB2 (Adrenoceptor Beta 2)

Correlation was shown between SNP rs2053044 (ADRB2, recessive model) and CDCP (chronic disabling comorbid neck and low back pain). The study strongly suggests that genetic variants in the ADRB2 gene coding for the beta-2-adrenergic receptor makes individuals predisposed to chronic musculoskeletal complaints [35].

Some relevant receptor-related gene studies that are not referenced in the text are listed in Table 1.

Table 1. Receptor-related genes.

Gene	Function/Pathway	Condition(s)	Citation	Number of Subjects/Geographic Region
DCC	Receptor for Netrin-1, as an axonal guidance molecule	LBP	Suri et al., 2018 [21]	$n = 168{,}000$
ESR1	Other/Estrogen receptor 1	LBP	Roh et al., 2013 [29]	$n = 192$, South Korea
ADRB2	Neurotransmission/beta-2 adrenergic receptor	TMD/LBP/Fibromyalgia LBP comorbid with neck pain	Diatchenko et al., 2006 [36]/Skouen et al. [35]/Vargas-Alarcon et al., 2009 [37]	$n = 1004$; Western Australian Pregnancy (Raine) Cohort
CNR2	Peripheral cannabinoid receptor; nociceptive transmission, inflammatory response, bone homeostasis	LBP/mechanical allodynia, neuroinflammation in CRPS1/Joint pain	Starkweather et al., 2017 [38]; Ramesh et al., 2018 [34]/Xu et al., 2016 [39]	$n = 62$ USA; $n = 84$ USA/animal model/animal model
OPRM1	Neurotransmission/Mu opioid receptor	LBP	Hasvik et al., 2014 [10], Omair et al. have not replicated the above (2015) [40]	$n = 118$ Caucasians, Norway

Abbreviations: TMD, temporomandibular disorder; LBP, low back pain; CRPS1, complex regional pain syndrome 1; DCC, deleted in colorectal carcinoma.

3.2. Enzymes

3.2.1. COMT (Catechol-O-Methyltransferase)

Catechol-O-Methyltransferase (COMT) is an enzyme that helps regulate adrenergic, nonadrenergic, and dopaminergic signaling through metabolizing catecholamines. Research has been done on a number of human and animal pain models to investigate the effects of decreased COMT enzyme activity on nociception. Peripheral pain sensitivity was found to be increased by low COMT activity in animal model data [41]. Low COMT activity in humans, however, attenuated spinal nociceptive activity and central sensitization [42]. Thus, it can be concluded that low COMT activity has a complex effect. A correlation between pain hypersensitivity and Met alleles producing low enzyme activity was often found in human pain models [43]. Pain sensitivity has been associated with a functional polymorphism reducing the enzyme activity in the gene encoding COMT, the COMT Val158Met SNP. Jacobsen et al. [44] examined COMT Val158Met SNP contribution to sciatica and discogenic subacute LBP. Degenerative disc disease (DDD) subjects' appearance of the Val158Met genotypes was measured against healthy controls. It was hoped that this SNP may help in predicting the advancement of pain and disability. There were no differences in the frequency of the COMT genotype between controls and newly diagnosed subjects. When patients' pain and disability were examined over time, a borderline significant rise in functionality measured with the ODI score and the McGill sensory score was found for patients who had a COMT Met/Met genotype. Furthermore, six months after inclusion, a significant relationship was observed between patients' COMT Met-allele, pain (VAS score), McGill sensory, and ODI scores. It was also found that Val158Met SNP may contribute to disc herniation symptoms; patients with Met/Met had the slowest recovery and most pain, followed by those with Val/Met, followed by those with Val/Val [44]. Baseline disability was found to be significantly related to two haplotypes ($p < 0.002$), age, sex, and smoking ($p \leq 0.002$), COMT SNPs rs6269 ($p = 0.007$), rs2075507 ($p = 0.009$), rs4818 in European adults ($p = 0.02$), and rs4633 ($p = 0.04$). There were no meaningful associations observed with clinical variables during the long-term follow up. Although this suggests that genetics plays a role in disability level in chronic LBP patients being considered for surgery, it was concluded that genetics does not affect the outcome of treatment in the long term [40]. A relationship between pain perception after lumbar discectomy and genetic polymorphism of the COMT enzyme was found by Rut et al. All of the subjects had a one-level symptomatic disc herniation from L3 to S1. The study tracked ODI to assess pain intensity and the patients' quality of life, as well as VAS to assess back and leg pain. At the one-year follow-up, patients with the rs4680 GG genotype and COMT rs4633 CC demonstrated significant improvement in LBP. Better clinical outcome was shown in ODI scores and VAS for patients with COMT haplotype related to low metabolic activity of the enzyme (A_C_C_G) after surgery. It is noted that the study was too small to draw conclusions about the relationship between genetic diversity in COMT and clinical outcome after lumbar discectomy. It is suggested by the authors that the COMT genotype could serve a purpose in determining which patients would benefit more from surgery e.g., selection of subjects for earlier surgery [45].

3.2.2. CASP9 (Caspase-9)

Caspase-9 (CASP-9) initiates apoptosis through signaling with the initiator caspase. CASP-9 influences the growth and progression of lumbar disc disease (LDD) [46]. The transcriptional activity of CASP-9 is intensified by polymorphism in the promoter region. This modulates the susceptibility to LDD [46]. Guo et al. studied the association between -712C/T (rs4645981) and CASP-9 -1263A/G (rs4645978) polymorphisms and discogenic LBP, finding that people with identified rs4645978 have a high probability of discogenic LBP. CASP-9 was found to be vital to regulating cell homeostasis through the cleavage of molecules concerned in apoptosis in mouse models, where the CASP-9 gene was made inoperative [47]. The apoptotic machinery within cells is engaged by numerous pro-apoptotic stimuli, leading to the generation of the apoptosome. The downstream CASP-9 cascade is then activated by the apoptosome with effector caspases, which leads to apoptosis [48]. Abnormal functioning apoptosomes are known to contribute to carcinogenesis, but may also play a role in various degenerative disorders [49,50]. Apoptosis inactivation is a hallmark of cancer, as it allows the survival of cells prone to genetic damage [51]. In contrast, apoptosis activation leads to cell reduction in the degenerated disc in LDD, particularly discogenic LBP. It is suggested by Guo et al. that the activity and/or frequency of CASP-9 could be greater in those who carry the -1263 GG genotype and that apoptosis of IVD cells may be abnormally enhanced in such individuals. Given that these disc cells possess and maintain a large extracellular matrix, the IVD being prone to degeneration with a reduced cell count is hardly surprising [52]. With advanced degeneration, radial tearing of the disc may occur [46].

3.2.3. GCH1 (GTP Cyclohydrolase 1)

According to Tegeder et al., GTP hydrolase (GCH1) is a key modulator of neuropathic and inflammatory pain [53]. It is an enzyme that limits the rate of synthesis of BH4 (tetrahydrobiopterin). Downstream, BH4 affects production of serotonin, nitric oxide, and catecholamines. The amount of BH4 increases in primary sensory neurons after axonal injury due to the upregulation of GCH1. Dorsal root ganglia (DRGs) also see increased levels of BH4 after peripheral inflammation due to greater GCH1 activity. In rats, preventing new BH4 synthesis led to attenuation of inflammatory and neuropathic pain, and stopped nerve injury-related nitric oxide production in the DRP, whereas depositing BH4 intrathecally was found to aggravate pain. A haplotype of GCH1 found in 15.4%

of the population was related to less pain after discectomy for persistent radicular low back pain in humans. Decreased pain sensitivity was shown in healthy test subjects homozygous for this haplotype. Leukocytes excited by forskolin in haplotype carriers saw less upregulated GCH1 than controls. In order to explore BH4's possible implications in human pain, studies [53,54] have evaluated the possible relationship of certain pain phenotypes with polymorphisms in GCH1. Serious neurological issues and DOPA-responsive dystonia occur if BH4 is significantly decreased or nonexistent in humans, which takes place in uncommon instances of mutations—nonsense, missense, insertion, or deletion mutations in coding areas of GTP cyclohydrolase or sepiapterin reductase genes [55,56]. Due to the dependency of serotonin and dopamine neurotransmitter-synthesizing enzymes on BH4, inadequate amounts of BH4 lead to deficiencies of these transmitters and therefore, neurological conditions. This study found no neurological conditions in homozygotes for the pain-protective haplotype. It was consequently suggested that the pain-protective haplotype contains a variation in a regulatory site, leading to deterioration in GTP cyclohydrolase function or production. To further support this finding, the constitutive frequency of GTP cyclohydrolase and BH4 production was found to be the same between non-carriers and carriers of the pain-protective haplotype. These findings showed that changes in the amount of essential enzyme cofactor BH4 affect the sensitivity of the pain system. Further, the risk of developing continuous neuropathic pain and responses of healthy humans to noxious stimuli were both found to be affected by SNPs in the gene for the enzyme GTP cyclohydrolase. Since a decreased susceptibility to developing continuous pain is associated with the pain-protective haplotype in GCH1, there is potential for a treatment that might avoid the initial onset or development of chronic pain. This potential treatment could decrease surplus de novo synthesis of BH4 in the DRG, but not constitutive amounts of BH4, by leaving the recycling pathway untouched or by focusing solely on induction of GTP cyclohydrolase. Additionally, a factor that provides predictions into the severity and length of pain would also be a helpful device in analyzing a patient's risk of chronic pain. The presence of BH4 in people suffering from inflammatory pain as well as peripheral neuropathy points to GCH1 upregulation as a result of overall injury to axons and thus, can predict the rate of chronic/postsurgical levels of pain [57,58].

3.2.4. MMP 1,2,3 (Matrix Metallopeptidases)

Matrix metalloproteinases (MMPs) have an effect on the development of LBP due to their direct involvement in the deterioration of the extracellular matrix in the IVD. The -1607 promoter polymorphism, which is a SNP for guanine insertion/deletion (G/D) of the MMP1 gene, significantly affects transcription level and promoter activity. Song et al. [59] demonstrated an association between degenerative disc disease in southern Chinese subjects and the -1607 promoter polymorphism of MMP1. Genotypic association on the presence of the D allele as well as D allelic were significantly associated with DDD. Genotypic and allelic association were demonstrated by further age stratification in the group of subjects over 40 years old. The D allele was not associated with Schmorl's nodes, disc bulges, or annular tears. Jacobsen et al. [60] have shown that inserting a SNP into the rs1799750 2G allele (promoter of MMP1) was associated with sciatica, LBP, and disability following lumbar disk herniation. These were measured by increased VAS scores, McGill pain questionnaire scores, and ODI scores. The presence of the rs1799750 2G allele is associated with the increase in in vitro MMP1 expression, but in clinical trials of patients with disk herniations, there were no differences in frequency of the allele when compared to pain-free controls. The MMP1 2G allele was not directly associated with disk degeneration in these patients. When compared to patients who were homozygous for the 2G allele, the patients who carried the 1G allele had less pain and were able to function better. The extracellular matrix within the IVD was prone to degradation where rs1799750 SNP was present because of increased MMP1 expression. Matrix degradation is thought to be principal in disk degeneration. As such, matrix metalloproteinase inhibitors have undergone clinical trials to try to treat neuropathic pain and multiple sclerosis. After nerve injury, the temporal and differential pattern of MMPs expression correlates with changes in concentrations of pro-inflammatory cytokines. This suggests that MMPs, besides being mediators for neuroinflammation, could also be directly associated with pain due to nerve damage. Blocking a single MMP with targeted treatments such as peptide inhibitors, monoclonal antibodies, and siRNAs can offer a better therapeutic approach while minimizing the adverse effects of broad-spectrum MMP inhibitors [61].

MMP2, matrix metalloproteinase-2, was demonstrated to contribute to the development of LDD. Amplified activity and expression of MMP2 were shown to be present in degenerative discs. There are reports of the polymorphism-1306C/T in the MMP-2 gene promoter influencing gene transcription and expression. LDD patients had a significantly greater prevalence of the MMP-2-1306CC genotype when compared to controls, as demonstrated by Don et al. [62]. CC-genotyped subjects had almost a three times greater risk for LDD development than did subjects who carried at least one T allele. On MR imaging, this genotype also corresponded with higher grade disc degeneration. Therefore, in young adults, the MMP-2-1306 C/T polymorphism may be a genetic risk factor linked to LDD susceptibility. Accelerated disc degeneration may result from increased expression of MMP-2 and subsequent tissue cleft formation and disc material resorption [62].

Matrix metalloproteinase-3 (MMP-3, stromelysin-1) has been implied in vertebral disc degeneration—specifically, 5a/6a polymorphism in the MMP3 promoter [63]. In elderly people, the 5A5A and 5A6A genotypes were associated with a notably larger number of degenerative IVDs and the degenerative scores were higher than in the 6A6A genotype. In younger people, there was no noted difference. This led to the conclusion that in the elderly, the 5A allele is a risk factor for accelerated lumbar disc changes. Omair et al. [64] found an association between improvement in pain at one year following lumbar fusion ($p = 0.03$) and with severe lumbar disc degeneration ($p = 0.006$) and MMP3 polymorphism rs72520913. Additionally, associations of severe degeneration with IL18RAP polymorphism rs1420100 and MMP3 polymorphism rs72520913 were observed in this study. The rs1420100 polymorphism was associated with more than one degenerated disc.

3.2.5. FAAH (Fatty Acid Amide Hydrolase)

In a study by Ramesh et al., subjects who experienced both acute and low back pain at baseline demonstrated elevated levels of CNR2 mRNA; however, only subjects who went on to develop chronic LBP exhibited elevated levels of FAAH and TRPV1 mRNA [34]. Modest yet significantly elevated FAAH and TRPV1 expression were observed in those who developed cLBP compared to the acute LBP group, suggesting a possible genetic interaction that may increase vulnerability to chronic pain. Two SNPs within FAAH, rs932816 and rs4141964, were associated with increased pain scores on the McGill pain questionnaire among patients with LBP and accounted for ~5% variance in the pain ratings. The FAAH SNP rs932816 was significantly associated with the overall increased average pain and interference of pain among LBP patients [34]. Ethanolamine (anandamide, AEA) is an endogenous cannabinoid. Most of its pharmacological effects are via binding and activation of CB (1) and CB (2) cannabinoid receptors, in the periphery and the CNS [65]. Elevated levels of FAAH mRNA could lead to lower AEA levels and thus, dysregulation of normal pain processing [66]. In a study by Schlosburg et al., mice treated with FAAH inhibitors and FAAH knockout mice were unable to hydrolyze AEA along with other non-cannabinoid lipid signaling molecules. The animals with compromised FAAH persistently demonstrated phenotypes that were anti-inflammatory and antinociceptive, with efficacy comparable to direct-acting cannabinoid receptor agonists like THC [65]. However, a study performed on 74 patients with knee osteoarthritis found a lack of analgesic effect of a potent and selective FAAH1 inhibitor PF-04457845, despite decreasing activity of FAAH by >96% and increasing levels of the four endogenous substrates (fatty acid amides) [67]. The apparent disconnect between the animal models and human subjects warrants further investigation.

Some relevant receptor-related gene studies that are not referenced in the text are listed in Table 2.

Table 2. Enzyme-related genes.

Gene	Function/Pathway	Condition(s)	Citation	Number of Subjects/Geographic Region
FAAH	hydrolyzes many primary and secondary fatty acid amides, including anandamide and oleamide as neuromodulators	cLBP	Ramesh et al., 2018 [34]	$n = 84$, USA
COMT	Neurotransmission/Catechol-O-methyltransferase	LBP	Rut et al., 2014 [45], Jacobsen et al., 2012 [44], Omair et al., 2013, 2015 [40,64]	$n = 176$, Poland/$n = 258$, Norway/$n = 93$, Norway (West Eur), $n = 371$, Europe
GCH	Guanosine triphosphate cyclohydrolase	LBP	Tegeder et al., 2006 [53]	Animal studies
MMP1	Protein degradation/matrix metalloproteinase	LBP	Song et al., 2008 [59] Jacobsen et al., 2013 [60]	$n = 691$, southern China; $n = 260$, Norway Eur White
MMP2	Protein degradation	LBP	Dong et al., 2007 [62]	$n = 162$, China
MMP3	Protein degradation	LBP	Takahashi et al., 2001 [63]	$n = 103$, Japan
CASP9	Apoptosis-mediating caspase	LBP	Guo et al., 2011 [46], Mu et al., 2013 [68]	$n = 154/216$ controls in China; $n = 305/587$ controls Chinese soldiers

Abbreviations: LBP, low back pain; cLBP, chronic low back pain.

3.3. Cytokines and Associated Receptors

3.3.1. IL18RAP (Interleukin 18 Receptor Accessory Protein); IL18R1 (Interleukin 18 Receptor 1); IL1A (Interleukin 1 Alpha)

Schistad et al. [69] reported that the C > T polymorphism rs1800587 in the interleukin-1α gene is associated with decreased pressure pain thresholds and increased pain intensity in patients with lumbar radicular pain. A pressure point threshold (PPT) was used to measure the pain severity for the gluteal muscles and VAS was used to measure the pain severity in the lower back and legs as the primary outcome. To determine the differences in genetic-makeup, a previously designed TaqMan assay was used for IL-1α rs1800587. By repeating analyses of variance with the different pain scores, the effect of the genotype was measured. After further analysis, the gene did have an effect on the scores in patients with symptomatic disk herniations. Patients who had CT/TT genotype had higher VAS pain scores for leg pain ($p = 0.002$) and lower PPT scores for the gluteus ($p = 0.016$ for both left and right side) compared to patients with the CC genotype during the 1-year follow-up. A study by Omair et al. [64] found that IL18RAP polymorphism rs1420100 was closely related to severe IVD degeneration in the lumbar segments (L4-L5 and L5-S1) and more than one degenerated IVD. Interestingly, SNPs rs917997 and rs1420106 from the same gene were linked to disequilibrium and with post treatment improvement in disability. The number of degenerated discs and degeneration severity associated with the rs1420100 SNP was confirmed by the study results of Videman et al. [70]. IL18RAP is important for IL18 signal transduction and ligand binding affinity, as it is a subunit of the IL18 receptor [71]. Secretion of interferon gamma (IFN-y) results from IL18R-induced activation of T cells and NK cells. The IFN activates macrophage cells to secrete Il-1 and TNF-alpha, leading to further production of cytokines and proteases and increased matrix degradation. The cells of herniated and degenerated discs secrete these proteases and cytokines [72–74]. This elucidates a link between inflammation and degeneration, and a viable pathway for back pain development. Significant associations with reduction in pain and improvement in disability were uncovered in association analysis of 5SNPs spanning the three genes (IL18RAP, IL18R1, IL1A).

3.3.2. GDF5 (Growth Differentiation Factor 5)

In the Chinese Han population, Mu et al. [68] found that the GDF5 polymorphism (+104T/C; rs143383) was found to be associated with susceptibility to symptomatic lumbar disc herniation (LDH). Type II collagen in the nucleus pulposus of the disc may be an important component in susceptibility to symptomatic LDH [68]. The +104T/C variant increases the risk of developing musculoskeletal diseases and is the most prevalent SNP for GDF5. The SNP rs143383 is associated with osteoarthritis according to recent studies with replication studies, confirming this finding in different ethnic populaces [75,76]. In the Han Chinese cohort, the polymorphic T allele was less frequent in the control group than the case group. These results agreed with those of Williams et al., who observed SNP rs143383 association with lumbar disc degeneration in a cohort of Northern Europeans [77]. In this study, T allele and TT genotype were identified as predisposing to the risk of symptomatic lumbar disc herniation in both sexes.

3.3.3. CCL2 (C-C Motif Chemokine Ligand 2)

Starkweather et al. [38] found chemokine (C-C motif) ligand 2 (CCL2) upregulation in the acute LBP group compared to no-pain controls. This gene has previously been shown in the oral surgery model of tissue injury and acute pain, with upregulation associated with pain intensity at three hours post op along with increased levels of proinflammatory cytokines [78].

Some relevant gene studies that are not referenced in the text are listed in Table 3.

Table 3. Genes related to cytokines and their associated receptors.

Gene	Function/Pathway	Condition(s)	Citation	Number of Subjects/ Geographic Region
CCL2	Chemotactic factor for monocytes and basophils	LBP	Starkweather et al., 2017 [38]	$n = 62$, USA
IL18R1 IL18RAP IL1A	Immune response/ Interleukin receptors	LBP	Omair et al., 2013 [64] Schistad et al., 2014 [69]	$n = 93$, Norway; $n = 121$, Norway
GDF5	Part of TGF-beta family, Cellular growth/Skeletal tissue differentiation	LBP	Mu et al., 2013 [79]	$n = 305/587$ controls Chinese soldiers

Abbreviations: LBP, low back pain.

3.4. Transcription Factors

3.4.1. SOX5 (SRY-Box 5)

Loci tagged by rs7833174 (CCDC26/GSDMC), rs4384683 (DCC), and rs12310519 (SOX5) across the genome were significantly associated with chronic back pain (CBP), as demonstrated by Suri et al. [21]. Among the examined traits related to CBP, the lead SNP rs12310519 in SOX5 was closely linked with degeneration in the IVDs in the lumbar region [21,80]. SOX genes are transcription factors which are involved in all developments of the embryo, as they determine the outcomes for many cell types [21]. As SOX5 and SOX6 genes have some of the same functions, they are able to coordinate well together in order to efficiently undergo chondrogenesis [81]. When SOX5 was inactive, small defects in cartilage and skeleton formation in mice were noted. When both SOX5 and SOX6 were inactive, the mice had severe chondrodysplasia [82]. SOX5 and SOX6 are vital in the formation of IVDs, the spinal column, and notochord development [81,83]. If SOX5 and/or SOX6 are not active, mice with a range of spinal developmental issues and abnormalities are noted [84].

3.4.2. CCDC26/GSDMC (CCDC26 Long Non-Coding RNA/Gasdermin C)

The lead SNP rs7833174 in CCDC26/GSDMC was known to mostly affect height and hip circumference in UKB (UK Biobank) [21]. It was also linked to radiographic hip osteoarthritis [85]. In a whole genome association study of Icelandic adults, all forms in CCFC26/GSDMC linked to CBP showed an interrelation with lumbar microdiscectomy for sciatica across phenotypes [86]. The effect direction was the same on other phenotypes as it was on CBP. For example, the T allele, which is associated with height increase, is also a prominent risk of osteoarthritis, CBP, and lumbar discectomy for sciatica [21]. Lumbar disc herniations bear some of the responsibility for causing forms of back pain [87]. Links between lumbar disc herniation and CBP can be clearly seen [88,89]. In the GSDM gene family, which is expressed in epithelial tissues, GASMC encodes for the protein Gasdermin C [21]. The role of GSDMC in lumbar disc herniation and sciatica is not known. In osteoarthritis-related cartilage and subchondral bone cartilage, it is usually linked to distinct methylation patterns [90,91]. After examining one variable genetic association for CBP at CCDC26/GSDMC across phenotypes, pleiotropy with radiographic hip OA at rs6470763 has been found [85]. These data suggest that there are links between variants at CCDC26/GSDMC and CBP [21].

3.4.3. PNOC (Prepronociceptin)

PNOC is the gene which encodes prepronociceptin, a precursor to nociceptin. Nociceptin helps the opioid receptor-like receptor (OPRL1) bind to other molecules. The OPRL1 can modulate nociceptive behavior and movement by acting as a transmitter in the brain. Prepronociceptin appears to induce upregulation of cytokines and IL-10 decreases the expression of PNOC [92]. In the study by Starkweather et al. [38], upregulation of PNOC was associated with mechanical sensitivity of the painful region in the acute LBP group, suggesting a role in contributing to peripheral sensitization.

All genes related to transcription factors, neurotransmission and other unknown functions are shown in Table 4.

Table 4. Genes related to transcription factors, neurotransmission, and other unknown functions.

Gene	Function/Pathway	Condition(s)	Citation	Number of Subjects/ Geographic Location
SOX5	Transcription factor, embryonic development	LBP	Suri et al., 2018 [21]	n = 168,000; worldwide
CCDC26/GSDMC	Non-coding/Codes gasdermin C; the N-terminal moiety promotes pyroptosis with unknown physiologic significance	LBP	Suri et al., 2018 [21]	n = 168,000; worldwide
PNOC	Codes prepronociceptin; nociceptin is a ligand of the opioid receptor-like receptor OPRL1; may modulate nociceptive and locomotor behavior	LBP	Starkweather et al., 2016 [38]	n = 62, CT USA

Abbreviations: LBP, low back pain.

3.5. Pharmacogenomics in Management of cLBP

An estimated 70,000–100,000 people die each year from opioid overdoses from all around the world [93]. Nearly half of all opioid overdose deaths were from opioids that were prescribed to those individuals. According to the U.S. Drug Enforcement Administration (DEA), the amount of opioid overdoses has reached an epidemic level [94]. When patients with chronic pain are prescribed with opioid medications, there is a higher risk of the treatment having a poor outcome in the long run. Opioid therapy can have severe side effects such as misuse, overdose, hyperalgesia, and death. As improving a patient's quality of life and functioning while avoiding adverse events is highly important, individualized therapies to treat chronic non-cancer pain are crucial [95]. In order for health care providers to be able to accurately diagnose and treat patients with chronic pain, they have to take into account variables like age, sex, ethnicity, lifestyle, comorbidities, and drugs that the patient may already be using. These factors combined with the contribution of genetics to the type of pain and efficacy and safety of drugs will ultimately impact the way that pharmacotherapy works.

The Human Pain Genetics Database (HPGDB) represents a large inventory of studies intended to summarize and reflect the association between genetic variations and different chronic pain conditions [96]. Interestingly, a specific phenotype category for which genetic associations were most frequently reported was analgesia. The Human Genome Research Project opened new opportunities for diagnosing diseases, developing drugs, and individualizing medicine. Personalized medicine in pain management has only been possible due to the advancements in research and technology, as well as the newly developed policies that empower patients [95]. Pharmacogenomics studies should help in discovering how an individual's genome affects their response to pharmacotherapy. As such, it is a pathway to individualized treatment and can impact pharmacotherapy to maximize efficacy and minimize adverse reactions and polypharmacy.

Cytochrome P450 (CYP450) is one of the most recognized superfamilies of enzymes responsible for inter-individual differences pertaining to drug effectiveness or adverse events profiles. Defined as membrane-associated proteins in the endoplasmic reticulum of cells, there are 57 genes identified coding for various CYP450 [97]. However, not all CYP types participate in drug metabolism. In the Caucasian population, a study associated four major CYP types (1A2, 2D6, 2C9, and 2C19) with 40.0% of drug metabolism [98] Moreover, in the same ethnic group, further analysis revealed 34 polymorphic alleles responsible for altered enzymatic activity. The authors also retrieved 199 non-synonymous SNPs with a prevalence of ≥1% in all genomes, irrespective of ethnicity (Figure 1). Prescribed analgesic drugs can have different effects on patients because of their genetic variations which contribute to the way they respond to the drugs, which is why pharmacogenomics plays a crucial role when dealing with pain management. Usually, the genetic variants in the CYP450 enzyme are what account for the different responses to drugs because of alteration to the protein structure and function. These variants are mostly known as single nucleotide polymorphisms [95]. The response to an analgesic medication therapy is highly dependent on prodrug metabolism, active component breakdown, and transport through cellular membranes [95].

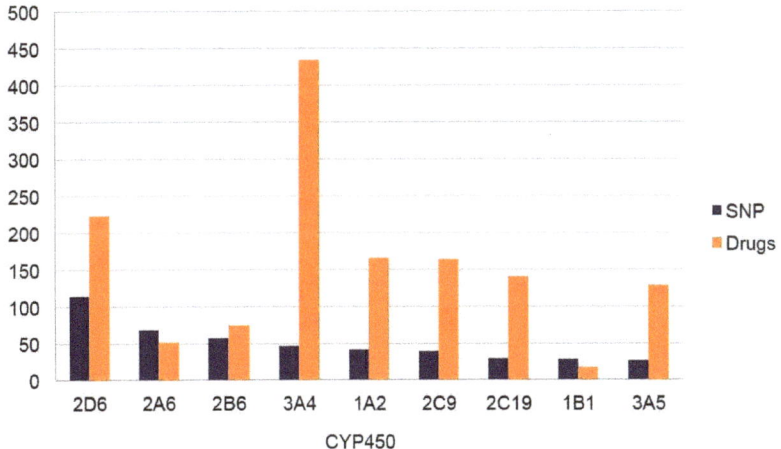

Figure 1. Number of known single nucleotide polymorphisms (SNPs) and drugs metabolized per cytochrome P450 (CYP) enzymes (modified from Preissner et al., 2013 [98]).

Nonsteroidal anti-inflammatory drugs (NSAIDs) represent a commonly used class of drugs for the initial treatment of cLBP. To a large extent, the biotransformation of NSAIDs is governed by cytochrome P450 isoforms, in particular by CYP2C9 [99]. Adjusted to CYP2C9 activity score, the Clinical Pharmacogenetics Implementation Consortium (CPIC) retrieved three distinct CYP2C9 phenotypes: poor metabolizers (PM), intermediate metabolizers (IM), and normal metabolizers (NM) [100]. PM and IM variants are linked with decreased metabolic clearance potential, which results in a prolonged plasma elimination half-life of NSAIDs. In addition, CYP2C9*3 was associated with decreased celecoxib, meloxicam, as well as S (+) and R (−) ibuprofen metabolism. The same genotype also rendered meloxicam with enhanced pharmacodynamic effects (increased inhibition of thromboxane B_2 formation). Gastroduodenal bleeding, a serious NSAID-related adverse event, has been found highly probable in CYP2C9*1/*3 and CYP2C9*1/*2 heterozygotes [101] A later study recognized the CYP2C9

359Leu (CYP2C9*3) allele as a risk factor for acute upper gastrointestinal bleeding in patients taking NSAIDs other than aspirin.

In chronic pain management, the CYP450 polymorphisms are also relevant in the metabolism of opioid drugs like codeine, tramadol, hydrocodone, and oxycodone. Their use, while common in pain management, can lead to unpredictable and sometimes dangerous consequences. Hepatic cytochrome P450 2D6 (CYP2D6) is pivotal for bioactivating codeine into morphine, and tramadol into O-desmethyltramadol. The clinical significance from CYP2D6 polymorphism would render an individual susceptible to variable outcomes to efficacy and safety profiles of codeine. Accordingly, CPIC guidelines have classified different patient phenotypes with respect to the CYP2D6 activity score [102]. The authors identified four such profiles: PM, IM, extensive metabolizer (EM (normal morphine formation)), and ultrarapid metabolizer (UM). PM variants can significantly reduce the activity of drug metabolism and lead to insufficient pain relief and lower drug clearance, requiring a reduction in the drug dose to avoid undesired adverse effects. For this phenotype, it is recommended to consider drugs such as morphine or use of a non-opioid [102]. Reduced codeine metabolism is also seen with IM, although not as pronounced as with PM, and therapy protocols in such phenotypes advocate for a trial of codeine as a first-line opioid analgesic. If no response is identified, second tier drugs would include morphine, use of a non-opioid, or tramadol. Finally, UM, as the least prevalent and most extensive metabolic-capable variant, has been described as being high risk for morphine toxicity; codeine should be avoided, and clinicians should instead opt for morphine or a non-opioid. Put into perspective, a retrospective cohort of 224 patients with CLBP treated with oxycodone or codeine were analyzed with respect to their CYP26D genotype [103]. There were statistically significant findings in regard to therapeutic failures at the haplotype (CYP2D6*6 (PM) and CYP2D6*9 (IM)) as well as diplotype level (CYP2D6 *1/*11 (EM), *4/*6 (PM), *41/*2N (UM)) with chronic opioid treatment ($p < 0.05$). Moreover, CYP2D6*2N patients exhibited increased risks of side effects. A prospective cohort study with 76 chronic pain patients receiving codeine or tramadol was conducted to assess the prevalence of CYP2D6 genotype among the cohort [104]. The authors analyzed the nine most common variants (CYP2D6 *2–6, *9, *10, *14, and *17), as well as those without polymorphic alleles (CYP2D6*1, wild type (wt)). The most common genotypes per se as well as adverse effects among such variants were identified, thus paving the path for a more personalized therapy.

Moreover, the link between hydromorphone and OPRM1 A118A genotypes (homozygous (AA) vs. heterozygous (AG)) was explored in 158 women receiving hydrocodone/acetaminophen postoperatively following Cesarean section [105]. Patients homozygous for the A118A allele had statistically significant pain relief associated with both the total dose of hydrocodone and serum hydromorphone level, while adverse events more commonly occurred in the heterozygous group. The CYP450 enzyme family is not the only one that affects pain management. A study with 231 opioid-naïve patients revealed that those with the COMT G472A-AA genotype (rs4680) and KCNJ6 A1032G-A allele (rs2070995) required higher dosing. When a higher pain intensity was present, they responded differently to opioid titration with higher pain intensity, thereby requiring higher dosing [106] The single-nucleotide polymorphisms in genes closely related to pain transmission and the metabolism of opioids may cause patients with cLBP to possibly be predisposed to excessive sensitivity and variation in the effects of opioid analgesics.

The management of different chronic pain conditions includes adjunct drugs such as antidepressants, muscle relaxants, and anticonvulsants. The three major CYP enzymes implicated in the metabolism of antidepressants are CYP1A2, CYP2D6, and CYP2C19; however, other enzymes are also involved as evidenced by the metabolism of amitriptyline (1A2, 2C9, 2C19, 2D6, 3A), bupropion (2B6), imipramine (1A2, 2C19, 2D6, 3A), venlafaxine (2D6, 3A), etc. [107–109]. Nevertheless, CYP2D6 isoenzyme has been most extensively studied in regards to antidepressant metabolism. Indeed, CYP2D6 phenotypes predispose to large differences in plasma drug concentrations and variable rates of adverse events [107,110]. The Royal Dutch Association of the Advancement of Pharmacy developed pharmacogenetics-based guidelines for a number of drugs including venlafaxine [111]. For PM and IM phenotypes, the recommendations were to select an alternate drug (e.g., citalopram, sertraline) or adjust dose and monitor O-desmethylvenlafaxine, a venlafaxine metabolite. In contrast, for the UM phenotype, it is recommended to titrate to a maximum of 150% of the normal dose or opt for one of the abovementioned alternative drugs. Of note, the efficacy and safety of venlafaxine has been associated with SNPs rs2032582 (G2677T) and rs1045642 (C3435T) within the ABCB1 gene that codes for membrane-bound P-glycoprotein (P-gp) [112–114] Genetic polymorphism for serotonin transporter 5-HT (5-HTTLPR), characterized by short (s) and long (l) variants, has been associated with the efficacy of another antidepressant, citalopram [115] Among l/l 5-HTTLPR homozygotes, citalopram significantly reduces pain-related responses in the cerebellum and in parts of the cerebral cortex, while the relationship between the 5-HTTLPR genotype and pain-related brain response was shown to be a good predictor of pain alleviating properties of citalopram. Duloxetine, a serotonin and norepinephrine reuptake inhibitor, is another antidepressant drug whose metabolism is amenable to certain CYP (primarily CYP1A2, but also CYP2D6 and CYP2C9) enzymes. For this reason, one should expect potentially toxic plasma levels of duloxetine in the case of concomitant administration of a strong CYP1A2 inhibitor [95].

The pharmacokinetic properties of a commonly used muscle relaxant, cyclobenzaprine, were the subject of investigation in four clinical studies [116]. It was shown that steady-state plasma concentrations of this drug were two-fold higher in the elderly population and those individuals with hepatic insufficiency, necessitating dose reduction in such patient groups. In addition, there is preclinical evidence that rendered the therapeutic plasma levels of cyclobenzaprine accountable for the initiation of serotonin syndrome, a potentially fatal condition characterized by altered mental status and autonomic instability [117].

The activity of some of the aforementioned CYP enzymes, such as CYP3A4, CYP2C9, and CYP2C19, may be affected by different anticonvulsants in a stimulating (phenytoin, carbamazepine) or inhibitory (oxcarbazepine, valproic acid) fashion, thus creating an environment for adverse drug reactions and drug–drug interactions [118]. In contrast, gabapentinoids (gabapentin, pregabalin) are neither activators/inhibitors of the cytochrome P450 system nor subject to hepatic metabolism [119,120], but are instead excreted in urine. This process is under the influence of organic cation transporters OCTN1 and OCT2 coded by SLC22A4 and SLC22A2 genes, respectively [121–123]. However, the genotype of an individual (e.g., OCTN1 polymorphism) was found to have a negligible role in gabapentin clearance and was much more affected by the renal function and absorption process [123].

3.5.1. Drug–Drug Interactions

An additional shortfall of current cLBP management is the unfortunate circumstance of polypharmacy use, and with it, drug–drug interactions (DDIs), where the toxicity and/or efficacy of one or all drugs is altered. If the metabolism of the used drugs (several opioids) goes through the cytochrome P450 (CYP450) pathways, the patient is possibly exposed to dangerous DDIs. The overall prevalence of DDIs among cLBP is 27% [124]. A large retrospective cohort analysis was conducted to assess for pharmacokinetic drug–drug interactions (pDDI) in 57,752 chronic non-cancer pain patients taking opioids [125] The authors matched the 9 most commonly prescribed opioids against 19 precipitant drugs capable of inducing CYP450-dependent metabolic effects changes, and sought for those pDDIs with a potential to induce adverse drug reactions (i.e., PDDI-major). In a decreasing order of frequency, the most prevalent pDDIs were caused from 3A inhibition, followed by 2D6 inhibition and 3A induction, while the leading precipitant drugs included fluconazole, followed by diltiazem, clarithromycin, and verapamil. The summary of the most common, CYP450-related, prescribed opioids and precipitant drugs in chronic non-cancer pain patients is shown in Figure 2. About 5.7% of the cohort was found to have been exposed to potential PDDI-major, and these had significantly higher healthcare costs vs. patients without a drug–drug interaction.

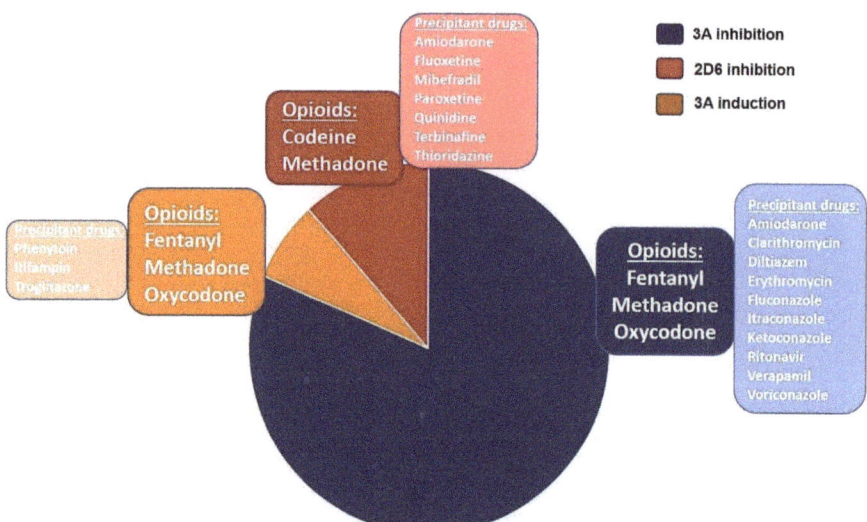

Figure 2. Most common CYP450-related pharmacokinetic drug–drug interactions between opioids and precipitant drugs (modified with permission from Pergolizzi et al. [125]).

3.5.2. Drug–Drug–Gene Interactions

Knowing a patient's genotyping as part of an overall clinical practice may lead to better outcomes. Pharmacogenomics and therapeutic drug monitoring can potentially minimize adverse events, while maximizing efficacy. The incidence of adverse events depends on a number of variables, including sex, age, comorbidities, genetic variations, etc. Indeed, a recent retrospective analysis in patients with known genetic polymorphisms in major drug metabolizing enzymes (CYP2D6, CYP2C9, and CYP2C19) revealed that drug–gene (DG) and drug–drug–gene (DDG) interactions accounted for 14.7% and 19.2% of adverse events [126]. DDG interactions have been classified into three categories: inhibitory, induction, and phenoconversion interactions [127]. Inhibitory and induction interactions assume altered metabolic and pharmacokinetic properties of the target drug, which can be influenced by the presence of another drug, genetic mutations of relevant enzymes, or their combination. Phenoconversion is related to opposing effects between the effect of the interacting drug and the genotype, which practically would make genetically susceptible individuals normalized by adding medications having opposite effects on metabolism. Moreover, drug–drug–gene interactions have also been proposed to influence drug transporters (i.e., drug–drug–transporters genes interaction), and subsequently, drug pharmacokinetics, in a similar fashion as with drug metabolizing enzymes. Storelli et al. managed to render physiologically based pharmacokinetic (PBPK) modeling appropriate to predict the influence of CYP2D6 genetic polymorphisms on DDIs [128]. The clinical significance behind PBPK simulations lies in personalized medicine—to help identify individuals susceptible to higher risk of DDIs and deliver a genotype-specific drug dose. Incorporating genetic analysis into clinical studies can help predict responses to different treatment options by identifying clinical and genetic factors. When the treating physician knows how a patient might respond to a given therapy, this can help them guide which therapies they might prescribe. This form of personalized medicine with incorporated biomarkers helps to drastically improve the effectiveness of current and future strategies in pain management [129].

4. Conclusions

Treatment of chronic low back pain (cLBP) should be multimodal. We hope that with future research, it will be possible to use genetic markers for identifying patients at risk for developing cLBP early. Additionally, genotyping may assist in directing treatment, predicting lack of efficacy with any particular approach, and facilitating decisions between conservative approaches or early escalations to more radical approaches such as surgery. Examining genetic markers could provide objective data for physicians treating cLBP, instead of relying upon more subjective measures such as numeric pain rating scales. Making a "pain profile" of a patient, which would include genetic markers, while being costly at present, could lead to minimizing healthcare costs in the future, by getting the patients the personalized treatment that they require early, and by minimizing inefficacious approaches. In order to deliver a more personalized therapy, further research is warranted to explore how an individual's genotype affects their responses to therapy. In particular, the focus should be on genetic polymorphisms in CYP450 and other enzymes crucial for affecting the metabolic profile of target drugs. Implementation of gene-focused pharmacotherapy has the potential to deliver select, more efficacious drugs and avoid unnecessary, polypharmacy-related adverse events in many painful conditions, including chronic low back pain.

Our review provides some targets for future research into pharmacogenomics. It is our hope that by obtaining additional knowledge regarding polymorphisms in these genes and their relationship to pharmacotherapy response, we will help guide future therapies, reduce overall healthcare costs, and prevent perpetuation of the opioid epidemic, among other benefits.

Author Contributions: Conceptualization, N.N.K. and V.S.; methodology, V.S.; investigation, V.S., F.J. and E.K.; resources, N.N.K.; data curation, V.S., F.J. and E.K.; writing—original draft preparation, V.S., F.J. and E.K.; writing—review and editing, N.N.K., and K.D.C.; visualization, E.K.; supervision, N.N.K. All authors have read and agreed to the published version of the manuscript.

Funding: This research received no external funding.

Conflicts of Interest: The authors declare no conflict of interest.

References

1. Manchikanti, L.; Singh, V.; Falco, F.J.; Benyamin, R.M.; Hirsch, J.A. Epidemiology of low back pain in adults. *Neuromodulation* **2014**, *17* (Suppl. 2), 3–10. [CrossRef] [PubMed]
2. Shmagel, A.; Foley, R.; Ibrahim, H. Epidemiology of Chronic Low Back Pain in US Adults: Data from the 2009-2010 National Health and Nutrition Examination Survey. *Arthritis Care Res.* **2016**, *68*, 1688–1694. [CrossRef] [PubMed]
3. Polderman, T.J.; Benyamin, B.; de Leeuw, C.A.; Sullivan, P.F.; Van Bochoven, A.; Visscher, P.M.; Posthuma, D. Meta-analysis of the heritability of human traits based on fifty years of twin studies. *Nat. Genet.* **2015**, *47*, 702–709. [CrossRef] [PubMed]
4. Ferreira, P.H.; Beckenkamp, P.; Maher, C.G.; Hopper, J.L.; Ferreira, M.L. Nature or nurture in low back pain? Results of a systematic review of studies based on twin samples. *Eur. J. Pain* **2013**, *17*, 957–971. [CrossRef]
5. Battie, M.C.; Videman, T.; Levalahti, E.; Gill, K.; Kaprio, J. Heritability of low back pain and the role of disc degeneration. *Pain* **2007**, *131*, 272–280. [CrossRef]
6. Rodriguez-Raecke, R.; Niemeier, A.; Ihle, K.; Ruether, W.; May, A. Structural brain changes in chronic pain reflect probably neither damage nor atrophy. *PLoS ONE* **2013**, *8*, e54475. [CrossRef]
7. Baliki, M.N.; Petre, B.; Torbey, S.; Herrmann, K.M.; Huang, L.; Schnitzer, T.J.; Fields, H.L.; Apkarian, A.V. Corticostriatal functional connectivity predicts transition to chronic back pain. *Nat. Neurosci.* **2012**, *15*, 1117–1119. [CrossRef]
8. Seminowicz, D.A.; Wideman, T.H.; Naso, L.; Hatami-Khoroushahi, Z.; Fallatah, S.; Ware, M.A.; Jarzem, P.; Bushnell, M.C.; Shir, Y.; Ouellet, J.A.; et al. Effective treatment of chronic low back pain in humans reverses abnormal brain anatomy and function. *J. Neurosci.* **2011**, *31*, 7540–7550. [CrossRef]
9. Zorina-Lichtenwalter, K.; Meloto, C.B.; Khoury, S.; Diatchenko, L. Genetic predictors of human chronic pain conditions. *Neuroscience* **2016**, *338*, 36–62. [CrossRef]
10. Hasvik, E.; Iordanova Schistad, E.; Grovle, L.; Julsrud Haugen, A.; Roe, C.; Gjerstad, J. Subjective health complaints in patients with lumbar radicular pain and disc herniation are associated with a sex—OPRM1 A118G polymorphism interaction: A prospective 1-year observational study. *BMC Musculoskelet. Disord.* **2014**, *15*, 161. [CrossRef]

11. Grovle, L.; Haugen, A.J.; Ihlebaek, C.M.; Keller, A.; Natvig, B.; Brox, J.I.; Grotle, M. Comorbid subjective health complaints in patients with sciatica: A prospective study including comparison with the general population. *J. Psychosom. Res.* **2011**, *70*, 548–556. [CrossRef] [PubMed]
12. Zubieta, J.K.; Dannals, R.F.; Frost, J.J. Gender and age influences on human brain mu-opioid receptor binding measured by PET. *Am. J. Psychiatry* **1999**, *156*, 842–848. [CrossRef] [PubMed]
13. Ray, R.; Ruparel, K.; Newberg, A.; Wileyto, E.P.; Loughead, J.W.; Divgi, C.; Blendy, J.A.; Logan, J.; Zubieta, J.-K.; Lerman, C. Human Mu Opioid Receptor (OPRM1 A118G) polymorphism is associated with brain mu-opioid receptor binding potential in smokers. *Proc. Natl. Acad. Sci. USA* **2011**, *108*, 9268–9273. [CrossRef] [PubMed]
14. Matsunaga, M.; Isowa, T.; Murakami, H.; Kasugai, K.; Yoneda, M.; Kaneko, H.; Ohira, H. Association of polymorphism in the human mu-opioid receptor OPRM1 gene with proinflammatory cytokine levels and health perception. *Brain Behav. Immun.* **2009**, *23*, 931–935. [CrossRef] [PubMed]
15. Way, B.M.; Taylor, S.E.; Eisenberger, N.I. Variation in the mu-opioid receptor gene (OPRM1) is associated with dispositional and neural sensitivity to social rejection. *Proc. Natl. Acad. Sci. USA* **2009**, *106*, 15079–15084. [CrossRef]
16. Milner, T.A.; Burstein, S.R.; Marrone, G.F.; Khalid, S.; Gonzalez, A.D.; Williams, T.J.; Schierberl, K.C.; Torres-Reveron, A.; Gonzales, K.L.; McEwen, B.S.; et al. Stress differentially alters mu opioid receptor density and trafficking in parvalbumin-containing interneurons in the female and male rat hippocampus. *Synapse* **2013**, *67*, 757–772. [CrossRef]
17. Nicholl, B.I.; Holliday, K.L.; Macfarlane, G.J.; Thomson, W.; Davies, K.A.; O'Neill, T.; Bartfai, G.; Boonen, S.; Casanueva, F.F.; Finn, J.D.; et al. Association of HTR2A polymorphisms with chronic widespread pain and the extent of musculoskeletal pain: Results from two population-based cohorts. *Arthritis Rheum.* **2011**, *63*, 810–818. [CrossRef]
18. Yildiz, S.H.; Ulasli, A.M.; Ozdemir Erdogan, M.; Dikici, Ö.; Terzi, E.S.A.; Dündar, Ü.; Solak, M. Assessment of Pain Sensitivity in Patients with Chronic Low Back Pain and Association with HTR2A Gene Polymorphism. *Arch. Rheumatol.* **2017**, *32*, 3–9. [CrossRef]
19. Kato, K.; Kikuchi, S.; Konno, S.; Sekiguchi, M. Participation of 5-hydroxytryptamine in pain-related behavior induced by nucleus pulposus applied on the nerve root in rats. *Spine* **2008**, *33*, 1330–1336. [CrossRef]
20. Kanayama, M.; Hashimoto, T.; Shigenobu, K.; Yamane, S. Efficacy of serotonin receptor blocker for symptomatic lumbar disc herniation. *Clin. Orthop. Relat. Res.* **2003**, *411*, 159–165. [CrossRef]
21. Suri, P.; Palmer, M.R.; Tsepilov, Y.A.; Freidin, M.B.; Boer, C.G.; Yau, M.S.; Evans, D.S.; Gelemanović, A.; Bartz, T.M.; Nethander, M.; et al. Genome-wide meta-analysis of 158,000 individuals of European ancestry identifies three loci associated with chronic back pain. *PLoS Genet.* **2018**, *14*, e1007601. [CrossRef]
22. Finci, L.; Zhang, Y.; Meijers, R.; Wang, J.H. Signaling mechanism of the netrin-1 receptor DCC in axon guidance. *Prog. Biophys. Mol. Biol.* **2015**, *118*, 153–160. [CrossRef] [PubMed]
23. Wu, C.H.; Yuan, X.C.; Gao, F.; Li, H.-P.; Cao, J.; Liu, Y.-S.; Yu, W.; Tian, B.; Meng, X.-F.; Shi, J.; et al. Netrin-1 Contributes to Myelinated Afferent Fiber Sprouting and Neuropathic Pain. *Mol. Neurobiol.* **2016**, *53*, 5640–5651. [CrossRef] [PubMed]
24. Dun, X.P.; Parkinson, D.B. Role of Netrin-1 Signaling in Nerve Regeneration. *Int. J. Mol. Sci.* **2017**, *18*, 491. [CrossRef] [PubMed]
25. Bu, G.; Hou, S.; Ren, D.; Wu, Y.; Shang, W.; Huang, W. Increased expression of netrin-1 and its deleted in colorectal cancer receptor in human diseased lumbar intervertebral disc compared with autopsy control. *Spine* **2012**, *37*, 2074–2081. [CrossRef]
26. Freemont, A.J.; Peacock, T.E.; Goupille, P.; Hoyland, J.A.; O'Brien, J.; Jayson, M.I. Nerve ingrowth into diseased intervertebral disc in chronic back pain. *Lancet* **1997**, *350*, 178–181. [CrossRef]
27. Pinheiro, M.B.; Ferreira, M.L.; Refshauge, K.; Colodro-Conde, L.; Carrillo, E.; Hopper, J.L.; Ordoñana, J.R.; Ferreira, P.H. Genetics and the environment affect the relationship between depression and low back pain: A co-twin control study of Spanish twins. *Pain* **2015**, *156*, 496–503. [CrossRef]
28. Okbay, A.; LifeLines Cohort Study; Baselmans, B.M.; De Neve, J.E.; Turley, P.; Nivard, M.G.; Fontana, M.A.; Meddens, S.F.W.; Linnér, R.K.; Rietveld, C.A.; et al. Genetic variants associated with subjective well-being, depressive symptoms, and neuroticism identified through genome-wide analyses. *Nat. Genet.* **2016**, *48*, 624–633. [CrossRef]

29. Roh, H.L.; Lee, J.S.; Suh, K.T.; Kim, J.I.; Lee, H.S.; Goh, T.S.; Park, S.H. Association between estrogen receptor gene polymorphism and back pain intensity in female patients with degenerative lumbar spondylolisthesis. *J. Spinal Disord. Tech.* **2013**, *26*, E53–E57. [CrossRef]
30. Lindberg, M.K.; Alatalo, S.L.; Halleen, J.M.; Mohan, S.; Gustafsson, J.A.; Ohlsson, C. Estrogen receptor specificity in the regulation of the skeleton in female mice. *J. Endocrinol.* **2001**, *171*, 229–236. [CrossRef]
31. Vidal, O.; Lindberg, M.K.; Hollberg, K.; Baylink, D.J.; Andersson, G.; Lubahn, D.B.; Mohan, S.; Gustafsson, J.-Å.; Ohlsson, C. Estrogen receptor specificity in the regulation of skeletal growth and maturation in male mice. *Proc. Natl. Acad. Sci. USA* **2000**, *97*, 5474–5479. [CrossRef] [PubMed]
32. Ushiyama, T.; Ueyama, H.; Inoue, K.; Nishioka, J.; Ohkubo, I.; Hukuda, S. Estrogen receptor gene polymorphism and generalized osteoarthritis. *J. Rheumatol.* **1998**, *25*, 134–137. [PubMed]
33. Racz, I.; Nadal, X.; Alferink, J.; Banos, J.E.; Rehnelt, J.; Martin, M.; Pintado, B.; Gutierrez-Adan, A.; Sanguino, E.; Manzanares, J.; et al. Crucial role of CB(2) cannabinoid receptor in the regulation of central immune responses during neuropathic pain. *J. Neurosci.* **2008**, *28*, 12125–12135. [CrossRef] [PubMed]
34. Ramesh, D.; D'Agata, A.; Starkweather, A.R.; Young, E.E. Contribution of Endocannabinoid Gene Expression and Genotype on Low Back Pain Susceptibility and Chronicity. *Clin. J. Pain* **2018**, *34*, 8–14. [CrossRef]
35. Skouen, J.S.; Smith, A.J.; Warrington, N.M.; O'Sullivan, P.; McKenzie, L.; Pennell, C.E.; Straker, L. Genetic variation in the beta-2 adrenergic receptor is associated with chronic musculoskeletal complaints in adolescents. *Eur. J. Pain* **2012**, *16*, 1232–1242. [CrossRef]
36. Diatchenko, L.; Anderson, A.D.; Slade, G.D.; Fillingim, R.B.; Shabalina, S.A.; Higgins, T.J.; Sama, S.; Belfer, I.; Goldman, D.; Max, M.B.; et al. Three major haplotypes of the beta2 adrenergic receptor define psychological profile, blood pressure, and the risk for development of a common musculoskeletal pain disorder. *Am. J. Med. Genet. B Neuropsychiatr. Genet.* **2006**, *141B*, 449–462. [CrossRef] [PubMed]
37. Vargas-Alarcon, G.; Fragoso, J.M.; Cruz-Robles, D.; Vargas, A.; Martinez, A.; Lao, J.I.; Garcia-Fructuoso, F.; Vallejo, M.; Martínez-Lavín, M. Association of adrenergic receptor gene polymorphisms with different fibromyalgia syndrome domains. *Arthritis Rheum.* **2009**, *60*, 2169–2173. [CrossRef]
38. Starkweather, A.R.; Ramesh, D.; Lyon, D.E.; Siangphoe, U.; Deng, X.; Sturgill, J.; Heineman, A.; Elswick, R.K., Jr.; Dorsey, S.G.; Greenspan, J.; et al. Acute Low Back Pain: Differential Somatosensory Function and Gene Expression Compared with Healthy No-Pain Controls. *Clin. J. Pain* **2016**, *32*, 933–939. [CrossRef]
39. Xu, J.; Tang, Y.; Xie, M.; Bie, B.; Wu, J.; Yang, H.; Foss, J.; Yang, B.; Rosenquist, R.W.; Naguib, M. Activation of cannabinoid receptor 2 attenuates mechanical allodynia and neuroinflammatory responses in a chronic post-ischemic pain model of complex regional pain syndrome type I in rats. *Eur. J. Neurosci.* **2016**, *44*, 3046–3055. [CrossRef]
40. Omair, A.; Mannion, A.F.; Holden, M.; Fairbank, J.; Lie, B.A.; Hägg, O.; Fritzell, P.; Brox, J.I. Catechol-O-methyltransferase (COMT) gene polymorphisms are associated with baseline disability but not long-term treatment outcome in patients with chronic low back pain. *Eur. Spine J.* **2015**, *24*, 2425–2431. [CrossRef]
41. Nackley, A.G.; Tan, K.S.; Fecho, K.; Flood, P.; Diatchenko, L.; Maixner, W. Catechol-O-methyltransferase inhibition increases pain sensitivity through activation of both beta2- and beta3-adrenergic receptors. *Pain* **2007**, *128*, 199–208. [CrossRef] [PubMed]
42. Jacobsen, L.M.; Eriksen, G.S.; Pedersen, L.M.; Gjerstad, J. Catechol-O-methyltransferase (COMT) inhibition reduces spinal nociceptive activity. *Neurosci. Lett.* **2010**, *473*, 212–215. [CrossRef] [PubMed]
43. Zubieta, J.K.; Heitzeg, M.M.; Smith, Y.R.; Bueller, J.A.; Xu, K.; Koeppe, R.A.; Stohler, C.S.; Goldman, D. COMT val158met genotype affects mu-opioid neurotransmitter responses to a pain stressor. *Science* **2003**, *299*, 1240–1243. [CrossRef] [PubMed]
44. Jacobsen, L.M.; Schistad, E.I.; Storesund, A.; Pedersen, L.; Rygh, L.; Røe, C.; Gjerstad, J. The COMT rs4680 Met allele contributes to long-lasting low back pain, sciatica and disability after lumbar disc herniation. *Eur. J. Pain* **2012**, *16*, 1064–1069. [CrossRef] [PubMed]
45. Rut, M.; Machoy-Mokrzynska, A.; Reclawowicz, D.; Słoniewski, P.; Kurzawski, M.; Droździk, M.; Safranow, K.; Morawska, M.; Białecka, M. Influence of variation in the catechol-O-methyltransferase gene on the clinical outcome after lumbar spine surgery for one-level symptomatic disc disease: A report on 176 cases. *Acta Neurochir.* **2014**, *156*, 245–252. [CrossRef] [PubMed]

46. Guo, T.M.; Liu, M.; Zhang, Y.G.; Guo, W.T.; Wu, S.X. Association between Caspase-9 promoter region polymorphisms and discogenic low back pain. *Connect. Tissue Res.* **2011**, *52*, 133–138. [CrossRef]
47. Kuida, K.; Haydar, T.F.; Kuan, C.Y.; Gu, Y.; Taya, C.; Karasuyama, H.; Su, M.S.-S.; Rakic, P.; Flavell, R.A. Reduced apoptosis and cytochrome c-mediated caspase activation in mice lacking caspase 9. *Cell* **1998**, *94*, 325–337. [CrossRef]
48. Srinivasula, S.M.; Ahmad, M.; Fernandes-Alnemri, T.; Alnemri, E.S. Autoactivation of procaspase-9 by Apaf-1-mediated oligomerization. *Mol. Cell.* **1998**, *1*, 949–957. [CrossRef]
49. Shivapurkar, N.; Reddy, J.; Chaudhary, P.M.; Gazdar, A.F. Apoptosis and lung cancer: A review. *J. Cell Biochem.* **2003**, *88*, 885–898. [CrossRef]
50. Sang, T.K.; Li, C.; Liu, W.; Rodriguez, A.; Abrams, J.M.; Zipursky, S.L.; Jackson, G.R. Inactivation of Drosophila Apaf-1 related killer suppresses formation of polyglutamine aggregates and blocks polyglutamine pathogenesis. *Hum. Mol. Genet.* **2005**, *14*, 357–372. [CrossRef]
51. Hanahan, D.; Weinberg, R.A. The hallmarks of cancer. *Cell* **2000**, *100*, 57–70. [CrossRef]
52. Zhao, C.Q.; Jiang, L.S.; Dai, L.Y. Programmed cell death in intervertebral disc degeneration. *Apoptosis* **2006**, *11*, 2079–2088. [CrossRef] [PubMed]
53. Tegeder, I.; Costigan, M.; Griffin, R.S.; Abele, A.; Belfer, I.; Schmidt, H.; Ehnert, C.; Nejim, J.; Marian, C.; Scholz, J.; et al. GTP cyclohydrolase and tetrahydrobiopterin regulate pain sensitivity and persistence. *Nat. Med.* **2006**, *12*, 1269–1277. [CrossRef] [PubMed]
54. Lotsch, J.; Klepstad, P.; Doehring, A.; Dale, O. A GTP cyclohydrolase 1 genetic variant delays cancer pain. *Pain* **2010**, *148*, 103–106. [CrossRef] [PubMed]
55. Ichinose, H.; Ohye, T.; Takahashi, E.; Seki, N.; Hori, T.-A.; Segawa, M.; Nomura, Y.; Endo, K.; Tanaka, H.; Tsuji, S.; et al. Hereditary progressive dystonia with marked diurnal fluctuation caused by mutations in the GTP cyclohydrolase I gene. *Nat. Genet.* **1994**, *8*, 236–242. [CrossRef]
56. Bonafe, L.; Thony, B.; Penzien, J.M.; Czarnecki, B.; Blau, N. Mutations in the sepiapterin reductase gene cause a novel tetrahydrobiopterin-dependent monoamine-neurotransmitter deficiency without hyperphenylalaninemia. *Am. J. Hum. Genet.* **2001**, *69*, 269–277. [CrossRef]
57. Bisgaard, T.; Klarskov, B.; Rosenberg, J.; Kehlet, H. Characteristics and prediction of early pain after laparoscopic cholecystectomy. *Pain* **2001**, *90*, 261–269. [CrossRef]
58. Bisgaard, T.; Rosenberg, J.; Kehlet, H. From acute to chronic pain after laparoscopic cholecystectomy: A prospective follow-up analysis. *Scand. J. Gastroenterol.* **2005**, *40*, 1358–1364. [CrossRef]
59. Song, Y.Q.; Ho, D.W.; Karppinen, J.; Kao, P.Y.P.; Fan, B.J.; Luk, K.D.K.; Yip, S.P.; Leong, J.C.Y.; Cheah, K.S.E.; Sham, P.C.; et al. Association between promoter -1607 polymorphism of MMP1 and lumbar disc disease in Southern Chinese. *BMC Med. Genet.* **2008**, *9*, 38. [CrossRef]
60. Jacobsen, L.M.; Schistad, E.I.; Storesund, A.; Pedersen, L.M.; Espeland, A.; Rygh, L.J.; Røe, C.; Gjerstad, J. The MMP1 rs1799750 2G allele is associated with increased low back pain, sciatica, and disability after lumbar disk herniation. *Clin. J. Pain* **2013**, *29*, 967–971. [CrossRef]
61. Dev, R.; Srivastava, P.K.; Iyer, J.P.; Dastidar, S.G.; Ray, A. Therapeutic potential of matrix metalloprotease inhibitors in neuropathic pain. *Expert Opin. Investig. Drugs* **2010**, *19*, 455–468. [CrossRef] [PubMed]
62. Dong, D.M.; Yao, M.; Liu, B.; Sun, C.Y.; Jiang, Y.Q.; Wang, Y.S. Association between the -1306C/T polymorphism of matrix metalloproteinase-2 gene and lumbar disc disease in Chinese young adults. *Eur. Spine J.* **2007**, *16*, 1958–1961. [CrossRef] [PubMed]
63. Takahashi, M.; Haro, H.; Wakabayashi, Y.; Kawa-uchi, T.; Komori, H.; Shinomiya, K. The association of degeneration of the intervertebral disc with 5a/6a polymorphism in the promoter of the human matrix metalloproteinase-3 gene. *J. Bone Jt. Surg. Br.* **2001**, *83*, 491–495. [CrossRef]
64. Omair, A.; Holden, M.; Lie, B.A.; Reikeras, O.; Brox, J.I. Treatment outcome of chronic low back pain and radiographic lumbar disc degeneration are associated with inflammatory and matrix degrading gene variants: A prospective genetic association study. *BMC Musculoskelet. Disord.* **2013**, *14*, 105. [CrossRef] [PubMed]
65. Schlosburg, J.E.; Kinsey, S.G.; Lichtman, A.H. Targeting fatty acid amide hydrolase (FAAH) to treat pain and inflammation. *AAPS J.* **2009**, *11*, 39–44. [CrossRef] [PubMed]
66. Piomelli, D.; Sasso, O. Peripheral gating of pain signals by endogenous lipid mediators. *Nat. Neurosci.* **2014**, *17*, 164–174. [CrossRef]

67. Huggins, J.P.; Smart, T.S.; Langman, S.; Taylor, L.; Young, T. An efficient randomised, placebo-controlled clinical trial with the irreversible fatty acid amide hydrolase-1 inhibitor PF-04457845, which modulates endocannabinoids but fails to induce effective analgesia in patients with pain due to osteoarthritis of the knee. *Pain* **2012**, *153*, 1837–1846.
68. Mu, J.; Ge, W.; Zuo, X.; Chen, Y.; Huang, C. A SNP in the 5′UTR of GDF5 is associated with susceptibility to symptomatic lumbar disc herniation in the Chinese Han population. *Eur. Spine J.* **2014**, *23*, 498–503. [CrossRef]
69. Schistad, E.I.; Jacobsen, L.M.; Roe, C.; Gjerstad, J. The interleukin-1alpha gene C > T polymorphism rs1800587 is associated with increased pain intensity and decreased pressure pain thresholds in patients with lumbar radicular pain. *Clin. J. Pain* **2014**, *30*, 869–874. [CrossRef]
70. Videman, T.; Saarela, J.; Kaprio, J.; Näkki, A.; Levälahti, E.; Gill, K.; Peltonen, L.; Battié, M.C. Associations of 25 structural, degradative, and inflammatory candidate genes with lumbar disc desiccation, bulging, and height narrowing. *Arthritis Rheum.* **2009**, *60*, 470–481. [CrossRef]
71. Puren, A.J.; Fantuzzi, G.; Dinarello, C.A. Gene expression, synthesis, and secretion of interleukin 18 and interleukin 1beta are differentially regulated in human blood mononuclear cells and mouse spleen cells. *Proc. Natl. Acad. Sci. USA* **1999**, *96*, 2256–2261. [CrossRef] [PubMed]
72. Cavanaugh, J.M. Neural mechanisms of lumbar pain. *Spine* **1995**, *20*, 1804–1809. [CrossRef] [PubMed]
73. Rannou, F.; Corvol, M.T.; Hudry, C.; Anract, P.; Dumontier, M.; Tsagris, L.; Revel, M.; Poiraudeau, S.; Serge, M.D. Sensitivity of anulus fibrosus cells to interleukin 1 beta. Comparison with articular chondrocytes. *Spine* **2000**, *25*, 17–23. [CrossRef] [PubMed]
74. Doita, M.; Kanatani, T.; Ozaki, T.; Matsui, N.; Kurosaka, M.; Yoshiya, S. Influence of macrophage infiltration of herniated disc tissue on the production of matrix metalloproteinases leading to disc resorption. *Spine* **2001**, *26*, 1522–1527. [CrossRef] [PubMed]
75. Valdes, A.M.; Spector, T.D.; Doherty, S.; Wheeler, M.; Hart, D.J.; Doherty, M. Association of the DVWA and GDF5 polymorphisms with osteoarthritis in UK populations. *Ann. Rheum. Dis.* **2009**, *68*, 1916–1920. [CrossRef]
76. Chapman, K.; Takahashi, A.; Meulenbelt, I.; Watson, C.; Rodríguez-López, J.; Egli, R.; Tsezou, A.; Malizos, K.N.; Kloppenburg, M.; Shi, D.; et al. A meta-analysis of European and Asian cohorts reveals a global role of a functional SNP in the 5′ UTR of GDF5 with osteoarthritis susceptibility. *Hum. Mol. Genet.* **2008**, *17*, 1497–1504. [CrossRef]
77. Williams, F.M.; Popham, M.; Hart, D.J.; De Schepper, E.; Bierma-Zeinstra, S.; Hofman, A.; Uitterlinden, A.G.; Arden, N.K.; Cooper, C.; Spector, T.D.; et al. GDF5 single-nucleotide polymorphism rs143383 is associated with lumbar disc degeneration in Northern European women. *Arthritis Rheum.* **2011**, *63*, 708–712. [CrossRef]
78. Zhang, L.; Stuber, F.; Stamer, U.M. Inflammatory mediators influence the expression of nociceptin and its receptor in human whole blood cultures. *PLoS ONE* **2013**, *8*, e74138. [CrossRef]
79. Mu, J.; Ge, W.; Zuo, X.; Chen, Y.; Huang, C. Analysis of association between IL-1beta, CASP-9, and GDF5 variants and low-back pain in Chinese male soldier: Clinical article. *J. Neurosurg. Spine* **2013**, *19*, 243–247. [CrossRef]
80. Williams, F.M.; Bansal, A.T.; van Meurs, J.B.; Bell, J.T.; Meulenbelt, I.; Suri, P.; Rivadeneira, F.; Sambrook, P.N.; Hofman, A.; Bierma-Zeinstra, S.; et al. Novel genetic variants associated with lumbar disc degeneration in northern Europeans: A meta-analysis of 4600 subjects. *Ann. Rheum. Dis.* **2013**, *72*, 1141–1148. [CrossRef]
81. Liu, C.F.; Lefebvre, V. The transcription factors SOX9 and SOX5/SOX6 cooperate genome-wide through super-enhancers to drive chondrogenesis. *Nucleic Acids Res.* **2015**, *43*, 8183–8203. [CrossRef] [PubMed]
82. Smits, P.; Li, P.; Mandel, J.; Zhang, Z.; Deng, J.M.; Behringer, R.R.; De Crombrugghe, B.; Lefebvre, V. The transcription factors L-Sox5 and Sox6 are essential for cartilage formation. *Dev. Cell* **2001**, *1*, 277–290. [CrossRef]
83. Liu, C.F.; Samsa, W.E.; Zhou, G.; Lefebvre, V. Transcriptional control of chondrocyte specification and differentiation. *Semin. Cell Dev. Biol.* **2017**, *62*, 34–49. [CrossRef] [PubMed]
84. Smits, P.; Lefebvre, V. Sox5 and Sox6 are required for notochord extracellular matrix sheath formation, notochord cell survival and development of the nucleus pulposus of intervertebral discs. *Development* **2003**, *130*, 1135–1148. [CrossRef] [PubMed]

85. Rodriguez-Fontenla, C.; Calaza, M.; Evangelou, E.; Valdes, A.M.; Arden, N.; Blanco, F.J.; Carr, A.; Chapman, K.; Deloukas, P.; Doherty, M.; et al. Assessment of osteoarthritis candidate genes in a meta-analysis of nine genome-wide association studies. *Arthritis Rheumatol.* **2014**, *66*, 940–949. [CrossRef]
86. Bjornsdottir, G.; Benonisdottir, S.; Sveinbjornsson, G.; Styrkarsdottir, U.; Thorleifsson, G.; Walters, G.B.; Bjornsson, A.; Olafsson, I.H.; Ulfarsson, E.; Vikingsson, A.; et al. Sequence variant at 8q24.21 associates with sciatica caused by lumbar disc herniation. *Nat. Commun.* **2017**, *8*, 14265. [CrossRef]
87. Truumees, E. A history of lumbar disc herniation from Hippocrates to the 1990s. *Clin. Orthop. Relat. Res.* **2015**, *473*, 1885–1895. [CrossRef]
88. Chou, D.; Samartzis, D.; Bellabarba, C.; Patel, A.; Luk, K.; Kisser, J.M.S.; Skelly, A.C. Degenerative magnetic resonance imaging changes in patients with chronic low back pain: A systematic review. *Spine* **2011**, *36*, S43–S53. [CrossRef]
89. Endean, A.; Palmer, K.T.; Coggon, D. Potential of magnetic resonance imaging findings to refine case definition for mechanical low back pain in epidemiological studies: A systematic review. *Spine* **2011**, *36*, 160–169. [CrossRef]
90. Zhang, Y.; Fukui, N.; Yahata, M.; Katsuragawa, Y.; Tashiro, T.; Ikegawa, S.; Lee, M.T.M. Genome-wide DNA methylation profile implicates potential cartilage regeneration at the late stage of knee osteoarthritis. *Osteoarthr. Cartil.* **2016**, *24*, 835–843. [CrossRef]
91. Zhang, Y.; Fukui, N.; Yahata, M.; Katsuragawa, Y.; Tashiro, T.; Ikegawa, S.; Lee, M.T.M. Identification of DNA methylation changes associated with disease progression in subchondral bone with site-matched cartilage in knee osteoarthritis. *Sci. Rep.* **2016**, *6*, 34460. [CrossRef] [PubMed]
92. Burston, J.J.; Sagar, D.R.; Shao, P.; Bai, M.; King, E.; Brailsford, L.; Turner, J.M.; Hathway, G.; Bennett, A.J.; Walsh, D.A.; et al. Cannabinoid CB2 receptors regulate central sensitization and pain responses associated with osteoarthritis of the knee joint. *PLoS ONE* **2013**, *8*, e80440. [CrossRef] [PubMed]
93. Rudd, R.A.; Seth, P.; David, F.; Scholl, L. Increases in Drug and Opioid-Involved Overdose Deaths—United States, 2010–2015. *Morb. Mortal. Wkly. Rep.* **2016**, *65*, 1445–1452. [CrossRef] [PubMed]
94. Kolodny, A.; Courtwright, D.T.; Hwang, C.S.; Kreiner, P.; Eadie, J.L.; Clark, T.W.; Alexander, G.C. The prescription opioid and heroin crisis: A public health approach to an epidemic of addiction. *Annu. Rev. Public Health* **2015**, *36*, 559–574. [CrossRef]
95. Knezevic, N.N.; Tverdohleb, T.; Knezevic, I.; Candido, K.D. The Role of Genetic Polymorphisms in Chronic Pain Patients. *Int. J. Mol. Sci.* **2018**, *19*, 1707. [CrossRef]
96. Meloto, C.B.; Benavides, R.; Lichtenwalter, R.N.; Wen, X.; Tugarinov, N.; Zorina-Lichtenwalter, K.; Chabot-Dore, A.-J.; Piltonen, M.H.; Cattaneo, S.; Verma, V.; et al. Human pain genetics database: A resource dedicated to human pain genetics research. *Pain* **2018**, *159*, 749–763. [CrossRef]
97. Nelson, D.R.; Zeldin, D.C.; Hoffman, S.M.; Maltais, L.J.; Wain, H.M.; Nebert, D.W. Comparison of cytochrome P450 (CYP) genes from the mouse and human genomes, including nomenclature recommendations for genes, pseudogenes and alternative-splice variants. *Pharmacogenetics* **2004**, *14*, 1–18. [CrossRef]
98. Preissner, S.C.; Hoffmann, M.F.; Preissner, R.; Dunkel, M.; Gewiess, A.; Preissner, S. Polymorphic cytochrome P450 enzymes (CYPs) and their role in personalized therapy. *PLoS ONE* **2013**, *8*, e82562. [CrossRef]
99. Yiannakopoulou, E. Pharmacogenomics of acetylsalicylic acid and other nonsteroidal anti-inflammatory agents: Clinical implications. *Eur. J. Clin. Pharmacol.* **2013**, *69*, 1369–1373. [CrossRef]
100. Theken, K.N.; Lee, C.R.; Gong, L.; Caudle, K.E.; Formea, C.M.; Gaedigk, A.; Klein, T.E.; Agúndez, J.A.; Grosser, T. Clinical Pharmacogenetics Implementation Consortium Guideline (CPIC) for CYP2C9 and Nonsteroidal Anti-Inflammatory Drugs. *Clin. Pharmacol. Ther.* **2020**, *108*, 191–200. [CrossRef]
101. Pilotto, A.; Seripa, D.; Franceschi, M.; Scarcelli, C.; Colaizzo, D.; Grandone, E.; Niro, V.; Andriulli, A.; Leandro, G.; Di Mario, F.; et al. Genetic susceptibility to nonsteroidal anti-inflammatory drug-related gastroduodenal bleeding: Role of cytochrome P450 2C9 polymorphisms. *Gastroenterology* **2007**, *133*, 465–471. [CrossRef] [PubMed]
102. Crews, K.R.; Gaedigk, A.; Dunnenberger, H.M.; Klein, T.E.; Shen, D.D.; Callaghan, J.T.; Kharasch, E.D.; Skaar, T.C. Clinical Pharmacogenetics Implementation Consortium (CPIC) guidelines for codeine therapy in the context of cytochrome P450 2D6 (CYP2D6) genotype. *Clin. Pharmacol. Ther.* **2012**, *91*, 321–326. [CrossRef]

103. Dagostino, C.; Allegri, M.; Napolioni, V.; D'Agnelli, S.; Bignami, E.; Mutti, A.; Van Schaik, R.H. CYP2D6 genotype can help to predict effectiveness and safety during opioid treatment for chronic low back pain: Results from a retrospective study in an Italian cohort. *Pharmgenomics Pers. Med.* **2018**, *11*, 179–191. [CrossRef] [PubMed]
104. Batistaki, C.; Chrona, E.; Kostroglou, A.; Kostopanagiotou, G.; Gazouli, M. CYP2D6 Basic Genotyping of Patients with Chronic Pain Receiving Tramadol or Codeine. A Study in a Greek Cohort. *Pain Med.* **2020**. [CrossRef] [PubMed]
105. Boswell, M.V.; Stauble, M.E.; Loyd, G.E.; Langman, L.; Ramey-Hartung, B.; Baumgartner, R.N.; Tucker, W.W.; Jortani, S.A. The role of hydromorphone and OPRM1 in postoperative pain relief with hydrocodone. *Pain Physician* **2013**, *16*, E227–E235. [PubMed]
106. Margarit, C.; Roca, R.; Inda, M.D.; Muriel, J.; Ballester, P.; Moreu, R.; Conte, A.L.; Nuñez, A.; Morales, M.; Peiró, A.M. Genetic Contribution in Low Back Pain: A Prospective Genetic Association Study. *Pain Pract.* **2019**, *19*, 836–847. [CrossRef]
107. Rodieux, F.; Piguet, V.; Berney, P.; Desmeules, J.; Besson, M. Pharmacogenetics and analgesic effects of antidepressants in chronic pain management. *Pers. Med.* **2015**, *12*, 163–175. [CrossRef]
108. Samer, C.F.; Lorenzini, K.I.; Rollason, V.; Daali, Y.; Desmeules, J.A. Applications of CYP450 testing in the clinical setting. *Mol. Diagn. Ther.* **2013**, *17*, 165–184. [CrossRef]
109. Staddon, S.; Arranz, M.J.; Mancama, D.; Mata, I.; Kerwin, R.W. Clinical applications of pharmacogenetics in psychiatry. *Psychopharmacology* **2002**, *162*, 18–23. [CrossRef]
110. Bertilsson, L.; Dahl, M.L.; Dalen, P.; Al-Shurbaji, A. Molecular genetics of CYP2D6: Clinical relevance with focus on psychotropic drugs. *Br. J. Clin. Pharmacol.* **2002**, *53*, 111–122. [CrossRef]
111. Swen, J.J.; Nijenhuis, M.; de Boer, A.; Grandia, L.; Maitland-van der Zee, A.H.; Mulder, H.; Rongen, G.A.P.J.M.; Van Schaik, R.H.N.; Schalekamp, T.; Touw, D.J.; et al. Pharmacogenetics: From bench to byte—An update of guidelines. *Clin. Pharmacol. Ther.* **2011**, *89*, 662–673. [CrossRef] [PubMed]
112. Chang, H.H.; Chou, C.H.; Yang, Y.K.; Lee, I.H.; Chen, P.S. Association between ABCB1 Polymorphisms and Antidepressant Treatment Response in Taiwanese Major Depressive Patients. *Clin. Psychopharmacol. Neurosci.* **2015**, *13*, 250–255. [CrossRef] [PubMed]
113. Singh, A.B.; Bousman, C.A.; Ng, C.H.; Byron, K.; Berk, M. ABCB1 polymorphism predicts escitalopram dose needed for remission in major depression. *Transl. Psychiatry* **2012**, *27*, e198. [CrossRef] [PubMed]
114. Suwala, J.; Machowska, M.; Wiela-Hojenska, A. Venlafaxine pharmacogenetics: A comprehensive review. *Pharmacogenomics* **2019**, *20*, 829–845. [CrossRef]
115. Ma, Y.; Wang, C.; Luo, S.; Li, B.; Wager, T.D.; Zhang, W.; Rao, Y.; Han, S. Serotonin transporter polymorphism alters citalopram effects on human pain responses to physical pain. *Neuroimage* **2016**, *135*, 186–196. [CrossRef]
116. Winchell, G.A.; King, J.D.; Chavez-Eng, C.M.; Constanzer, M.L.; Korn, S.H. Cyclobenzaprine pharmacokinetics, including the effects of age, gender, and hepatic insufficiency. *J. Clin. Pharmacol.* **2002**, *42*, 61–69. [CrossRef]
117. Mestres, J.; Seifert, S.A.; Oprea, T.I. Linking pharmacology to clinical reports: Cyclobenzaprine and its possible association with serotonin syndrome. *Clin. Pharmacol. Ther.* **2011**, *90*, 662–665. [CrossRef]
118. Perucca, E. Clinically relevant drug interactions with antiepileptic drugs. *Br. J. Clin. Pharmacol.* **2006**, *61*, 246–255. [CrossRef]
119. Ben-Menachem, E. Pregabalin pharmacology and its relevance to clinical practice. *Epilepsia* **2004**, *45* (Suppl. 6), 13–18. [CrossRef]
120. Honarmand, A.; Safavi, M.; Zare, M. Gabapentin: An update of its pharmacological properties and therapeutic use in epilepsy. *J. Res. Med. Sci.* **2011**, *16*, 1062–1069.
121. Koepsell, H. The SLC22 family with transporters of organic cations, anions and zwitterions. *Mol. Asp. Med.* **2013**, *34*, 413–435. [CrossRef] [PubMed]
122. Koepsell, H.; Lips, K.; Volk, C. Polyspecific organic cation transporters: Structure, function, physiological roles, and biopharmaceutical implications. *Pharm. Res.* **2007**, *24*, 1227–1251. [CrossRef] [PubMed]
123. Yamamoto, P.A.; Benzi, J.R.L.; Azeredo, F.J.; Dach, F.; Ianhez Junior, E.; Zanelli, C.F.; De Moraes, N.V. Pharmacogenetics-based population pharmacokinetic analysis of gabapentin in patients with chronic pain: Effect of OCT2 and OCTN1 gene polymorphisms. *Basic Clin. Pharmacol. Toxicol.* **2019**, *124*, 266–272. [CrossRef] [PubMed]

124. Pergolizzi, J.V., Jr.; Labhsetwar, S.A.; Puenpatom, R.A.; Joo, S.; Ben-Joseph, R.H.; Summers, K.H. Prevalence of exposure to potential CYP450 pharmacokinetic drug-drug interactions among patients with chronic low back pain taking opioids. *Pain Pract.* **2011**, *11*, 230–239. [CrossRef] [PubMed]
125. Pergolizzi, J.V.; Ma, L.; Foster, D.R.; Overholser, B.R.; Sowinski, K.M.; Taylor, R., Jr.; Summers, K.H. The prevalence of opioid-related major potential drug-drug interactions and their impact on health care costs in chronic pain patients. *J. Manag. Care Spec. Pharm.* **2014**, *20*, 467–476. [CrossRef]
126. Verbeurgt, P.; Mamiya, T.; Oesterheld, J. How common are drug and gene interactions? Prevalence in a sample of 1143 patients with CYP2C9, CYP2C19 and CYP2D6 genotyping. *Pharmacogenomics* **2014**, *15*, 655–665. [CrossRef]
127. Malki, M.A.; Pearson, E.R. Drug-drug-gene interactions and adverse drug reactions. *Pharm. J.* **2020**, *20*, 355–366. [CrossRef]
128. Storelli, F.; Desmeules, J.; Daali, Y. Physiologically-Based Pharmacokinetic Modeling for the Prediction of CYP2D6-Mediated Gene-Drug-Drug Interactions. *CPT Pharmacomet. Syst. Pharmacol.* **2019**, *8*, 567–576. [CrossRef]
129. Trescot, A.M.; Faynboym, S. A review of the role of genetic testing in pain medicine. *Pain Physician* **2014**, *17*, 425–445.

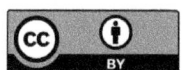

© 2020 by the authors. Licensee MDPI, Basel, Switzerland. This article is an open access article distributed under the terms and conditions of the Creative Commons Attribution (CC BY) license (http://creativecommons.org/licenses/by/4.0/).

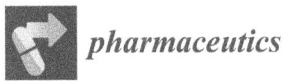

Article

Frequency of CYP3A5 Genetic Polymorphisms and Tacrolimus Pharmacokinetics in Pediatric Liver Transplantation

Jefferson Antonio Buendía [1,*], Esteban Halac [2], Andrea Bosaleh [3], María T. Garcia de Davila [3], Oscar Imvertasa [2] and Guillermo Bramuglia [4]

1. Department of Pharmacology and Toxicology, Faculty of Medicine, University of Antioquia, Medellin 050010, Colombia
2. Liver Transplant Service, J.P. Garrahan Hospital, Buenos Aires C1245AAM, Argentina; ehalac@gmail.com (E.H.); imventarzaoscar@gmail.com (O.I.)
3. Pathology Service, J.P. Garrahan Hospital, Buenos Aires C1245AAM, Argentina; apbosaleh@yahoo.com.ar (A.B.); gdedavila@gmail.com (M.T.G.d.D.)
4. Faculty of Pharmacy and Biochemistry, University of Buenos Aires, Buenos Aires C1113, Argentina; gfbramuglia@gmail.com
* Correspondence: jefferson.buendia@udea.edu.co or jefferson.buendia@gmail.com

Received: 11 December 2018; Accepted: 16 April 2019; Published: 22 September 2020

Abstract: The evidence available in the pediatric population is limited for making clinical decisions regarding the optimization of tacrolimus (TAC) in pharmacotherapy. The objective of this study was to estimate the frequency of CYP3A5 genetic polymorphisms and their relationship with tacrolimus requirements in the pediatric population. This was a longitudinal cohort study with a two-year follow-up of 77 patients under 18 years old who underwent a liver transplant during the period 2009–2012 at the J.P. Garrahan Pediatric Hospital. Tacrolimus levels from day five up to two years after the transplant were obtained from hospital records of routine therapeutic drug monitoring. The genotyping of CYP3A5 (CYP3A5*1/*3 or *3/*3) was performed in liver biopsies from both the donor and the recipient. The frequency of CYP3A5*1 expression for recipients was 37.1% and 32.2% for donors. Patients who received an expresser organ showed lower Co/dose, especially following 90 days after the surgery. The role of each polymorphism is different according to the number of days after the transplant, and it must be taken into account to optimize the benefits of TAC therapy during the post-transplant induction and maintenance phases.

Keywords: tacrolimus; CYP3A5; liver transplant; pharmacokinetics

1. Introduction

Tacrolimus (TAC) is a calcineurin inhibitor widely used in solid organ transplantation. TAC has a narrow therapeutic margin and a large intra- and inter-individual variability [1,2]. Incidence of rejection and adverse effects remain as problems despite therapeutic drug monitoring of TAC [3]. There is growing interest in developing markers that will allow for an individual treatment with TAC. Within this group of potential biomarkers, we find the single nucleotide polymorphisms of CYP3A5 [3–5]. This enzyme has a highly polymorphic expression with at least 11 single nucleotide polymorphisms (SNPs) documented [3]. The most studied SNP is the transition from adenine to guanine at the position 6986-intron 3-CYP3A5 gene (rs776746), also known as CYP3A5*1. This allele is associated with high levels of CYP3A5-mRNA and fully functional CYP3A5-protein [6,7]. The Caucasian population expresses CYP3A5*1 between 10–40%, while the Asian population expresses it between 50–70% [8]. CYP3A5*1 (homozygotes and heterozygotes) expressers require much higher daily doses of TAC as well as more time to reach its desired serum levels. Furthermore, expressers have three times the risk of acute rejection within the first month after transplant than non-expressers [9].

After a liver transplant, the simultaneous expression of CYP3A5*1 in both the intestine and the implanted liver may occur [3]. In previous studies in the adult population, we showed that this interaction does occur. The expression of CYP3A5*1 present in the liver donor has a great impact on TAC levels adjusted by dose in long-term concentrations, while the expression of this SNP in the receiver also has a great impact, but only after transplantation [8]. However, its kinetics and pharmacodynamics are very different when comparing pediatric and adult populations. This can be explained by the greater variability of specific enzymes, which are acquired by the child during growth and alter the clinical response to TAC [3]. The evidence available in the pediatric population is limited for making clinical decisions regarding the therapeutic optimization of TAC. Thus, it is essential to generate more information to optimize and customize monitoring strategies for liver transplants in this population. The objective of this study was to estimate the frequency of CYP3A5 genetic polymorphisms and their relationship with pharmacokinetics in pediatric liver transplantation.

2. Materials and Methods

A longitudinal study was conducted in 77 patients under 18 years old after liver transplantation during the period 2009–2012 at the J.P. Garrahan Pediatric Hospital (JPGPH).

Patients with full or partial liver grafts from either living or cadaveric donors were included. All patients were receiving tacrolimus with or without steroids and with or without mofetil mycophenolate (MMF). We excluded HIV infected patients who suffered an early death before receiving an immunosuppressive regimen with TAC immediately after surgery and patients with partial or total loss of medical records.

2.1. Dosage and Treatment Scheme

Patient information was collected immediately after the liver transplantation. The immunosuppression scheme used on the subjects according to the Clinical Practice Guidelines of JPGPH for patients after liver transplantation is described below. During the induction phase, all patients received basiliximab. Patients who weighed less than 30 kg received a 10 mg/dose, and those who weighed more than 30 kg received a 20 mg/dose. Both doses were administered as an intravenous bolus, the first one within 8 h after reperfusion of the graft and the second one on the fourth day after surgery. TAC was dispensed in the maintenance phase, which started 24 h after reperfusion. The initial oral regimen was 0.1 mg/kg/day every 12 h. After, the dose of TAC was adjusted to tacrolimus blood levels, liver parameters, kidney function, and the viral load of Epstein Barr Virus (EBV) [10]. In patients without infectious activity (viral load less than 4000 copies/μg DNA) and a creatinine clearance less than the expected range for their age, the initial desired TAC blood levels were 8–12 ng/mL during the first month after transplantation and then 5, 6, 7, and 8 ng/mL until a year after transplantation had passed [10]. We proceeded with a quick immunosuppression reduction in those patients with viral loads above 4000 copies/μg DNA in two consecutive samples or clinical evidence of EBV infection. No antiviral therapy was implemented. In patients who developed renal toxicity, regardless of viral load, monitoring of TAC was decreased to 25%. In those cases, MMF was added as rescue therapy with an initial dose of 20 mg/kg/day, and then it was increased up to 40 mg/kg/day after a week of treatment.

2.2. Monitoring and Quantification of Tacrolimus Blood Levels

TAC levels from day five up to the second year after the transplant were obtained from hospital records of routine therapeutic drug monitoring. The values recorded correlated to monitoring blood levels from samples drawn prior to the morning dose or Co (concentration measured in $t = 0$ before the first dose of the drug).

The quantification of TAC was performed by chemiluminescence immunoassay by Abbott's Architect i1000 according to the manufacturer's instructions. The low quantification limit was 2.0 ng/mL, and linearity was observed between 2–30 ng/mL. The variation coefficient for quality control samples was lower than 6%.

2.3. Collected Information

Demographic information (date of birth, gender), anthropometric data (weight, height), indication of transplant, post-transplantation follow-up time, current medication and doses, concomitant medications, amount of transplanted graft, amount of postsurgical days, and data related to the donor type were collected. We registered clinical laboratory results including hematology (hemoglobin, hematocrit, red blood cells, white cells and platelets, prothrombin time (PT), activated partial thromboplastin time (aPTT), and thrombin time (TT) and clinical chemistry results (creatinine, urea nitrogen, total and direct bilirubin, alkaline phosphatase, alanine aminotransferase (GPT or ALT), aspartate aminotransferase (GOT or AST), gamma glutamyl transpeptidase (GGT), and albumin.

2.4. DNA Isolation and Genotyping

The genotyping of CYP3A5 was performed in liver biopsies of both the donor and the recipient. The donor's DNA was obtained from liver biopsies or surgical specimens obtained from the pathology service at the JPGPH. Each of them was tissue-fixed in formalin-buffer, embedded in paraffin, and sectioned 10 microns thick.

DNA extraction was performed using commercial kits QIAamp DNA Blood Kit and QIAamp DNA FFPE Tissue following the manufacturer's instructions. We obtained from 20 to 100 ng DNA in each case. CYP3A5*3 (rs776746) polymorphism was detected by PCR and directly sequenced. Patients with variants CYP3A5*1/*1 or CYP3A5*1/*3 were called "expressers", while those with variants CYP3A5*3/*3 were called "non-expressers".

2.5. Ethical Aspects

A proper informed consent was signed by a parent or legal guardian before starting any specific evaluations. The study was approved by the office of Teaching and Research at the JPGPH (Code 740 21/08/12) and by the Ethics Committee of the Faculty of Pharmacy and Biochemistry, at the University of Buenos Aires (Code 930 21/03/14).

2.6. Statistical Analysis

We compared daily doses of TAC, Co (TAC levels before the morning dose), and Co/dose (concentration adjusted by dose) according to CYP3A5*1 allele expression between donors and recipients. All values were expressed as mean ± standard deviation. The U Mann-Whitney test was used to determine differences among continuous variables in the groups. The chi-square test was used to analyze differences among discrete variables. All analyses were performed using STATA 11.0$^©$ (Lakeway Drive, College Station, TX, USA).

3. Results

We evaluated 77 pediatric patients medicated with TAC during the first two years after transplantation. Table 1 shows the characteristics of the population studied. We observed 45 patients (58.44%) with adverse events associated with tacrolimus, 51 patients (66.23%) had at least one acute cellular rejection episode, and eight patients died (10.39%) during follow-up.

Table 1. Characteristics of the studied population (n = 77).

Feature	n (%)
Female	46 (59.74)
Age at transplantation (years, ±SD)	5.32 (5.42)
Weight (kg, ±DE)	21.84(17.89)
Origin	
Argentina	64(83.11)
Bolivia	2(2.60)
Paraguay	9(11.69)
Other	2(2.59)
Primary disease	
Biliary atresia	32(41.55)
Fulminant hepatitis	16(20.77)
Autoimmune hepatitis	11(14.28)
Hepatoblastoma	8(10.38)
Others	10(12.98)
Kind of Donor	
Cadaveric	55(71.42)
Live	22(28.57)
Kind of Graft	
Full	26(33.76)
Technical variant	51(66.23)

CYP3A5*1 expression was 37.1% in recipients and 32.2% in donors. There were no statistically significant deviations in the distribution of polymorphisms according to the Hardy-Weinberg principle ($p > 0.05$).

A total of 3670 blood concentrations of TAC were analyzed during the study period with a mean of 47.8 samples per patient. We observed a greater difference in expresser recipients compared with non-expressers, especially in the first two weeks after surgery, and those differences tended to reduce over time (Figure 1).

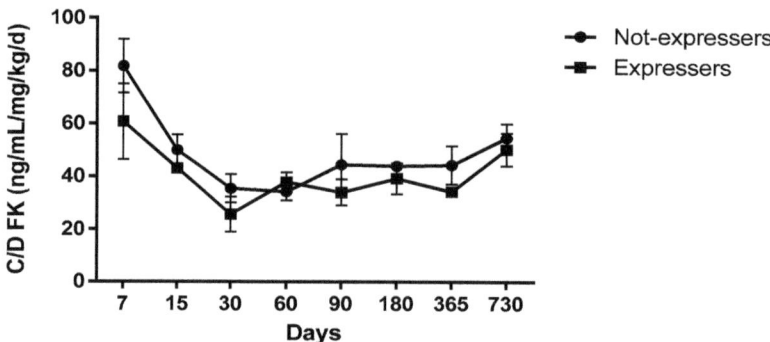

Figure 1. Co/dose of tacrolimus (TAC) according to the recipient genotype.

When we adjusted the dose by concentrations according to the genotype of the donor, those who received an expresser organ showed a lower Co/dose, especially 90 days after surgery (Figure 2). A statistically significant reduction of 0.00063 ng/mL mg/kg/day in the Co/dose was observed compared with those receiving a non-expresser organ ($p = 0.001$).

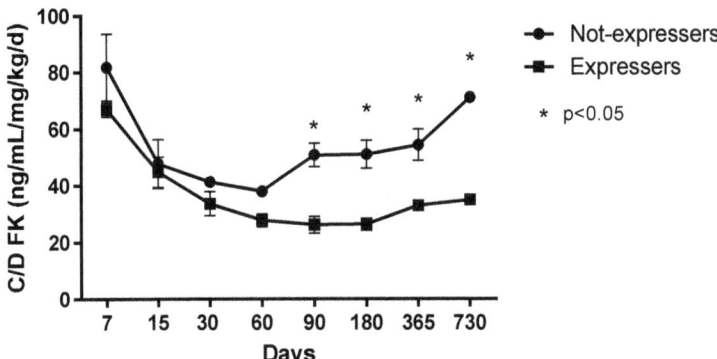

Figure 2. Co/dose of TAC according to the donor genotype.

4. Discussion

CYP3A5 polymorphisms have a differential impact in the pharmacokinetics of tacrolimus according to its expression in donors and recipients. In contrast to previous studies, this is the first study in pediatric patients that evaluates the effect of polymorphisms on TAC pharmacokinetics in the long term. Other studies considered shorter periods and generally did not include the Hispanic population.

Patients with CYP3A5 allele A (CYP3A5*1 or wild type) have a normal splicing of all 13 exons in this gene. This results in a normal transcript and a production of high levels of mRNA, which in turn expresses the enzyme metabolizing TAC. Patients with allele G (CYP3A5*3) have a point mutation (A/G) resulting in the insertion of an inappropriate 3B "exon" within the transcript. This new exon introduces an early termination codon, leading to a non-functional protein fragment [11]. The frequency of expressers (CYP3A5*1) in our study was reported to be intermediate within the ranges of Asian (33% to 66%) and Caucasian (9% to 15%) populations. These estimates were consistent with previous results in studies in Argentinean renal transplant patients, which reported values ranging from 9% to 27% [12–14]. These differences between Caucasian and Asian frequencies reveal the genetic diversity present in Latin America as a result of the colonial era, as well as the African (slaves in the 19th century) and post-independence immigrants (the majority coming from Spain, Italy, France, and eastern Europe) [15].

Similar results have been found in studies focused on the frequency of variations in other genes related to anti-neoplastic metabolism [16]. Continuing to build this pharmacogenetic map in Latin America will improve the understanding of the variations in the metabolism and the effect of various drugs without the need to extrapolate results obtained from other populations.

In liver transplant patients, both donors and recipients carrying the CYP3A5 polymorphisms are associated with changes in the pharmacokinetics of TAC. Nevertheless, the role of each polymorphism is different according to the number of days after transplantation. We have shown that the recipient CYP3A5 genotype plays a more important role than the donor genotype. Recipients with CYP3A5*1 achieved lower blood concentrations of TAC and lower dose-adjusted concentrations despite the medical pharmacotherapeutic follow-up (based on adjusting the blood concentrations to the reference therapeutic margins). These findings were consistent with a recent study of 64 post-transplant children with a one year follow-up [17]. It was shown that lower dose-adjusted ($p < 0.05$) concentrations were required in patients who were expressers, without any correlation with donor genotype, especially in the first seven days after transplantation [17].

To recognize the role played by the recipient CYP3A5 genotype in the first weeks after transplantation, it is essential to avoid excessive dose increases in patients who are expressers of this genotype [18].

On the other hand, the donor genotype alters the kinetics of TAC, significantly increasing with time after transplantation. The effect of CYP3A5 expression on the recipient is an increased hepatic clearance of the liver implanted with the polymorphism. This tendency was evidenced in our study, where a reduction of dose-adjusted concentrations was documented as statistically significant 60 to 90 days after surgery. This observation might be related to the time needed by the organ to recover from the ischemia and reperfusion injuries, regeneration, and graft growth as months after transplantation pass [19]. Our results indicate the importance of knowing the genotype present in the organ before being transplanted. During the ambulatory follow-up, it is a priority to select patients with greater hepatic clearance who will get a lower concentration and who may require different medical follow-up to avoid sub-immunosuppression.

Our study has limitations primarily due to its retrospective nature. Among them, some are due to the misclassification of patients either by memory bias or problems with recording information in clinical histories (by omission or incorrect recording). These biases could be minimized by always obtaining information from primary registers (physical or electronic medical history) and double-checking with other clinical records (nursing records and hospital pharmacy records). Additionally, we only analyzed concentrations per patient at time 0 (C0) given the fact that we used hospital therapeutic monitoring data, and for TAC, this concentration is used for clinical monitoring of these drugs. Also, the effect of other variables on the pharmacokinetics of TAC, such as age, drug interaction, and length of the event related to dose-adjusted concentrations, were not evaluated and should be analyzed in further studies.

In conclusion, patients after liver transplantation—both donors and recipients—carrying CYP3A5 polymorphisms are susceptible to suffering changes in TAC pharmacokinetics. However, the role of each polymorphism is different according to the number of days after transplantation, and it must be taken into account to optimize the benefits of TAC therapy during the post-transplant induction and maintenance phases.

Author Contributions: All authors contributed equally in the revision, drafting, and writing of this article.

Funding: This research received no external funding.

Acknowledgments: We would like to thank the University of Antioquia, Fundación Investigar, Buenos Aires Argentina, Paula Schaiquevich, Natalia Riva, and the pharmacokinetics laboratory at the JPGPH.

Conflicts of Interest: The authors declare no conflict of interest.

References

1. Undre, N.; Stevenson, P.; Schäfer, A. Pharmacokinetics of tacrolimus: Clinically relevant aspects. *Transplant. Proc.* **1999**, *31*, 21–24. [CrossRef]
2. Wallemacq, P.; Armstrong, V.W.; Brunet, M.; Haufroid, V.; Holt, D.W.; Johnston, A.; Kuypers, D.; Le Meur, Y.; Marquet, P.; Oellerich, M.; et al. Opportunities to Optimize Tacrolimus Therapy in Solid Organ Transplantation: Report of the European Consensus Conference. *Ther. Drug Monit.* **2009**, *31*, 139–152. [CrossRef] [PubMed]
3. Staatz, C.E.; Tett, S.E. Clinical pharmacokinetics and pharmacodynamics of tacrolimus in solid organ transplantation. *Clin. Pharmacokinet.* **2004**, *43*, 623–653. [CrossRef] [PubMed]
4. Wang, L.; McLeod, H.L.; Weinshilboum, R.M. Genomics and drug response. *N. Engl. J. Med.* **2011**, *364*, 1144–1153. [CrossRef] [PubMed]
5. Hesselink, D.A.; van Schaik, R.H.; van der Heiden, I.P.; van der Werf, M.; Gregoor, P.J.; Lindemans, J.; Weimar, W.; van Gelder, T. Genetic polymorphisms of the CYP3A4, CYP3A5, and MDR-1 genes and pharmacokinetics of the calcineurin inhibitors cyclosporine and tacrolimus. *Clin. Pharmacol. Ther.* **2003**, *74*, 245–254. [CrossRef]
6. Buendía, J.A.; Otamendi, E.; Kravetz, M.C.; Cairo, F.; Ruf, A.; de Davila, M.; Powazniak, Y.; Nafissi, J.; Lazarowski, A.; Bramuglia, G.; et al. Combinational Effect of CYP3A5 and MDR-1 Polymorphisms on Tacrolimus Pharmacokinetics in Liver Transplant Patients. *Exp. Clin. Transplant* **2015**, *13*, 441–448.
7. Lamba, J.K.; Lin, Y.S.; Schuetz, E.G.; Thummel, K.E. Genetic contribution to variable human CYP3A-mediated metabolism. *Adv. Drug Deliv. Rev.* **2002**, *54*, 1271–1294. [CrossRef]

8. Buendia, J.A.; Bramuglia, G.; Staatz, C.E. Effects of combinational CYP3A5 6986A>G polymorphism in graft liver and native intestine on the pharmacokinetics of tacrolimus in liver transplant patients: a meta-analysis. *Ther. Drug Monit.* **2014**, *36*, 442–447. [CrossRef] [PubMed]
9. Rojas, L.E.; Herrero, M.J.; Boso, V.; García-Eliz, M.; Poveda, J.L.; Librero, J.; Aliño, S.F. Meta-analysis and systematic review of the effect of the donor and recipient CYP3A5 6986A>G genotype on tacrolimus dose requirements in liver transplantation. *Pharmacogenet. Genom.* **2013**, *23*, 509–517. [CrossRef] [PubMed]
10. Allen, U.; Farmer, D.; Shemesh, E.; Kelly, D.A.; Bucuvalas, J.C.; Alonso, E.M.; Karpen, S.J.; Green, M.; McDonald, R.A. Long-term medical management of the pediatric patient after liver transplantation: 2013 practice guideline by the American Association for the Study of Liver Diseases and the American Society of Transplantation. *Liver Transplant.* **2013**, *19*, 798–825.
11. Kuehl, P.; Zhang, J.; Lin, Y.; Lamba, J.; Assem, M.; Schuetz, J.; Watkins, P.B.; Daly, A.; Wrighton, S.A.; Hall, S.D.; et al. Sequence diversity in CYP3A promoters and characterization of the genetic basis of polymorphic CYP3A5 expression. *Nat. Genet.* **2001**, *27*, 383–391. [CrossRef]
12. Lavandera, J.; Parera, V.; Rossetti, M.V.; Batlle, A.; Buzaleh, A.M. Identificación de polimorfismos del CYP3A5 y CYP2B6 en infección por VIH asociada a Porfiria Cutánea Tardía en la población Argentina. In Proceedings of the Reunion Cienfitica anual de la Sociedad Argentina de Investigación Clínica (SAIC), Buenos Aires, Argentina, 1 August 2010; Sociedad Argentina de Investigación Clínica (SAIC): Buenos Aires, Argentina, 2010.
13. Larriba, J.; Imperiali, N.; Groppa, R.; Giordani, C.; Algranatti, S.; Redal, M. Pharmacogenetics of Immunosuppressant Polymorphism of CYP3A5 in Renal Transplant Recipients. *Transplant. Proc.* **2010**, *42*, 257–259. [CrossRef]
14. Ferraris, J.R.; Argibay, P.F.; Costa, L.; Jimenez, G.; Coccia, P.A.; Ghezzi, L.F.; Ferraris, V.; Belloso, W.H.; Redal, M.A.; Larriba, J.M. Influence of CYP3A5 polymorphism on tacrolimus maintenance doses and serum levels after renal transplantation: Age dependency and pharmacological interaction with steroids. *Pediatr. Transplant.* **2011**, *15*, 525–532. [CrossRef]
15. Arrieta, O.; Cardona, A.F.; Bramuglia, G.F.; Gallo, A.; Campos-Parra, A.D.; Serrano, S.; Castro, M.; Avilés, A.; Amorin, E.; Kirchuk, R.; et al. Genotyping Non-small Cell Lung Cancer (NSCLC) in Latin America. *J. Thorac. Oncol.* **2011**, *6*, 1955–1959. [CrossRef] [PubMed]
16. Roco, A.M.P.; Quinones, L.A.; García-Martín, E.M.; Squicciarini, V.P.; Miranda, C.E.P.; Garay, J.M.; Farfán, N.P.; Saavedra, I.N.P.; Caceres, D.D.M.; Ibarra, C.; et al. Frequencies of 23 functionally significant variant alleles related with metabolism of antineoplastic drugs in the chilean population: comparison with caucasian and asian populations. *Front. Genet.* **2012**, *3*, 229. [CrossRef]
17. Xue, F.; Han, L.; Chen, Y.; Xi, Z.; Li, Q.; Xu, N.; Xia, Y.; Streicher, K.; Zhang, J.; Xia, Q. CYP3A5 genotypes affect tacrolimus pharmacokinetics and infectious complications in Chinese pediatric liver transplant patients. *Pediatr. Transplant.* **2014**, *18*, 166–176. [CrossRef] [PubMed]
18. Chen, S.-Y.; Li, J.-L.; Meng, F.-H.; Wang, X.-D.; Li, J.; Liu, L.-S.; Wang, C.-X.; Chen, S.; Li, J.; Meng, F.; et al. Individualization of tacrolimus dosage basing on cytochrome P450 3A5 polymorphism—A prospective, randomized, controlled study. *Clin. Transplant.* **2013**, *27*, E272–E281. [CrossRef] [PubMed]
19. Starkel, P.; Laurent, S.; Petit, M.; Berge, V.V.D.; Lambotte, L.; Horsmans, Y. Early down-regulation of cytochrome P450 3A and 2E1 in the regenerating rat liver is not related to the loss of liver mass or the process of cellular proliferation. *Liver Int.* **2000**, *20*, 405–410. [CrossRef] [PubMed]

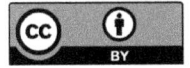

© 2020 by the authors. Licensee MDPI, Basel, Switzerland. This article is an open access article distributed under the terms and conditions of the Creative Commons Attribution (CC BY) license (http://creativecommons.org/licenses/by/4.0/).

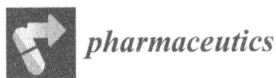

Article

Whole Transcription Profile of Responders to Anti-TNF Drugs in Pediatric Inflammatory Bowel Disease

Sara Salvador-Martín [1,†], Bartosz Kaczmarczyk [1,†], Rebeca Álvarez [2], Víctor Manuel Navas-López [3], Carmen Gallego-Fernández [4], Ana Moreno-Álvarez [5], Alfonso Solar-Boga [5], Cesar Sánchez [6], Mar Tolin [6], Marta Velasco [7], Rosana Muñoz-Codoceo [7], Alejandro Rodriguez-Martinez [8], Concepción A. Vayo [9], Ferrán Bossacoma [10], Gemma Pujol-Muncunill [11], María J. Fobelo [12], Antonio Millán-Jiménez [13], Lorena Magallares [14], Eva Martínez-Ojinaga [14], Inés Loverdos [15], Francisco J. Eizaguirre [16], José A. Blanca-García [17], Susana Clemente [18], Ruth García-Romero [19], Vicente Merino-Bohórquez [20], Rafael González de Caldas [21], Enrique Vázquez [2], Ana Dopazo [2], María Sanjurjo-Sáez [1] and Luis A. López-Fernández [1,*]

1. Pharmacy Department, Instituto de Investigación Sanitaria Gregorio Marañón, Hospital General Universitario Gregorio Marañón, 28007 Madrid, Spain; sara.salvador@iisgm.com (S.S.-M.); bkackmar@ucm.es (B.K.); maria.sanjurjo@salud.madrid.org (M.S.-S.)
2. Genomics Unit, Spanish Nacional Center for Cardiovascular Diseases (CNIC), 28029 Madrid, Spain; ralvarez@cnic.es (R.Á.); enrique.vazquez@cnic.es (E.V.); adopazo@cnic.es (A.D.)
3. Pediatric Gastroenterology and Nutrition Unit, Hospital Regional Universitario de Málaga, IBIMA Multidisciplinary Group for Pediatric Research, 29010 Málaga, Spain; victorm.navas.sspa@juntadeandalucia.es
4. Pharmacy Department, Hospital Regional Universitario de Málaga, 29010 Málaga, Spain; carmen.gallego.sspa@juntadeandalucia.es
5. Pediatric Gastroenterology Unit, Department of Pediatrics, A Coruña University Hospital, 15006 A Coruña, Spain; ana.moreno.alvarez@sergas.es (A.M.-Á.); alfonso.solar.boga@sergas.es (A.S.-B.)
6. Gastroenterology Unit, Instituto de Investigación Sanitaria Gregorio Marañón, Hospital General Universitario Gregorio Marañón, 28007 Madrid, Spain; cesar.sanchez.sanchez@salud.madrid.org (C.S.); mariamar.tolin@salud.madrid.org (M.T.)
7. Department of Pediatric Gastroenterology, Hospital Infantil Universitario Niño Jesús, 28009 Madrid, Spain; mvelasco@salud.madrid.org (M.V.); rosana.munoz@salud.madrid.org (R.M.-C.)
8. Pediatric Gastroenterology, Hepatology and Nutrition Unit, Hospital Universitario Virgen del Rocio, 41013 Seville, Spain; alejandro.rodriguez.m.sspa@juntadeandalucia.es
9. Pharmacy Service, Hospital Universitario Virgen del Rocio, 41013 Seville, Spain; concepcion.alvarezvayo.sspa@juntadeandalucia.es
10. Fundació Sant Joan de Déu, Fundació Salut Emporda, 08950 Barcelona, Spain; fbossacoma@sjdhospitalbarcelona.org
11. Department of Pediatric Gastroenterology, Hepatology and Nutrition, Hospital Sant Joan de Déu, 08950 Barcelona, Spain; gpujol@sjdhospitalbarcelona.org
12. Pharmacy Service, Hospital Virgen de Valme, 41014 Sevilla, Spain; mariaj.fobelo.sspa@juntadeandalucia.es
13. Pediatric Gastroenterology Unit, Hospital Virgen de Valme, 41014 Sevilla, Spain; amillan1@us.es
14. Department of Pediatric Gastroenterology, University Hospital La Paz, 28046 Madrid, Spain; lorena.magallares@salud.madrid.org (L.M.); eva.martinezojinaga@salud.madrid.org (E.M.-O.)
15. Pediatric Gastroenterology, Hepatology and Nutrition Unit, Hospital de Sabadell, Corporació Sanitària Universitària Parc Taulí, 08208 Barcelona, Spain; iloverdos@tauli.cat
16. Pediatric Gastroenterology Unit, Hospital Universitario Donostia, 20014 San Sebastián, Spain; franciscojavier.eizaguirrearocena@osakidetza.eus
17. Pediatric Gastroenterology Unit, Hospital Puerta del Mar, 11009 Cadiz, Spain; digestivo_infantil.hpm.sspa@juntadeandalucia.es
18. Pharmacy Unit, Hospital Universitario Vall d'Hebrón, 08035 Barcelona, Spain; sclemente@vhebron.net

[19] Pediatric Gastroenterology Unit, Hospital Infantil Miguel Servet, 50009 Zaragoza, Spain; rgarciarom@salud.aragon.es
[20] UGC Pharmacy Department, Hospital Virgen de la Macarena, 41009 Sevilla, Spain; vicente.merino.sspa@juntadeandalucia.es
[21] Pediatric Gastroenterology Unit, Hospital Reina Sofía, 14004 Córdoba, Spain; rgonzalezdecaldasmarchal@gmail.com
* Correspondence: luis.lopez@iisgm.com
† These authors contributed equally to this work.

Received: 5 November 2020; Accepted: 6 January 2021; Published: 8 January 2021

Abstract: Background: Up to 30% of patients with pediatric inflammatory bowel disease (IBD) do not respond to anti-Tumor Necrosis Factor (anti-TNF) therapy. The aim of this study was to identify pharmacogenomic markers that predict early response to anti-TNF drugs in pediatric patients with IBD. Methods: An observational, longitudinal, prospective cohort study was conducted. The study population comprised 38 patients with IBD aged < 18 years who started treatment with infliximab or adalimumab (29 responders and nine non-responders). Whole gene expression profiles from total RNA isolated from whole blood samples of six responders and six non-responders taken before administration of the biologic and after two weeks of therapy were analyzed using next-generation RNA sequencing. The expression of six selected genes was measured for purposes of validation in all of the 38 patients recruited using qPCR. Results: Genes were differentially expressed in non-responders and responders (32 before initiation of treatment and 44 after two weeks, Log2FC (Fold change) >0.6 or <−0.6 and p value < 0.05). After validation, *FCGR1A*, *FCGR1B*, and *GBP1* were overexpressed in non-responders two weeks after initiation of anti-TNF treatment (Log2FC 1.05, 1.21, and 1.08, respectively, p value < 0.05). Conclusion: Expression of the *FCGR1A*, *FCGR1B*, and *GBP1* genes is a pharmacogenomic biomarker of early response to anti-TNF agents in pediatric IBD.

Keywords: biomarker; gene expression; infliximab; adalimumab; ulcerative colitis; Crohn disease; inflammatory bowel disease

1. Introduction

Inflammatory bowel disease (IBD), which includes ulcerative colitis (UC) and Crohn disease (CD), is a multifactorial autoimmune disorder in which a quarter of patients are diagnosed when aged under 18 years [1,2]. IBD, when diagnosed in children, is linked with more extensive disease and greater complications compared to patients whose disease first appears in adulthood [3]. Since children with pediatric IBD (pIBD) have to take current therapy for longer, treatment must be optimized.

The use of biological therapy, such as anti-Tumor Necrosis Factor (anti-TNF) agents, has dramatically changed the treatment of autoimmune disease, including IBD. The use of these drugs is often linked to more severe symptoms of pIBD [4]. The only anti-TNFs approved for pIBD are infliximab (IFX) and adalimumab (ADL). However, treatment with biological drugs very often fails. Thus, up to 41% of children with moderate to severe CD and treated with IFX do not achieve clinical remission [5].

Mucosal healing is the best outcome in pIBD. However, given that pIBD is a chronic disease whose response cannot be monitored using regular biopsies, the use of non-invasive biomarkers is highly recommended.

Trough serum anti-TNF levels and antidrug antibodies, among other serological biomarkers, are usually measured in IBD to monitor anti-TNF treatment response [6,7]. However, neither can be measured prior to starting or during the first two weeks of anti-TNF treatment. Trough serum anti-TNF levels as soon as six weeks after initiation of treatment were recently reported to predict remission [8]. No earlier biomarkers have been identified to date.

Identification of genomic biomarkers could be useful to identify groups of pIBD patients who are less likely to respond in early stages of treatment or even before initiation. The mRNA levels in some genes have been identified as pharmacogenomic biomarkers of the activity of anti-TNF drugs in the inflamed tissues of adults diagnosed with IBD or other autoimmune disorders [9–13]. However, these biomarkers are identified using invasive techniques that are not suitable for monitoring. In addition, pharmacogenomic biomarkers of response to anti-TNF drugs have not been extensively investigated in pIBD. Identification of biomarkers in blood facilitates monitoring. In a recent comparison with healthy people, several genes were differentially expressed in the blood of children, but not adults, diagnosed with IBD during an active phase of the illness [14]. On the other hand, some studies in adults have revealed the usefulness of biomarkers of gene expression from whole blood in the assessment of response to anti-TNF agents [15,16].

In the present study, we analyzed whole gene expression profiles using next-generation sequencing of RNA in whole blood from children diagnosed with IBD. Differential gene expression before and after two weeks of treatment with IFX or ADL was analyzed with the aim of identifying very early biomarkers of response to IFX or ADL in pIBD.

2. Materials and Methods

2.1. Patient Samples

This study was prospective and multicentric and recruited 38 IBD patients aged < 18 years between March 2017 and May 2019, (30 with CD and eight with UC, 17 treated with ADL and 21 with IFX) [17]. The groups analyzed were matched for age and sex. Patients with a confirmed diagnosis of inflammatory bowel disease, aged between 1–17 years, and who had started treatment with infliximab (5 mg/kg, 0–2–6 weeks) or adalimumab (160/80 mg in those patients weighing more than 40 kg and 80/40 mg for those weighing 40 kg or less) were included.

Age, sex, type of IBD, anti-TNF drug, and specific disease activity scores, such as Pediatric Crohn Disease Activity Index (PCDAI) and Pediatric Ulcerative Colitis Activity Index (PUCAI), were collected to measure anti-TNF response, which was defined as a decrease of at least 15 points in PCDAI or PUCAI from the start of treatment to weeks 14 (IFX) or 26 (ADL). Study data were collected and managed using Research Electronic Data Capture (REDCap) tools hosted at Hospital General Universitario Gregorio Marañón, Madrid, Spain [18].

2.2. Ethics Statement

This study was approved by the Ethics Committee of Hospital General Universitario Gregorio Marañón with the number LAL-TNF-2019-01. Written, informed consent was obtained from the patients and parents or legal guardians.

2.3. Extraction of Total RNA from Whole Blood

Blood samples were collected in Paxgene tubes (PreAnalytics, Hombrechtikon, Switzerland) and whole blood RNA was extracted using PAXgene Blood RNA kit (PreAnalytics) at two different points: before the first administration of ADL or IFX (week 0) and after two weeks of the first administration of the drug (week 2) following manufacturer's recommendations. The total RNA concentration was measured by spectrophotometry, and the integrity of RNA was verified by electrophoresis. Only RNA samples with an RNA integrity number > 7 were used.

2.4. RNA Sequencing

The quality and integrity of each RNA sample were checked using both a Bioanalyzer and a Nanodrop device before proceeding to the RNA sequencing (RNAseq) protocol. Poly A+ RNA from 100 nanograms of total RNA was reverse transcribed and barcoded RNAseq libraries were constructed using NEBNext Ultra II Directional RNA Library Prep Kit (New England Biolabs) following manufacturer's recommendations. The quality of each RNA sample library was checked using a Bioanalyzer and a Qubit.

Libraries were sequenced at 13 pM on a HiSeq 2500 (Illumina, San Diego, CA, USA) single-read flow cell (1 × 60) and processed with RTA v1.18.66.3. FastQ files for each sample were obtained using bcl2fastq v2.20.0.422 software (Illumina).

Sequencing reads were aligned to the human reference transcriptome (GRCh38 v91) and quantified with RSem v1.3.1 (Li and Dewey 2011). Raw counts were normalized using transcripts per million and the trimmed mean of M values, transformed into log2 expression (log2[rawCount+1]), were compared to calculate fold-change and corrected p value. Only those genes expressed with at least one count in at least 12 samples were taken into account. As there are no gene expression changes with an associated Benjamini and Hochberg-adjusted p value < 0.05, we considered candidates to be confirmed as such by qPCR genes with |log2FC| > 0.6 and a non-adjusted p value < 0.05. The RNAseq data have been deposited with the accession number GSE159034 in the Gene Expression Omnibus database (https://www.ncbi.nlm.nih.gov/geo/query/acc.cgi?acc=GSE159034) [19].

2.5. Quantitative Reverse Transcription-Polymerase Chain Reaction (qRT-PCR)

Total RNA was reverse transcribed and amplified, and relative expression of *GBP1, GBP5, IGHG2, GNLY, FCGR1A, FCGR1B, ACTB,* and *RPL4* was quantified, as described in Salvador-Martín [17]. *ACTB* and *RPL4* were used for normalization and three technical replicates were used for each sample. The oligonucleotide sequences used for gene amplification are shown in Table 1. Primer pair efficiency was used for correction and relative expression calculated using the $2^{-\Delta\Delta Ct}$ method.

Table 1. Oligonucleotide sequences used for PCR amplification.

	Forward (5'-3')	Reverse (5'-3')
GBP1	TTCTCCAGAGGAAGGTGGAA	TTTTCTTCATTAGCCCAATTGTT
GBP5	CAAAGTCGGCAAGCAAATTTAT	GGTGTCTGCCTCCTCAGATT
IGHG2	CAGGACTCTACTCCCTCAGCA	GCACTCGACACAACATTTGC
GNLY	AGGGTGACCTGTTGACCAAA	CAGCATTGGAAACACTTCTCTG
FCGR1A	CACTGCAAAGAGACGCTTCA	AGGCAAGATCTGGACTCTATGG
FCGR1B	TGTCAGGAACAAAAAGAAGAACA	GATGGCCACCAACTGAGC
ACTB	CTGTGCTGTGGAAGCTAAGT	GATGTCCACGTCACACTTCA
RPL4	AGGCCAGGAATCACAAGCTC	AGGCCAGGAATCACAAGCTC

2.6. Statistical Analysis

Individual gene expression analyses at t = 0 and t = 2 weeks were performed using ExpressionSuite v1.1 (Applied Biosystems, Foster City, CA, USA), using the responder sample (D005) as relative quantification 1 in both times of comparison. Comparison of gene expression changes from t = 0 to t = 2 in responder versus non-responders was performed using GraphPad Prism (GraphPad Software, San Diego, CA, USA), using the responder sample (D005) at t = 2 as relative quantification 1. The mean relative quantification on the triplicated samples was used for expression and the unpaired t test applied for analyzing responder versus non-responder groups. P values were corrected using the false discovery rate with a confidence level of 95%. Categorical and numerical variables were compared using the *t* test and the Fisher exact test, respectively. For all tests, a *p* value < 0.05 was considered as statistically significant.

The statistical review was performed by a biomedical statistician.

The positive predictive value (PPV), negative predictive value (NPV), sensitivity, specificity, and diagnostic odds ratios for relative expression of *GBP1*, *FCGR1A*, and *FCGR1B* were calculated as described elsewhere [20]. The + and − likelihood ratios were calculated with a 95% confidence interval (CI).

3. Results

3.1. Patients' Characteristics

Thirty-eight patients (29 responders and nine non-responders) met the inclusion criteria and were included in the study. The failure rate was 23.7%. The characteristics of both groups of patients are summarized in Table 2.

Table 2. Characteristics of patients.

Characteristic	Overall (n = 38)	Responders (n = 29)	Non-Responders (n = 9)	p Value
Gender				
Male, n (%)	20 (52.6%)	15 (51.7%)	5 (55.6%)	1
Female, n (%)	18 (47.4%)	14 (48.3%)	4 (44.4%)	
Age (years)				
At diagnosis, median (IQR, range)	10.5 (4.55, 0.7–17)	10.5 (4.63, 2–17)	10.2 (7.5, 0.7–13)	0.137
At start of treatment, median (IQR, range)	11.9 (4.15, 1.1–17)	12.2 (4.6, 3.5–17)	11.5 (6, 1.1–14.1)	0.263
Type of IBD				
CD, n (%)	30 (78.9%)	22 (75.9%)	8 (88.9%)	0.650
UC, n (%)	8 (21.1%)	7 (24.1%)	1 (11.1%)	
Type of Anti-TNF				
Infliximab, n (%)	21 (55.3%)	14 (48.3%)	7 (77.8%)	0.148
Adalimumab, n (%)	17 (44.7%)	15 (51.7%)	2 (22.2%)	
PCDAI at start of treatment, median (IQR, range)	28.75 (25.63, 5–60)	32.5 (31.25, 5–60)	16.25 (11.25, 7.5–30)	0.045 **
PUCAI at start of treatment, median (IQR, range)	47.5 (35, 5–60) *	50 (40, 5–60)	45 *	-
CRP at start of treatment, median (IQR, range)	14.09 (28.54, 0.4–110.9)	22.3 (32.19, 0.4–110.9)	8.45 (17.94, 4–27.5)	0.042 **
FC at start of treatment, median (IQR, range)Concomitant immunomodulator at start of treatment	1800 (2253, 27–9543)	2000 (2288, 27–9543)	1207.5 (1432, 130–3167)	0.106
Azathioprine, n (%)	26 (68.4%)	22 (75.9%)	4 (44.4%)	
Methotrexate, n (%)	4 (10.5%)	4 (13.8%)	0	0.006 **
None, n (%)	8 (21.1%)	3 (10.3%)	5 (55.56%)	

IBD, inflammatory bowel disease; CD, Crohn disease; UC, ulcerative colitis; IQR, interquartile range; PCDAI, Pediatric Crohn Disease Activity Index; PUCAI, Pediatric Ulcerative Colitis Activity Index; CRP, C-reactive protein; FC, fecal calprotectin. * IQR not applicable. ** *p* value < 0.05.

Patients were mainly male (52.6%; median age at diagnosis, 10.5 years), diagnosed with CD (78.9%), and treated with IFX (55.3%). The statistical differences between both groups were in the PCDAI and C-reactive protein (CRP) levels at initiation of treatment (16.25 in non-responders versus 32.5 in responders [p = 0.045] and 8.45 in non-responders versus 22.3 in responders [p = 0.042]) and in the concomitant immunomodulator at initiation of treatment.

The demographic and clinical variables of the six responders and six non-responders selected for RNAseq were more homogeneous than those of the total population (Supplementary Materials Table S1). In these patients only PCDAI was statistically significant between both groups (p = 0.025).

3.2. Differential Gene Expression Using RNAseq in the Response of Anti-TNF Agents Prior to Starting Treatment

Twenty genes were overexpressed and two downregulated in non-responders versus responders (Log2FC [Fold change] > 0.6 or <−0.6 and p value < 0.05) immediately prior to the first administration of the anti-TNF agent (Table 3). For this analysis, the relative expression of the whole transcriptome using RNAseq was measured in six responders and six non-responders. Responders were used as the reference group.

Table 3. List of genes expressed differentially between responders (R) and non-responders (NR) prior to initiation of anti-TNF treatment.

Gene Name	Mean TPM R	Mean TMM+1 R	Log2 R	Mean TPM NR	Mean TMM+1 NR	Log2 NR	Fold Change (Log2)	p Value
HK2	46.41	5.98	2.56	26.02	3.69	1.89	−0.67	0.0254
DNAJC13	32.18	4.19	2.07	16.19	2.67	1.42	−0.65	0.0107
TSPAN33	13.53	2.47	1.31	25.58	3.77	1.91	0.61	0.0096
MAP3K7CL	15.98	2.73	1.45	30.07	4.16	2.06	0.61	0.0110
TRBC2	171.80	17.93	4.16	245.97	27.67	4.79	0.63	0.0180
MT-CO3	1097.32	120.77	6.92	1767.21	187.72	7.55	0.64	0.0136
CCL4	6.51	1.61	0.69	14.43	2.53	1.34	0.65	0.0276
DDX11L10	3.54	1.39	0.47	12.37	2.18	1.13	0.65	0.0495
MT-ND4L	132.36	15.82	3.98	227.85	25.23	4.66	0.67	0.0392
MT-ATP6	1024.97	115.51	6.85	1739.84	186.20	7.54	0.69	0.0253
MT-CYB	868.49	99.71	6.64	1494.58	162.26	7.34	0.70	0.0382
ACRBP	11.09	2.30	1.20	25.66	3.76	1.91	0.71	0.0020
TREML1	13.74	2.71	1.44	31.99	4.50	2.17	0.73	0.0297
MT-ND1	1094.43	126.98	6.99	1989.71	212.16	7.73	0.74	0.0423
HLA-C	1809.25	194.04	7.60	2990.89	325.05	8.34	0.74	0.0080
HLA-H	80.05	9.74	3.28	140.43	16.50	4.04	0.76	0.0361
AP001189.1	10.66	2.32	1.21	26.74	3.92	1.97	0.76	0.0221
MT-ATP8	107.65	13.26	3.73	202.76	22.62	4.50	0.77	0.0251
MT-ND2	865.51	99.05	6.63	1596.88	169.80	7.41	0.78	0.0168
SH3BGRL2	8.73	2.04	1.03	24.59	3.54	1.82	0.80	0.0294
IFITM3	327.49	37.05	5.21	594.78	65.05	6.02	0.81	0.0181
KLRD1	37.29	4.30	2.11	61.96	7.61	2.93	0.82	0.0491
TUBB1	76.43	10.11	3.34	163.15	17.92	4.16	0.83	0.0259
GP1BB	22.65	3.79	1.92	53.23	6.71	2.75	0.83	0.0172
IFITM1	373.17	43.37	5.44	727.55	77.03	6.27	0.83	0.0459
OASL	23.87	3.31	1.73	50.93	5.98	2.58	0.85	0.0423
PF4	23.49	3.63	1.86	60.29	7.32	2.87	1.01	0.0049
EPSTI1	41.88	4.57	2.19	83.41	9.27	3.21	1.02	0.0344
MYL9	11.02	2.41	1.27	38.53	5.20	2.38	1.11	0.0269
CCL5	122.76	13.85	3.79	276.24	30.37	4.92	1.13	0.0002
MYOM2	2.67	1.23	0.30	15.28	2.86	1.52	1.22	0.0377
GNLY	62.70	6.77	2.76	191.26	21.55	4.43	1.67	0.0409

TPM, transcripts per million; TMM, trimmed mean of M values; R, responder; NR, non-responder.

The most overexpressed gene in non-responders was GNLY (2.8 fold). The most downregulated gene in the same patients was DNAJC13 (2.4 fold).

3.3. Differential Gene Expression in Response to Anti-TNF Agents at Week 2 Post-Treatment

Twenty-six genes were overexpressed in non-responders and 16 were downregulated in responders (Log2FC [Fold change] >0.6 or <−0.6 and p value < 0.05) at two weeks post-treatment with anti-TNFs (Table 4). Responders were used as the reference group.

Table 4. List of genes expressed differentially between responders (R) and non-responders (NR) after two weeks of anti-TNF treatment.

Gene Name	Mean TPM R	Mean TMM+1 R	Log2 R	Mean TPM NR	Mean TMM+1 NR	Log2 NR	Fold Change (Log2)	p Value
IGHG1	492.65	54.71	5.77	98.10	11.26	3.49	−2.28	0.0394
IGKV3-20	92.59	11.12	3.47	37.71	4.50	2.17	−1.30	0.0096
IGHG2	163.72	19.68	4.30	71.31	8.06	3.01	−1.29	0.0372
IGHA1	510.70	57.75	5.85	254.62	25.75	4.69	−1.17	0.0268
IGKC	1398.17	155.23	7.28	669.09	70.45	6.14	−1.14	0.0159
IGKV1-39	45.72	5.83	2.54	18.16	2.83	1.50	−1.04	0.0313
IGKV2D-28	35.88	5.17	2.37	15.11	2.54	1.34	−1.03	0.0061
IGHV4-59	14.97	2.63	1.40	5.01	1.45	0.54	−0.86	0.0272
IGKV1-5	42.43	5.66	2.50	21.94	3.14	1.65	−0.85	0.0380
IGHV3-74	12.98	2.48	1.31	4.11	1.40	0.49	−0.82	0.0091
IGKV3-11	32.50	4.50	2.17	15.11	2.56	1.36	−0.81	0.0070
IGKV3-15	39.70	5.50	2.46	21.91	3.14	1.65	−0.81	0.0300
IGKV1-12	15.46	2.63	1.40	6.00	1.59	0.67	−0.72	0.0095
IGHV3-7	16.04	2.85	1.51	7.78	1.74	0.80	−0.72	0.0146
IGHV3-48	8.96	1.95	0.97	2.03	1.20	0.26	−0.70	0.0459
IGLV1-44	28.69	4.13	2.05	15.36	2.54	1.35	−0.70	0.0272
RARRES3	27.27	4.05	2.02	46.58	6.15	2.62	0.60	0.0327
RHBDF2	46.64	6.02	2.59	75.71	9.17	3.20	0.61	0.0281
IGFLR1	22.43	3.47	1.80	40.98	5.39	2.43	0.63	0.0070
APOL2	67.33	8.64	3.11	117.78	13.65	3.77	0.66	0.0385
TYMP	266.66	30.75	4.94	451.43	48.71	5.61	0.66	0.0444
IL1B	29.29	4.23	2.08	53.16	6.72	2.75	0.67	0.0226
DNAJC25-GNG10	26.40	3.93	1.98	51.09	6.29	2.65	0.68	0.0397
GZMA	14.86	2.62	1.39	29.03	4.20	2.07	0.68	0.0493
IRF1	307.23	35.90	5.17	538.82	58.4	5.87	0.70	0.0295
HLA-C	1710.59	197.19	7.62	2939.53	323.41	8.34	0.71	0.0096
HLA-H	77.17	9.96	3.32	139.23	16.44	4.04	0.72	0.0378
APOL6	93.85	11.01	3.46	166.82	18.54	4.21	0.75	0.0205
DHRS9	17.27	2.75	1.46	35.50	4.73	2.24	0.78	0.0197
UBE2L6	91.58	11.15	3.48	168.82	19.24	4.27	0.79	0.0272
ODF3B	26.61	3.85	1.95	56.06	6.92	2.79	0.84	0.0273
GBP2	200.76	23.37	4.55	393.53	42.06	5.39	0.85	0.0118
SECTM1	128.31	15.52	3.96	252.39	28.29	4.82	0.87	0.0484
FCGR1CP	4.89	1.47	0.56	18.76	3.13	1.65	1.09	0.0313
SERPING1	20.09	3.07	1.62	56.06	6.79	2.76	1.14	0.0293
MYOM2	2.43	1.27	0.34	14.53	2.80	1.48	1.14	0.0389
GBP1	84.92	9.85	3.30	208.64	22.49	4.49	1.19	0.0201
ANKRD22	3.24	1.34	0.42	19.72	3.11	1.64	1.22	0.0382
FCGR1B	33.63	4.77	2.25	106.67	12.48	3.64	1.39	0.0293
FCGR1A	27.68	4.15	2.05	93.02	10.90	3.45	1.39	0.0212
BATF2	6.67	1.69	0.76	36.71	4.89	2.29	1.53	0.0201
GBP5	130.99	14.13	3.82	393.84	41.43	5.37	1.55	0.0373

TPM, transcripts per million; TMM, trimmed mean of M values; R, responder; NR, non-responder.

The most overexpressed gene in non-responders was GBP5 (2.4 fold). The most downregulated gene in the same patients was IGLV1-44 (2.4 fold).

3.4. Functional in Silico Analysis

Functional analysis of differentially expressed genes was performed using Ingenuity Pathways Analysis (IPA, Qiagen, Germany).

Developmental disorder (p value range 1.96×10^{-2} to 9.23×10^{-15}), cell-to-cell signaling interaction (p value range 1.96×10^{-2} to 4.30×10^{-9}), and hematological system development and function (p value range 1.96×10^{-2} to 4.30×10^{-9}) were found to be the most significant disease and biofunctions represented by all of the selected genes prior to initiation of treatment (Supplementary Materials Table S2).

Figure 1 shows the main network generated by IPA and based on known interactions between the genes expressed differentially between responders and non-responders prior to initiation of anti-TNF treatment. The main diseases and functions associated with this network were developmental disorder, hereditary disorder, and metabolic disease.

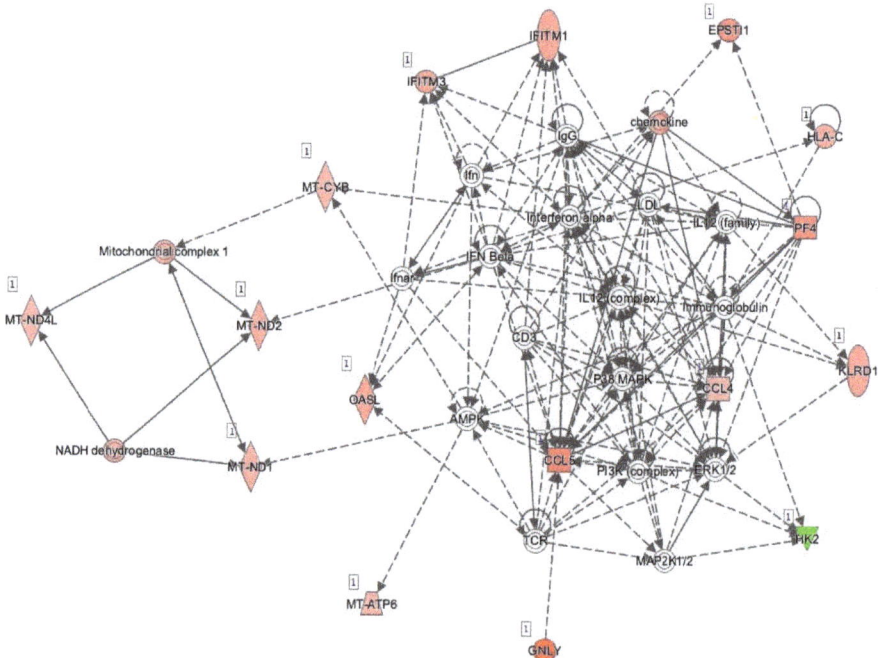

Figure 1. Network of differentially expressed genes prior to initiation of anti-TNF therapy based on interactions using Ingenuity Pathway Analysis. Red, genes overexpressed in non-responders vs. responders; green, genes downregulated in non-responders vs. responders.

The results for all of the genes selected after two weeks of anti-TNF treatment showed inflammatory response (p value range 1.30×10^{-2} to 5.74×10^{-23}), cellular function and maintenance (p value range 1.19×10^{-2} to 5.11×10^{-19}), and humoral immune response (p value range 1.23×10^{-2} to 5.74×10^{-23}) to be the most significant disease and biofunctions represented by the selected genes after two weeks of treatment (Supplementary Materials Table S3)

The most informative network generated by IPA and based on known interactions between the genes differentially expressed between responders and non-responders after two weeks of anti-TNF treatment is represented in Figure 2. The top disease and functions associated with this network were consistent with those obtained for all of the selected genes, namely, cellular function and maintenance, humoral immune response, and inflammatory response. For this reason, we decided to select most of the genes for validation from among the genes that were differentially expressed after two weeks of treatment.

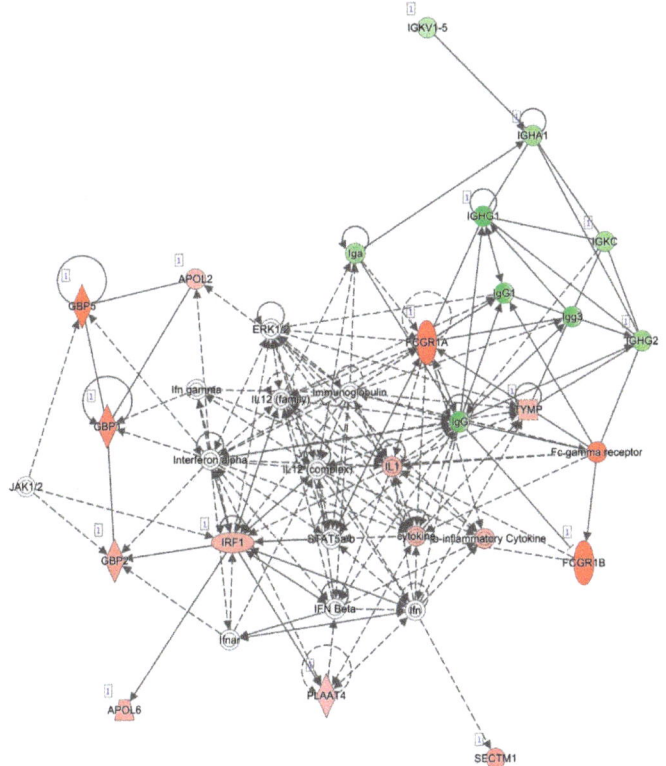

Figure 2. Network of differentially expressed genes after two weeks of anti-TNF treatment based on interactions using IPA. Red, genes overexpressed in non-responders vs. responders; green, genes downregulated in non-responders vs. responders.

3.5. Validation of Differentially Expressed Genes by qRT-PCR

Eight genes were selected from the RNAseq analyses for validation by real-time PCR (one differentially expressed at T0 and seven at T2). Semiquantitative real-time PCR was performed to assess RNA from patients' blood prior to treatment and after two weeks of treatment (Figure 3). None of the genes studied was expressed differentially between responders and non-responders before initiation of anti-TNF treatment.

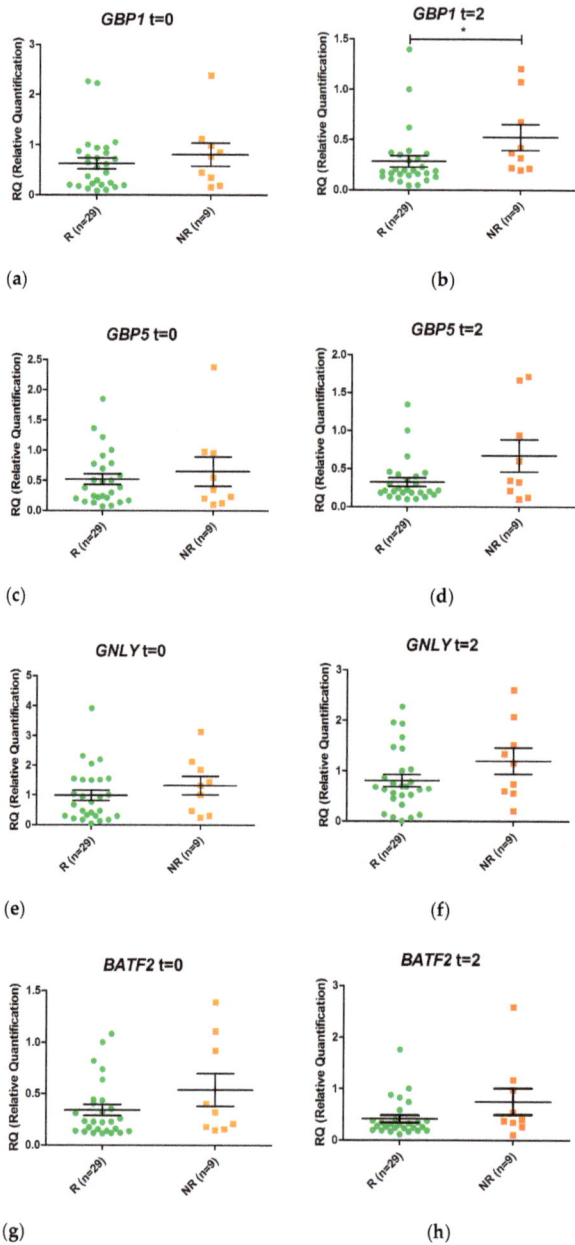

Figure 3. *Cont.*

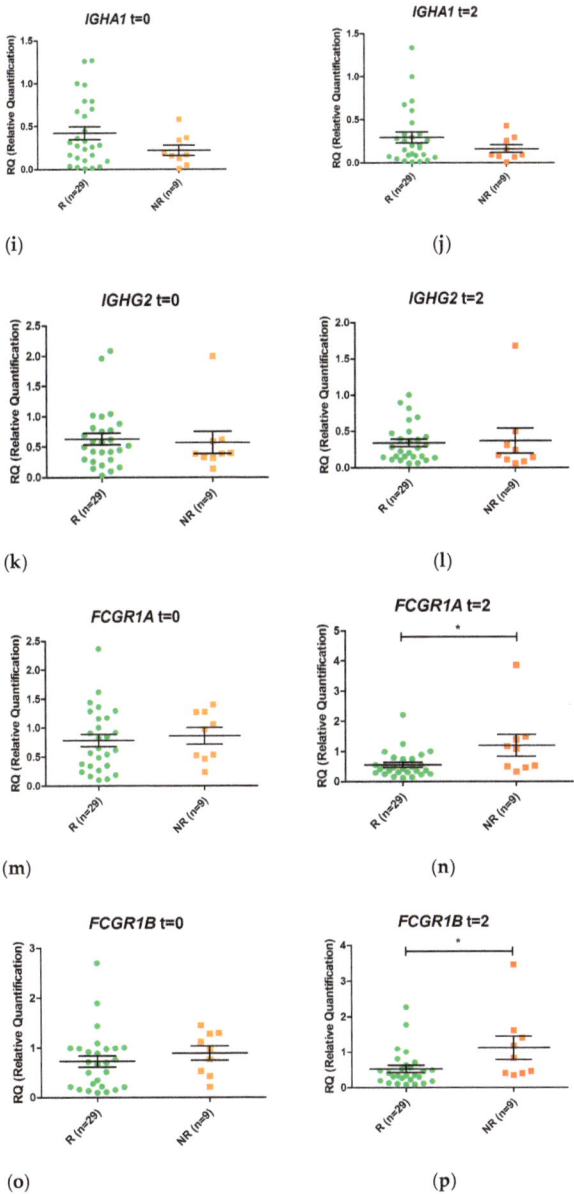

Figure 3. Relative expression levels of the genes *GBP1* (**a,b**), *GBP5* (**c,d**), *GNLY* (**e,f**), *BATF2* (**g,h**), *IGHA1* (**i,j**), *IGHG2* (**k,l**), *FCGR1A* (**m,n**), and *FCGR1B* (**o,p**) in responders (R, green) and non-responders (NR, orange) at time 0 ($t = 0$) and at two weeks ($t = 2$) after initiation of anti-TNF therapy. Expression values were normalized to the *ACTB* and *RPL4* genes. Values are expressed as mean (horizontal line) and standard error of the mean (SEM); *n*, sample size; * p value < 0.05 vs. control (unpaired *t* test).

GBP1 was overexpressed in non-responders compared with responders after two weeks of treatment (LogFC = 1.08, *p* value 0.006, False Discovery Rate (FDR) 0.032). In addition, *FCGR1A* and *FCGR1B* were also induced 1.05 fold more in non-responders (*p* value = 0.006, FDR 0.035) and 1.21 fold more in responders (*p* value = 0.005; FDR 0.032) (in LogFC). No other statistically significant changes were detected.

A comparison of the results for changes in gene expression using RNAseq and qRT-PCR (Table 5) revealed a good correlation, mainly in the data on genes selected after two weeks of anti-TNF treatment (R^2 = 0.83). The differences were statistically significant using both techniques in three cases.

Table 5. Correlation between RNAseq and qRT-PCR for selected genes.

Gene	Log2FC NR/R T0 RNAseq	Log2FC NR/R T0 qPCR	Log2FC NR/R T2 RNAseq	Log2FC NR/R T2 qPCR
GBP1	0.69	0.49	1.19 *	1.08 *
GBP5	0.95	0.19	1.55 *	0.78
GNLY	1.67 *	0.54	1.35	1.15
BATF2	1.16	0.48	1.53 *	0.55
IGHA1	−0.76	−0.67	−1.17 *	−0.34
IGHG2	−0.29	−0.01	−1.29 *	−0.23
FCGR1A	0.22	0.39	1.39 *	1.05 *
FCGR1B	0.25	0.66	1.39 *	1.21 *

* *p* value < 0.05.

3.6. Prediction of Response to Anti-TNF Therapy Based on Expression of GBP1, FCGR1A, and FCGR1B after Two Weeks of Treatment

Expression of *GBP1*, *FCGR1A*, and *FCGR1B* mRNA at T2 was higher in non-responders than in responders (Figure 4). The PPV, NPV, sensitivity, specificity, diagnostic odds ratio, positive likelihood ratio (+LR), and negative likelihood ratio (−LR) are presented in Table 6. The best diagnostic odds ratio corresponds to *FCGR1B* expression

3.7. Differences in Gene Expression between Responders and Non-Responders during the First Two Weeks of Anti-TNF Therapy

Changes in gene expression from T0 to T2 were measured for the eight selected genes when responders and non-responders were compared (Figure 4). Only FCGR1A changed its expression during the first two weeks of treatment (*p* value < 0.05). An increase in FCGR1A expression was observed in non-responders, while a decrease was observed in responders. Similar trends were observed for GBP1 and FCGR1B, although the differences were not statistically significant.

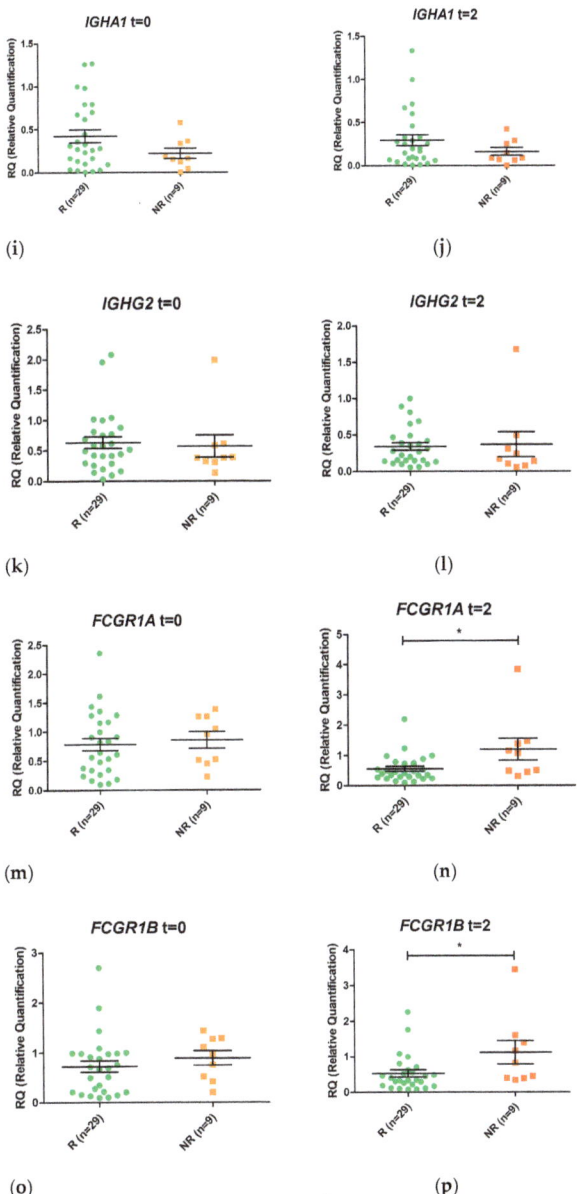

Figure 4. Schematic representation of the ratio between relative expression levels at week 2 (T2) and week 0 (T0) (T2/T0) of the genes *GBP1* (**a**), *GBP5* (**b**), *GNLY* (**c**), *BATF2* (**d**), *IGHA1* (**e**), *IGHG2* (**f**), *FCGR1A* (**g**), and *FCGR1B* (**h**) in responders (R) and non-responders (NR). Expression values were normalized to the *ACTB* and *RPL4* genes. Values are expressed as mean (horizontal line) and standard error of the mean (SEM); *n*, sample size; * p value < 0.05 vs. control (unpaired *t* test).

Table 6. Diagnostic values of *GBP1*, *FCGR1A*, and *FCGR1B* expression after two weeks of anti-TNF treatment.

	GBP1 [1]	FCGR1A [1]	FCGR1B [1]
Sensitivity	67%	78%	89%
Specificity	70%	63%[1]	52%
PPV	43%	41%	38%
NPV	86%	89%	93%
Diagnostic odds ratio	4.75	5.95	8.61
+LR	2,25	2.1	1.84
−LR	0.47	0.35	0.21

[1] Relative expression cut-off: *GBP1* = 0.3, *FCGR1A* = 0.5, and *FCGR1B* = 0.39.

4. Discussion

The use of biologic drugs such as anti-TNF agents has dramatically transformed the treatment of autoimmune diseases, including IBD. However, more than 20% of patients do not respond correctly to this therapy [6]. The identification of the patients in whom therapy is more likely to fail in early stages or even before initiation would enable therapy to be personalized. The benefits of personalization in terms of safety and efficacy are of particular interest in children, who are necessarily treated for longer. Finding specific biomarkers for children is necessary since genetics has a more important role in pIBD than in adult disease. Consequently, several gene polymorphisms have been involved in susceptibility to pIBD or to very-early-onset ulcerative colitis [21,22]. The serum levels of proteins, such as clusterin and ceruloplasmin, also differ between children and adults with IBD [23]. As for response, genetic polymorphisms in genes such as *ATG16L1*, *CDKAL1*, *ICOSLG*, *BRWD1*, and *HLA-DQA1* have been associated with the response to anti-TNF treatment in children [24]. In contrast, several genes associated with expression and response to anti-TNF response have been identified only in adults with IBD [9,10,13]. Our group recently showed expression of *SMAD7* in blood to be a biomarker of the response to anti-TNF agents two weeks after initiation of treatment [17]. To our knowledge, ours is the first study to assess whole gene expression profile by RNAseq in pIBD using biomarkers of response to anti-TNF agents. We identified putative gene networks and pathways involved in early response in pIBD and validated *GBP1*, *FCGR1A*, and *FCGR1B* as potential pharmacogenomic markers. Although we are still at a very early stage, the identification of these non-invasive biomarkers in pediatric IBD could revolutionize the selection of biological drug treatment in these patients in the future.

Humoral immune response, inflammatory response, and maintenance of cellular function were associated with the differentially expressed genes in responders and non-responders after two weeks of anti-TNF treatment. These diseases and biofunctions are clearly associated with IBD and indicate that our strategy could be helpful for identifying biomarkers of response to anti-TNF agents [25,26]. However, since these diseases and biofunctions are too extensive and provide little information in terms of prediction, we decided to focus on the differentially expressed genes verified by qPCR.

Certainly, only three out of eight genes were statistically validated. However, the correlation between log2 ratios (RNAseq) and relative quantification (RT-qPCR) was as high as $R^2 = 0.83$. This value was lower than those found in other works with ideal conditions for comparison [27]. Nevertheless, it was similar or even higher than the values found in other works with more variable samples, such as tissues from living organisms [28,29].

We found that expression of *GBP1* mRNA was upregulated in the peripheral blood cells of non-responders after two weeks of anti-TNF treatment. GBP1 is an interferon-stimulated, guanylate-binding protein involved in defense against pathogens and inflammation; its levels are elevated in the mucosa of patients with active disease [30]. The fact that this gene was overexpressed in non-responders after two weeks of treatment suggests a higher likelihood of inflammation and a higher risk of treatment failure.

Similarly, GBP1 was identified as differentially expressed in colitis-susceptible mice and in colitis-resistant mice [31].

Our results also revealed greater expression of the *FCGR1A* and *FCGR1B* genes in non-responders after two weeks of anti-TNF treatment. FCRG1A, also known as CD64, is upregulated in adults and children diagnosed with clinically active IBD [32] and has been related to calprotectin level [33]. FCRG1A and FCGR1B are expressed on the surface of neutrophils and have been suggested to be potential therapeutic targets [34]. Furthermore, both ADL and IFX are less effective in the peripheral blood mononuclear cells of adult IBD patients who express elevated levels of CD64 [35]. Here, we demonstrated a similar usefulness of these genes as biomarkers of response to anti-TNF drugs in children with IBD.

There are several limitations of this study. First, the sample size is small for a study of these characteristics [12,16]. Second, our results do not distinguish between the two drugs administered to patients, infliximab and adalimumab. Thus, although the mechanism of action of both drugs is similar, we cannot rule out a differential effect. Third, it is necessary to define the role of the PCDAI index in the causality of the response to anti-TNFs. Finally, the comparison with other works is complicated by differences in the study population, as well as in the evaluation criteria of the response [9,13].

Future research will require more studies involving larger populations to confirm our findings. Single-cell RNAseq might be useful to rule out the effect of mixed-cell populations. In addition, a larger sample size could help to differentiate biomarkers by anti-TNF drug and by type of pIBD. In spite of these limitations, the identification of *GBP1, FCGR1A,* and *FCGR1B* as blood biomarkers of response to anti-TNF agents shows great potential for the personalization of therapy in pIBD.

5. Conclusions

We identified the expression levels of *GBP1, FCGR1A1,* and *FCGR1B1* genes as potential biomarkers of response to treatment with IFX and ADL in children with IBD.

Supplementary Materials: The following are available online at http://www.mdpi.com/1999-4923/13/1/77/s1, Table S1: Characteristics of patients selected for RNAseq. Table S2: Top diseases and biofunctions of genes expressed differentially between responders and non-responders before initiation of anti-TNF treatment. Table S3: Top diseases and biofunctions of genes expressed differentially between responders and non-responders two weeks after initiation of anti-TNF treatment.

Author Contributions: L.A.L.-F. conceived and designed the research. S.S.-M., B.K., and R.Á. performed the experiments; S.S.-M., B.K., R.Á., V.M.N.-L., C.G.-F., A.M.-Á., A.S.-B., C.S., M.T., M.V., R.M.-C., A.R.-M., C.A.V., F.B., G.P.-M., M.J.F., A.M.-J., L.M., E.M.-O., I.L., F.J.E., J.A.B.-G., S.C., R.G.-R., V.M.-B., R.G.d.C., E.V., A.D., and M.S.-S. participated in data acquisition and curation. S.S.-M., B.K., and L.A.L.-F. wrote the original draft. L.A.L.-F. obtained funds. All authors revised, read, and approved the final manuscript. All authors have read and agreed to the published version of the manuscript.

Funding: This research was funded by Instituto de Salud Carlos III (grants numbers PI16/00559 and PI19/00792), Consejería de Educación y Deporte de la Comunidad de Madrid (grant number PEJ16/MED/AI-1260), and by the Gregorio Marañón Health Research Institute (grant number PRE-2018-2). The study was cofunded by European Regional Develompment Funds (FEDER) from the European Commission, "A way of making Europe".

Institutional Review Board Statement: The study was conducted according to the guidelines of the Declaration of Helsinki and approved by the Institutional Review Board (or Ethics Committee) of Hospital Gregorio Marañón (protocol code FG-2019-02 and date of approval 07/10/2019).

Informed Consent Statement: Informed consent was obtained from all subjects involved in the study.

Data Availability Statement: The RNAseq data have been deposited with the accession number GSE159034 in the Gene Expression Omnibus database (https://www.ncbi.nlm.nih.gov/geo/query/acc.cgi?acc=GSE159034) [19].

Acknowledgments: We would like to thank the patients and their parents for their participation in the study. Thanks to Xandra García-González and Alicia López Salvador for English revision of the manuscript.

Conflicts of Interest: The authors declare no conflict of interest. The funders had no role in the design of the study, in the collection, analyses, or interpretation of data, in the writing of the manuscript, or in the decision to publish the results.

References

1. Gu, P.; Feagins, L.A. Dining with Inflammatory Bowel Disease: A Review of the Literature on Diet in the Pathogenesis and Management of IBD. *Inflamm. Bowel Dis.* **2019**. [CrossRef] [PubMed]
2. Kuhnen, A. Genetic and Environmental Considerations for Inflammatory Bowel Disease. *Surg. Clin. N. Am.* **2019**, *99*, 1197–1207. [CrossRef] [PubMed]
3. Sawczenko, A.; Sandhu, B.K. Presenting features of inflammatory bowel disease in Great Britain and Ireland. *Arch. Dis. Child.* **2003**, *88*, 995–1000. [CrossRef] [PubMed]
4. Henderson, P.; van Limbergen, J.E.; Wilson, D.C.; Satsangi, J.; Russell, R.K. Genetics of childhood-onset inflammatory bowel disease. *Inflamm. Bowel Dis.* **2011**, *17*, 346–361. [CrossRef]
5. Hyams, J.; Crandall, W.; Kugathasan, S.; Griffiths, A.; Olson, A.; Johanns, J.; Liu, G.; Travers, S.; Heuschkel, R.; Markowitz, J.; et al. Reach Study Group Induction and Maintenance Infliximab Therapy for the Treatment of Moderate-to-Severe Crohn's Disease in Children. *Gastroenterology* **2007**, *132*, 863–873. [CrossRef]
6. Hendy, P.; Hart, A.; Irving, P. Anti-TNF drug and antidrug antibody level monitoring in IBD: A practical guide. *Frontline Gastroenterol.* **2016**, *7*, 122–128. [CrossRef]
7. Kelly, O.B.; Donnell, S.O.; Stempak, J.M.; Steinhart, A.H.; Silverberg, M.S. Therapeutic Drug Monitoring to Guide Infliximab Dose Adjustment is Associated with Better Endoscopic Outcomes than Clinical Decision Making Alone in Active Inflammatory Bowel Disease. *Inflamm. Bowel Dis.* **2017**, *23*, 1202–1209. [CrossRef]
8. Courbette, O.; Aupiais, C.; Viala, J.; Hugot, J.-P.; Roblin, X.; Candon, S.; Louveau, B.; Chatenoud, L.; Martinez-Vinson, C. Trough Levels of Infliximab at W6 Are Predictive of Remission at W14 in Pediatric Crohn Disease. *J. Pediatr. Gastroenterol. Nutr.* **2019**, *70*, 310–317. [CrossRef]
9. Arijs, I.; Li, K.; Toedter, G.; Quintens, R.; Van Lommel, L.; Van Steen, K.; Leemans, P.; De Hertogh, G.; Lemaire, K.; Ferrante, M.; et al. Mucosal gene signatures to predict response to infliximab in patients with ulcerative colitis. *Gut* **2009**, *58*, 1612–1619. [CrossRef]
10. Arijs, I.; Quintens, R.; Van Lommel, L.; Van Steen, K.; De Hertogh, G.; Lemaire, K.; Schraenen, A.; Perrier, C.; Van Assche, G.; Vermeire, S.; et al. Predictive value of epithelial gene expression profiles for response to infliximab in Crohn's disease. *Inflamm. Bowel Dis.* **2010**, *16*, 2090–2098. [CrossRef]
11. Julià, A.; Erra, A.; Palacio, C.; Tomas, C.; Sans, X.; Barceló, P.; Marsal, S. An eight-gene blood expression profile predicts the response to infliximab in rheumatoid arthritis. *PLoS ONE* **2009**, *4*, e7556. [CrossRef]
12. Nakamura, S.; Suzuki, K.; Iijima, H.; Hata, Y.; Lim, C.R.; Ishizawa, Y.; Kameda, H.; Amano, K.; Matsubara, K.; Matoba, R.; et al. Identification of baseline gene expression signatures predicting therapeutic responses to three biologic agents in rheumatoid arthritis: A retrospective observational study. *Arthritis Res. Ther.* **2016**, *18*, 159. [CrossRef]
13. Toedter, G.; Li, K.; Marano, C.; Ma, K.; Sague, S.; Huang, C.C.; Song, X.-Y.; Rutgeerts, P.; Baribaud, F. Gene Expression Profiling and Response Signatures Associated with Differential Responses to Infliximab Treatment in Ulcerative Colitis. *Am. J. Gastroenterol.* **2011**, *106*, 1272–1280. [CrossRef]
14. Ostrowski, J.; Dabrowska, M.; Lazowska, I.; Paziewska, A.; Balabas, A.; Kluska, A.; Kulecka, M.; Karczmarski, J.; Ambrozkiewicz, F.; Piatkowska, M.; et al. Redefining the Practical Utility of Blood Transcriptome Biomarkers in Inflammatory Bowel Diseases. *J. Crohn Colitis* **2019**, *13*, 626–633. [CrossRef]
15. Verstockt, B.; Verstockt, S.; Dehairs, J.; Ballet, V.; Blevi, H.; Wollants, W.-J.; Breynaert, C.; Van Assche, G.; Vermeire, S.; Ferrante, M. Low TREM1 expression in whole blood predicts anti-TNF response in inflammatory bowel disease. *EBioMedicine* **2019**. [CrossRef]

16. Toonen, E.J.M.; Gilissen, C.; Franke, B.; Kievit, W.; Eijsbouts, A.M.; den Broeder, A.A.; van Reijmersdal, S.V.; Veltman, J.A.; Scheffer, H.; Radstake, T.R.D.J.; et al. Validation Study of Existing Gene Expression Signatures for Anti-TNF Treatment in Patients with Rheumatoid Arthritis. *PLoS ONE* **2012**, *7*, e33199. [CrossRef]
17. Salvador-Martín, S.; Raposo-Gutiérrez, I.; Navas-López, V.M.; Gallego-Fernández, C.; Moreno-álvarez, A.; Solar-Boga, A.; Muñoz-Codoceo, R.; Magallares, L.; Martínez-Ojinaga, E.; Fobelo, M.J.; et al. Gene signatures of early response to anti-TNF drugs in pediatric inflammatory bowel disease. *Int. J. Mol. Sci.* **2020**, *21*, 3364. [CrossRef]
18. Harris, P.A.; Taylor, R.; Thielke, R.; Payne, J.; Gonzalez, N.; Conde, J.G. Research electronic data capture (REDCap)—A metadata—Driven methodology and workflow process for providing translational research informatics support. *J. Biomed. Inform.* **2009**, *42*, 377–381. [CrossRef]
19. Edgar, R.; Domrachev, M.; Lash, A.E. Gene Expression Omnibus: NCBI gene expression and hybridization array data repository. *Nucleic Acids Res.* **2002**, *30*, 207–210. [CrossRef]
20. Glas, A.S.; Lijmer, J.G.; Prins, M.H.; Bonsel, G.J.; Bossuyt, P.M.M. The diagnostic odds ratio: A single indicator of test performance. *J. Clin. Epidemiol.* **2003**, *56*, 1129–1135. [CrossRef]
21. Gazouli, M.; Pachoula, I.; Panayotou, I.; Mantzaris, G.; Chrousos, G.; Anagnou, N.P.; Roma-Giannikou, E. NOD2/CARD15, ATG16L1 and IL23R gene polymorphisms and childhood-onset of Crohn's disease. *World J. Gastroenterol.* **2010**, *16*, 1753–1758. [CrossRef] [PubMed]
22. Moran, C.J.; Walters, T.D.; Guo, C.-H.; Kugathasan, S.; Klein, C.; Turner, D.; Wolters, V.M.; Bandsma, R.H.; Mouzaki, M.; Zachos, M.; et al. IL-10R polymorphisms are associated with very-early-onset ulcerative colitis. *Inflamm. Bowel Dis.* **2013**, *19*, 115–123. [CrossRef] [PubMed]
23. Vaiopoulou, A.; Gazouli, M.; Papadopoulou, A.; Anagnostopoulos, A.K.; Karamanolis, G.; Theodoropoulos, G.E.; M'Koma, A.; Tsangaris, G.T. Serum protein profiling of adults and children with Crohn disease. *J. Pediatr. Gastroenterol. Nutr.* **2015**, *60*, 42–47. [CrossRef]
24. Dubinsky, M.C.; Mei, L.; Friedman, M.; Dhere, T.; Haritunians, T.; Hakonarson, H.; Kim, C.; Glessner, J.; Targan, S.R.; McGovern, D.P.; et al. Genome wide association (GWA) predictors of anti-TNF α therapeutic responsiveness in pediatric inflammatory bowel disease. *Inflamm. Bowel Dis.* **2010**, *16*, 1357–1366. [CrossRef]
25. Li, N.; Shi, R.-H. Updated review on immune factors in pathogenesis of Crohn's disease. *World J. Gastroenterol.* **2018**, *24*, 15–22. [CrossRef]
26. Tatiya-Aphiradee, N.; Chatuphonprasert, W.; Jarukamjorn, K. Immune response and inflammatory pathway of ulcerative colitis. *J. Basic Clin. Physiol. Pharmacol.* **2018**, *30*, 1–10. [CrossRef]
27. Everaert, C.; Luypaert, M.; Maag, J.L.V.; Cheng, Q.X.; Dinger, M.E.; Hellemans, J.; Mestdagh, P. Benchmarking of RNA-sequencing analysis workflows using whole-transcriptome RT-qPCR expression data. *Sci. Rep.* **2017**, *7*, 1559. [CrossRef]
28. Li, Y.; Zhang, L.; Li, R.; Zhang, M.; Li, Y.; Wang, H.; Wang, S.; Bao, Z. Systematic identification and validation of the reference genes from 60 RNA-Seq libraries in the scallop Mizuhopecten yessoensis. *BMC Genom.* **2019**, *20*, 288. [CrossRef]
29. Zhang, Z.; Duan, Y.; Wu, Z.; Zhang, H.; Ren, J.; Huang, L. PPARD is an Inhibitor of Cartilage Growth in External Ears. *Int. J. Biol. Sci.* **2017**, *13*, 669–681. [CrossRef]
30. Britzen-Laurent, N.; Herrmann, C.; Naschberger, E.; Croner, R.S.; Sturzl, M. Pathophysiological role of guanylate-binding proteins in gastrointestinal diseases. *World J. Gastroenterol.* **2016**, *22*, 6434–6443. [CrossRef]
31. De Buhr, M.F.; Mahler, M.; Geffers, R.; Hansen, W.; Westendorf, A.M.; Lauber, J.; Buer, J.; Schlegelberger, B.; Hedrich, H.J.; Bleich, A. Cd14, Gbp1, and Pla2g2a: Three major candidate genes for experimental IBD identified by combining QTL and microarray analyses. *Physiol. Genom.* **2006**, *25*, 426–434. [CrossRef]
32. Minar, P.; Haberman, Y.; Jurickova, I.; Wen, T.; Rothenberg, M.E.; Kim, M.-O.; Saeed, S.A.; Baldassano, R.N.; Stephens, M.; Markowitz, J.; et al. Utility of neutrophil Fc γ receptor I (CD64) index as a biomarker for mucosal inflammation in pediatric Crohn's disease. *Inflamm. Bowel Dis.* **2014**, *20*, 1037–1048. [CrossRef]
33. Tillinger, W.; Jilch, R.; Jilma, B.; Brunner, H.; Koeller, U.; Lichtenberger, C.; Waldhor, T.; Reinisch, W. Expression of the high-affinity IgG receptor FcRI (CD64) in patients with inflammatory bowel disease: A new biomarker for gastroenterologic diagnostics. *Am. J. Gastroenterol.* **2009**, *104*, 102–109. [CrossRef]

34. Muthas, D.; Reznichenko, A.; Balendran, C.A.; Bottcher, G.; Clausen, I.G.; Karrman Mardh, C.; Ottosson, T.; Uddin, M.; MacDonald, T.T.; Danese, S.; et al. Neutrophils in ulcerative colitis: A review of selected biomarkers and their potential therapeutic implications. *Scand. J. Gastroenterol.* **2017**, *52*, 125–135. [CrossRef]
35. Wojtal, K.A.; Rogler, G.; Scharl, M.; Biedermann, L.; Frei, P.; Fried, M.; Weber, A.; Eloranta, J.J.; Kullak-Ublick, G.A.; Vavricka, S.R. Fc γ receptor CD64 modulates the inhibitory activity of infliximab. *PLoS ONE* **2012**, *7*, e43361. [CrossRef]

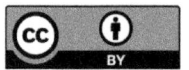

© 2021 by the authors. Licensee MDPI, Basel, Switzerland. This article is an open access article distributed under the terms and conditions of the Creative Commons Attribution (CC BY) license (http://creativecommons.org/licenses/by/4.0/).

MDPI
St. Alban-Anlage 66
4052 Basel
Switzerland
Tel. +41 61 683 77 34
Fax +41 61 302 89 18
www.mdpi.com

Pharmaceutics Editorial Office
E-mail: pharmaceutics@mdpi.com
www.mdpi.com/journal/pharmaceutics

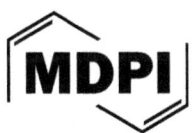

www.ingramcontent.com/pod-product-compliance
Lightning Source LLC
LaVergne TN
LVHW070635100526
838202LV00012B/813